COGNITIVE AND BEHAVIORAL THEORIES IN CLINICAL PRACTICE

Cognitive and Behavioral Theories in Clinical Practice

Edited by
Nikolaos Kazantzis
Mark A. Reinecke
Arthur Freeman

Foreword by Frank M. Dattilio

THE GUILFORD PRESS
New York   London

© 2010 The Guilford Press
A Division of Guilford Publications, Inc.
72 Spring Street, New York, NY 10012
www.guilford.com

Printed in the United States of America

This book is printed on acid-free paper.

Last digit is print number: 9 8 7 6 5 4 3 2 1

Library of Congress Cataloging-in-Publication Data

Cognitive and behavioral theories in clinical practice / edited by Nikolaos
Kazantzis, Mark A. Reinecke, and Arthur Freeman.
       p. cm. — (1st ed.)
   Includes bibliographical references and index.
   ISBN 978-1-60623-342-9 (hardcover : alk. paper)
   1. Cognitive therapy.   I. Kazantzis, Nikolaos, 1973–   II. Reinecke, Mark A.
III. Freeman, Arthur, 1942–
   RC489.C63C6228 2010
   616.89′1425—dc22
                                                    2009027695

I dedicate my work on this volume to the friends and colleagues who have contributed to its contents. Understanding their scientific advances will improve our understanding and our practices as clinicians. I also dedicate this work to my parents, Evangelos and Margaret, and my sister, Katerina, with love.

—N. K.

Change and growth are constants in life. I dedicate my work on this book to mental health professionals who, through their thoughtful practice, help others to change, to become more hopeful, and to approach the adversities of life with wisdom and resilience. I also dedicate this work to Marsha and Gracie, with love.

—M. A. R.

My father died when I was quite young. It left me adrift and confused. It was my good fortune to have an older brother who served, for many years, as both my anchor and my compass. Though he was a teenager and very much as lost as I, he was someone whom I could look up to and emulate. I am what I am today because of his steady presence. I dedicate my work on this volume to Dr. Stanley P. Freeman, Professor of Dentistry at Columbia University School of Dentistry, and to Sharon, whom Dr. Freeman married 50 years ago, thereby giving me a wonderful and loving older sister.

—A. F.

About the Editors

Nikolaos Kazantzis, PhD, recently assumed a faculty position at La Trobe University in Victoria, Australia, where he teaches and supervises clinical psychology and cognitive-behavioral therapy. From 2000 to 2008, he served on the staff at Massey University in New Zealand. Dr. Kazantzis's clinical and research interests focus on enhancing the use of therapeutic homework assignments in cognitive-behavioral therapy. He has published over 70 scholarly articles and book chapters and has frequently presented professional workshops for international audiences. His books for practitioners include *Using Homework Assignments in Cognitive Behavior Therapy* and *Handbook of Homework Assignments in Psychotherapy.*

Mark A. Reinecke, PhD, is Professor of Psychiatry and Behavioral Sciences and Chief of the Division of Psychology at Northwestern University's Feinberg School of Medicine. He serves on the staff of Northwestern Memorial Hospital and Children's Memorial Hospital in Chicago. Dr. Reinecke is a Distinguished Fellow and former president of the Academy of Cognitive Therapy and a Diplomate of the American Board of Professional Psychology (ABPP) in Clinical Psychology and Clinical Child and Adolescent Psychology. His research and clinical interests focus on understanding and treating depression and suicide among children and adolescents. Dr. Reinecke was a principal investigator on the Treatment of Adolescents with Depression Study (TADS). He has authored or edited seven books, including *Cognitive Therapy across the Lifespan, Comparative Treatments of Depression, Cognitive Therapy with Children and Adolescents,* and *Personality Disorders in Childhood and Adolescence.*

Arthur Freeman, EdD, ScD, is Visiting Professor in the Department of Psychology at Governors State University, University Park, Illinois. He is also

Director of Training at the Sheridan Shores Care and Rehabilitation Center in Chicago and Clinical Professor at the Philadelphia College of Osteopathic Medicine. Dr. Freeman is a Distinguished Founding Fellow of the Academy of Cognitive Therapy and a Diplomate of the American Board of Professional Psychology (ABPP) in Clinical Psychology, Behavioral Psychology, and Family Psychology. His research and clinical interests focus on understanding and treating chronic and complex psychological disorders, notably personality disorders. Dr. Freeman has published over 150 chapters, articles, and reviews and 70 books, including *Cognitive Therapy of Personality Disorders, Cognitive-Behavioral Strategies in Crisis Intervention, Personality Disorders in Childhood and Adolescence*, and *Cognitive and Behavioral Theories in Clinical Practice* (with Drs. Nikolaos Kazantzis and Mark Reinecke). He has lectured at conferences, congresses, and at academic venues in 40 countries and throughout the United States. His work has been translated from English into 15 other languages.

Contributors

Steven M. Brunwasser, BA, Department of Psychology, University of Michigan, Ann Arbor, Michigan

Prudence Cuper, BA, Department of Psychology and Neurosciences, Duke University, Durham, North Carolina

Raymond A. DiGiuseppe, PhD, ABPP, Department of Psychology, St. John's University, Queens, New York

Sona Dimidjian, PhD, Department of Psychology, University of Colorado at Boulder, Boulder, Colorado

Thomas J. D'Zurilla, PhD, Department of Psychology, Stony Brook University, Stony Brook, New York

Thomas Ehring, PhD, Department of Clinical Psychology, University of Amsterdam, Amsterdam, The Netherlands

Paul M. G. Emmelkamp, PhD, Department of Clinical Psychology, University of Amsterdam, Amsterdam, The Netherlands

Catherine Eubanks-Carter, PhD, Psychotherapy Research Program, Beth Israel Medical Center, New York, New York

Arthur Freeman, EdD, ScD, ABPP, Department of Psychology, Governors State University, University Park, Illinois

Steven C. Hayes, PhD, Department of Psychology, University of Nevada, Reno, Reno, Nevada

Nikolaos Kazantzis, PhD, School of Psychological Science, La Trobe University, Melbourne, Victoria, Australia

Blair V. Kleiber, BS, Department of Psychology, University of Colorado at Boulder, Boulder, Colorado

Peter M. Lewinsohn, PhD, Oregon Research Institute, Eugene, Oregon

Thomas R. Lynch, PhD, School of Psychology, University of Exeter, Exeter, United Kingdom

Christopher R. Martell, PhD, ABPP, private practice and Department of Psychology, University of Washington, Seattle, Washington

J. Christopher Muran, PhD, Derner Institute for Advanced Psychological Studies, Adelphi University, Garden City, New York, and Psychotherapy Research Program, Beth Israel Medical Center, New York, New York

Arthur M. Nezu, PhD, ABPP, Department of Psychology, Drexel University, Philadelphia, Pennsylvania

Christine Maguth Nezu, PhD, ABPP, Department of Psychology, Drexel University, Philadelphia, Pennsylvania

Nansook Park, PhD, Department of Psychology, University of Michigan, Ann Arbor, Michigan

Christopher Peterson, PhD, Department of Psychology, University of Michigan, Ann Arbor, Michigan

Mark B. Powers, PhD, Department of Clinical Psychology, University of Amsterdam, Amsterdam, The Netherlands

Mark A. Reinecke, PhD, ABPP, Division of Psychology, Feinberg School of Medicine, Northwestern University, Chicago, Illinois

Anthony Ryle, DM (Oxford), Fellow, Royal College of Psychiatrists, retired; formerly Consultant Psychotherapist, St. Thomas's Hospital, London, United Kingdom

Jeremy D. Safran, PhD, Department of Psychology, New School for Social Research, New York, New York

Jan Scott, MB, BS, PhD, FRCPsych, Institute of Neuroscience, Newcastle University, Newcastle Upon Tyne, United Kingdom, and Psychological Treatments Research, Institute of Psychiatry, London, United Kingdom

Zindel V. Segal, PhD, University of Toronto, Center for Addiction and Mental Health—Clarke Division, Toronto, Ontario, Canada

Thomas J. Waltz, PhD, Department of Psychology, University of Nevada, Reno, Reno, Nevada

Foreword

In his groundbreaking book *Cognitive Therapy of Depression* (which first appeared 30 years ago), Aaron T. Beck wrote in the Preface that although the initial findings of his empirical studies seemed to support his belief in the specific psychodynamic factors of depression, later experiments presented a number of unexpected findings that appeared to contradict his beginning hypothesis. The new information led Beck to evaluate critically the psychoanalytic theory of depression and ultimately the entire structure of psychoanalysis. Beck went on to state that the marked discrepancy between laboratory findings and clinical theory led to an "agonizing reappraisal" of his own belief system, at which point he began to change his thinking and develop his cognitive theory of depression.

Because of its strong theoretical and scientific foundation, Beck's cognitive therapy became one of the best-supported treatments in the armamentaria of psychotherapeutic approaches, yielding more empirical outcome studies than any other therapeutic modality in history. As a result of the dual emphasis on theory and clinical practice, cognitive therapy and the cognitive-behavioral therapies have been instrumental in setting the tone for the evidence-based treatments that now dominate the psychotherapy landscape, and that have established an age of "accountability" for many providers of treatment. In the early years of psychotherapy, many modalities had little, if any, theory behind them. The behaviorists were the exception, always maintaining an emphasis on reliable theoretical underpinnings. Surprisingly, however, although the professional literature calls for therapy to be built on a solid scientific foundation, the growth of "fringe psychotherapies" continues at a rapid pace. For a variety of reasons, these therapies are attractive to many mental health professionals. Unfortunately, many of these unsubstantiated, untested, and otherwise questionable assessment and treatment interventions threaten the integrity of the field. What is more, despite the availability of well-replicated, evidence-based treatments backed by sound theory, many practitioners in the field tend to rely solely on their own experience and clinical judgment rather than to draw from treatments that are scientifically scaffolded. This issue raises many dilemmas for clinicians of mental health treatment all along the spectrum, from treatment failure to the question of whether it is ethical to use approaches that have not been scientifically tested.

Recently, the introduction of what are known as the "third-wave behavior therapies" has further complicated the situation. Although there is some empirical evidence to support these approaches, some are under scrutiny because of the failure to fulfill the requirement of empirically supported treatments. Additionally, it is unclear whether many of the third-wave treatments can be considered independent from the basic genre of cognitive-behavioral therapy. Although some of the treatments attempt to provide innovative contributions, many of them simply rest on traditional models and wrap them in new paper.

A recent comprehensive meta-analysis has indicated that many published studies supporting the third-wave approaches used significantly less stringent research methodology than that used in studies published on cognitive-behavioral therapy during concurrent years. The meta-analysis further indicates that the mean effect size in these third-wave approaches was moderate for some studies, and that none of the third-wave therapies met the required criteria for empirically validated treatment. Such findings raise the question of how firmly the therapies are supported by any kind of theoretical foundation. Clearly, this volume comes at a critical juncture in our profession.

The editors of this volume have gathered a distinguished group of authors to offer perspectives on a variety of modalities. Every chapter provides sufficient material for readers to discern aptly whether the given approach is sufficiently grounded in a theoretical formulation to support the efficacy of the authors' claims.

The theoretical foundation is the backbone of any good psychotherapeutic approach, because all practitioners need a roadmap to guide them in working with the vast array of problems that clients bring to treatment. The interventions employed should tie into the basic theory from which they are delivered, providing a clinical justification for using techniques that are in keeping with the theoretical foundation. Yet, as Emmelkamp, Ehring, and Powers outline in the excellent first chapter in this volume, the emphasis on theory historically has waxed and waned over the years, resulting in an infatuation with "evidence-based treatments" and a relative neglect of "philosophy and theory." If we examine the basic proponents of the traditional cognitive-behavioral therapies, we find a solid relationship between theory and application that is ongoing. Most theoretical foundations are constructed from observation of human behaviors and lead to the generation of a hypothesis that is later scrutinized by rigorous empirical testing. Beck emphasizes in his Preface that if the empirical data do not support the hypothesis, then the hypothesis must be reconsidered or reformulated to match the result. In essence, the "proof of the pudding is in the eating"; that is, when a significant number of study outcomes are consistent with the proposed theory, credence can be given to the original hypothesis about the theory in general. However, in cases in which this methodology is bypassed and the results fall short of the anticipated outcome, the theorists must be honest about the result. It is also important that theorists identify when their approach is a recapitulation of a former theory rather than completely original. This is essential to the integrity of the field and the dignity of the individual. The editors of this book have attempted to present chapters that offer foundational perspectives on different theories. Readers can compare them and draw their own conclusions about which theories are reformulations of existing work, which rest on a weak foundation, and which are truly innovative approaches that are also solidly grounded. Such discernment is, by definition, thought provoking.

A strong focus on theory is essential in the field to avoid some of the problems posed by pure evidence-based approaches and to enable clinicians to rely on a roadmap that ties into that basic theory. Ideally, the preferred modality will have a sound, reliable theory behind it that is then bolstered by ongoing clinical observation and practice.

FRANK M. DATTILIO, PHD, ABPP
Department of Psychiatry
Harvard Medical School

Preface

What Is This Thing Called Theory?
How Is It Relevant for Practice?

Theory provides undergirding to effective case formulation, clinical practice, and research. The art and science of psychotherapy without theory is like a stool missing one of its supporting legs—shaky and unreliable.

We are introduced to theory during our training. University-based clinical psychology and psychiatry programs generally aim to span a range of psychotherapy models. We learn about the history of psychotherapy. We learn about the paradigms that have guided methods of scientific inquiry and that ultimately guide our practices as clinicians. We learn about the philosophical and theoretical assumptions within each approach.

We also learn about evidence-based practice. In fact, there are at least two overarching training approaches or models for basing psychotherapy practice on evidence. Programs based on the "Boulder model" seek to prepare practitioners to undertake ongoing research alongside their clinical work (i.e., as producers of research). The "Vail model," on the other hand, is premised upon the notion that training prepares practitioners to undertake practice that has been empirically substantiated (i.e., as consumers of research). Because research itself is theoretically based, our training was theoretically dependent on the model of training to which we were exposed. This raises the question: What do clinicians actually practice once they graduate?

Several large-scale surveys of practitioner populations have been conducted. These have generally sought to identify which theoretical models clinicians use in their work, along with other practice-relevant issues. The results of these surveys have shown that a wide variety of therapeutic models are actually used, and very few clinicians report a "pure-form" practice of therapy (i.e., practicing a single therapeutic model with all clients). These data might have inherent limitations because they are the result of nonrepresentative samples and the data collection methods were based on self-report. However, similar findings have been obtained among clinicians in many countries despite differences in training, work settings, and patient populations. If these data are accepted, then they support our subjective impression that practitioners rarely identify with a single theoretical orientation or model.

This book has been designed and written by those who practice psychotherapy. It illustrates a broad range of current behavior and cognitive therapy models through their application in practice. Each chapter provides the reader with a succinct overview of the model, including a brief outline of its history, philosophical and theoretical assumptions, and the state of the empirical evidence, with a focus on demonstrating the clinical application using a case study. All of our contributors have closely followed these guidelines, and in so doing mark the leading edge of knowledge regarding each model.

The book starts with a compelling Foreword (by Frank M. Dattilio), followed by a critical review of philosophy, psychology, and the causes and treatments of mental disorders (Chapter 1; Paul M. G. Emmelkamp, Thomas Ehring, and Mark B. Powers); Cognitive Therapy (Chapter 2; Jan Scott and Arthur Freeman); problem-solving therapy (Chapter 3; Arthur M. Nezu, Christine Maguth Nezu, and Thomas J. D'Zurilla); rational-emotive behavior therapy (Chapter 4; Raymond A. DiGiuseppe); acceptance and commitment therapy (Chapter 5; Thomas J. Waltz and Steven C. Hayes); behavioral activation therapy (Chapter 6; Christopher R. Martell, Sona Dimidjian, and Peter M. Lewinsohn); dialectical behavior therapy (Chapter 7; Thomas R. Lynch and Prudence Cuper); cognitive analytic therapy (Chapter 8; Anthony Ryle); positive psychology and therapy (Chapter 9; Nansook Park, Christopher Peterson, and Steven M. Brunwasser); mindfulness-based cognitive therapy (Chapter 10; Sona Dimidjian, Blair V. Kleiber, and Zindel V. Segal); and emotion-focused/interpersonal cognitive therapy (Chapter 11; Jeremy D. Safran, Catherine Eubanks-Carter, and J. Christopher Muran). We are grateful that such experienced, knowledgeable, and esteemed colleagues have contributed to this book. The participation of such a fine group speaks volumes about the importance of theory in practice.

For clinicians, putting these chapters side by side provides a valuable resource for the application of behavioral and cognitive theories. As with any advance or progress, there are discussions about what works, how, and why—and these controversies are useful in the context of psychotherapy practice. They encourage debate, generate new ideas and perspectives, and ultimately contribute to the evolution of psychotherapy.

NIKOLAOS KAZANTZIS
MARK A. REINECKE
ARTHUR FREEMAN

Contents

CHAPTER 1

Philosophy, Psychology, Causes, and Treatments of Mental Disorders

Paul M. G. Emmelkamp
Thomas Ehring
Mark B. Powers

> However interesting, plausible, and appealing a theory may be,
> it is techniques, not theories that are actually used on people.
> —PERRY LONDON, *The Modes and Morals*
> *of Psychotherapy* (1963, p. 33)

In this chapter, we briefly review the role of theory in the historical course of behavioral and cognitive therapy, which has increased and decreased over the years. In addition, we discuss the different views on the role of theory and their implications in clinical practice.

HISTORICAL ANALYSIS

Learning Theories

Although behavior therapy and behaviorism appear to be strongly related, the relationship between these two movements is far from unequivocal. Behaviorism is an important movement in experimental psychology, originating at the start of the 20th century. The American psychologist John B. Watson is usually considered the "father" of behaviorism, although it seems more likely that he functioned as a catalyst or charismatic leader of a larger societal movement (Kanfer, 1990). The onset of behavior therapy, however, occurred much later, in the 1950s. Behavior therapy started in response to the operative psychodynamic view of problem behavior. The discontent with the then-prevailing—notoriously unreliable—psychodiagnostic assessment and the effects of psychotherapy was another important impetus.

In 1952, the British psychologist Hans Eysenck caused a major stir with his empirical review claiming that the effects of traditional psychotherapy did not exceed those of no treatment at all. As an effective alternative, Eysenck mentioned behavior therapy based on modern learning theory. At the time, only a few British psychologists and psychiatrists were experimenting with this method, following the South African psychiatrist Joseph Wolpe. A similar development occurred more or less simultaneously in the United States. While Wolpe and the British group based their work predominantly on classical conditioning principles, in the United States the emphasis was on the application of operant conditioning principles in the treatment of dysfunctional behavior.

Classical Conditioning

Two major theoretical developments can be considered as the roots of behavior therapy. First, the classical conditioning paradigm established by Ivan Pavlov stimulated many psychologists to conceptualize psychopathological disorders in terms of learning processes. The most famous example of the use of the classical conditioning paradigm was the study on the development of specific phobias by Watson and Rayner (1920) in the 8-month-old "Little Albert." This study was pivotal in shaping the behavioral conceptualization of the development of phobias. Another important study from the 1920s was Jones's (1924) account of "Little Peter." The major contribution of the Little Albert and Little Peter cases was to emphasize the powerful role of learning in the acquisition of clinically relevant fears.

Although behavior theorists held that specific phobias are acquired through a process of conditioning, in which conditioned stimulus (CS) and unconditioned stimulus (UCS) are paired, the conditioning model of fear acquisition does not seem to be tenable in their original forms (e.g., Emmelkamp, 1982) and need broader reconceptualization within vulnerability–stress models. Recollection of traumatic experiences linked with the first phobic reactions has been reported in many specific phobias, but also nonphobic individuals report having experienced traumatic events in these situations. Research to date suggests that, apart from conditioning experiences, modeling and negative information transmission are also important factors in the etiology of specific phobias (Muris & Merckelbach, 2001). Furthermore, many factors other than the experienced pairings of CS and

UCS can affect the strength of the association between these events, including beliefs and expectancies about possible danger associated with a particular CS, and culturally transmitted information about the CS–UCS contingency (Davey, 1997).

Clinicians such as Eysenck and Wolpe held that classical conditioning processes could also be used to develop therapeutic procedures to extinguish anxiety and fears. For example, systematic desensitization was based on objectively derived principles of counterconditioning. Similarly, flooding and other exposure-based treatments were derived from experimental work on classical conditioning (Emmelkamp, 1982). The assumption was that if anxiety disorders were learned through a process of classical conditioning, then fear and anxiety could be remedied through applying procedures that effectively disrupted the learned CS–UCS association and extinguished the learned emotional response. Applications have not been limited to emotional disorders. Behavioral procedures based on classical conditioning have been used in the treatment of addictions as well (e.g., aversion therapy, cue exposure).

Operant Conditioning

Apart from the use of classical conditioning procedures in both the conceptualization of psychopathology and the development of treatment procedures, operant conditioning paradigms were also influential. Not all psychopathological conditions could easily be understood in terms of classical conditioning, and other disorders' etiology could be more easily explained by reference to the nature of the consequences of behavior. In the operant conditioning approach the emphasis is on the functional relationships between problem behavior and environmental contingencies.

A clinically important by-product of the operant approach is a behavioral assessment technique known as *behavioral analysis* or *functional analysis.* This functional analysis of problem behavior is an idiosyncratic approach that enables the clinician to identify reinforcers that maintain inadequate behavior, characteristic of the psychological dysfunction. The term *functional analysis* was used by Skinner (1953) to denote empirical demonstrations of "cause-and-effect relations" between environment and behavior. Nowadays, the term is used more widely to describe a wide range of procedures that are different in a number of ways (Hanley, Iwata, & McCord, 2003). In the United States functional analysis of problem behavior is still primarily used in the context of operant conditioning. In Europe, the term *functional analysis* is used much more broadly as a more general strategy to analyze patients' problems using not only operant conditioning but also classical conditioning and cognitive mediators.

Cognitive Models

Cognitive-behavioral therapy (CBT) is a general classification of psychotherapy including many different cognitive-behavioral approaches, such as rational-emotive behavior therapy (REBT; Ellis), cognitive therapy (CT; Beck), rational behavior therapy (Maultsby), self-instructional training and stress inoculation (Meichenbaum), schema-focused therapy (Young), meta-cognitive therapy (MCT; Wells), and—to some extent—dialectical behavior therapy (DBT; Linehan). Albert Ellis (1975) should be credited for developing the first comprehensive, primarily cognitively oriented psychotherapy. Although his work is based on Stoic philosophers, including Epictetus and Marcus Aurelius, it should be acknowledged that others also have contributed to the development of Ellis's thinking, be it positive or negative. From a sociology of science point of view, the development of Ellis's thoughts about therapy was negatively influenced on the one hand by his psychodynamic training. Disillusionment with the failure of psychodynamic therapies to provide a scientifically solid conceptualization of psychopathological disorders and therapeutic processes led to the development of rational-emotive therapy. On the other hand, Ellis was influenced in a positive way by publications of more behaviorally oriented psychologists, including Dollard and Miller's (1950) seminal attempts to interpret psychoanalysis into learning theory terms and Kelly's (1955) work on personal construct psychology.

Another important scholar is Aaron T. Beck (1976) who developed CT. Although there are more commonalities than differences between Ellis's and Beck's conceptualizations of the role of cognitive processes in psychopathology and how to target these in treatment, some differences exist in what each hold as the crucial cognitions. For example, whereas cognitive therapy is organized around the concepts of automatic thoughts and schemas, REBT is organized around the concept of rational and irrational beliefs. In the last decades, disorder-specific cognitive models and treatments have been developed for, among others, anxiety disorders (Clark, 1999), mood disorders (Beck, Rush, Shaw, & Emery, 1979), and personality disorders (Beck & Freeman, 1990).

If CT is aimed at changing cognition, it makes sense to base CT on the wealth of data provided by basic cognitive psychology (David & Szentagotai, 2006). Unfortunately, the terms used by Beck and Ellis to describe the cognitive processes are only loosely related to what is going on in the world of cognitive psychology. As noted by Hayes, Luoma-Bond, Masuda, and Lillis (2006) terms such as *cognitive disputation*, *empirical tests*, and *collaborative empiricism* are commonsense practical procedures that are generated clinically rather than derived from basic cognitive science: "The link between cognitive therapy and basic cognitive science continues to be weak. Looking at the array of popular techniques developed in CBT, none are known to have emerged directly from the basic cognitive science laboratories" (Hayes et al., 2006, p. 4). However, in recent years, a closer link between basic cognitive science and disorder-specific cognitive therapies is emerging (see Clark, 2004).

Third-Generation CBT

The history of CBT has recently been described as including three generations, namely, traditional behavior therapy, the addition of cognitive methods (CT or CBT), and the most recent third generation of contextualistic approaches (Hayes, 2004a, 2004b; Hayes et al., 2006). The contextualistic approach focuses on the function of behavior rather than the form. As described by the authors in this volume, acceptance and commitment therapy (ACT; Waltz & Hayes, Chapter 5) and mindfulness-based cognitive therapy (MBCT; Dimidjian, Kleiber, & Segal, Chapter 10) emerged in part from frustration with Beck's cognitive model of therapy for depression. Hayes (2004b) defined third-generation approaches as follows:

> Grounded in an empirical, principle-focused approach, the third wave of behavioral and cognitive therapy is particularly sensitive to the context and functions of psychological phenomena, not just their form, and thus tend to emphasize contextual and experiential change strategies in addition to more direct and didactic ones. These treatments tend to seek the construction of broad, flexible and effective repertoires over an eliminative approach to narrowly defined problems, and to emphasize the relevance of the issues they examine for clinicians as well as clients. (Hayes, 2004b, p. 658)

There is some discrepancy over which treatments are included in this "third wave." For example, Hayes et al. (2006) list ACT, DBT (Linehan, 1993), MBCT (Segal, Williams, & Teasdale, 2001), and MCT (Wells, 2000). Given the previous listed contextual treatments one may also consider adding a number of other approaches, including cognitive-behavioral analysis system of psychotherapy (CBASP; McCullough, 2000), integrated behavioral couple therapy (IBCT; Christensen & Jacobson, 2000), and functional-analytic psychotherapy (FAP; Kohlenberg & Tsai, 2007). The unifying theme among these third-generation approaches is the focus on controlling behavior while accepting negative affect. In addition, some authors suggest that these methods are more grounded in basic science. For example, ACT claims to be fundamentally different from other versions of behavioral and cognitive therapies. ACT is based on a contemporary behavioral analytic understanding of the behavior–environment functional relations involved in language, which is rooted in relational frame theory (RFT) and the functional analysis of rule-governed behavior (Hayes, Brownstein, Zettel, Haas, & Greenway,

1986). This approach is supported empirically both by a functional analysis of the social context for psychological distress and behavior change, and basic behavioral principles and the molar behavioral dynamics derived from basic behavioral analytic research. Overall, these approaches show relatively large effect sizes in clinical trials (Öst, 2008; Powers, Zum Vörde Sive Vörding, & Emmelkamp, 2009), and there is preliminary evidence that they work through the proposed mediators (Forman, Herbert, Moitra, Yeomans, & Geller, 2007; Lundgren, Dahl, & Hayes, 2008). For example, Forman et al. (2007) found that changes in "observing" and "describing" mediated outcome for cognitive therapy, but "experiential avoidance," "acting with awareness," and "acceptance" mediated outcomes for ACT. However, there remains much debate on whether they are truly a "new wave" or simply modifications to existing CBT (Hofmann & Asmundson, 2008), and it remains to be shown whether they are more effective than first- or second-wave CBT (Öst, 2008; Powers et al., 2009).

STATE OF THE ART OF THEORY IN COGNITIVE-BEHAVIORAL INTERVENTIONS

In the historical overview, the different waves or phases of CBT were organized according to their underlying theories. This reflects the fact that the CBT movement has always emphasized the role of theory, and basic research supporting this theory. However, over the years the emphasis has continuously shifted toward more eclectic approached and/or the use of empirically supported treatments regardless of their precise theoretical background, which we briefly describe in this chapter.

Eclectic Approaches

A number of professionals are less strict in attending to one specific theory of change but are more eclectic and use whatever technique comes in handy. The roots of this approach go back to Arnold Lazarus, who called for technical eclecticism (Lazarus, 1967). The forerunners of behavior therapy, Eysenck and Wolpe, did not welcome this approach. For example, Eysenck (1970) stated that this approach would lead to "nothing but a mishmash of theories, a huggermugger of procedures, a gallimaufry of therapies, and a charivaria of activities having no proper rationale, and incapable of being tested or evaluated" (p. 145). Rather than having a scientific discourse on the pros and the cons of technical eclecticism, Lazarus's call for eclecticism led to personal consequences. In Lazarus's own words: " Eysenck, as editor-in-chief of *Behaviour Research and Therapy*, expelled me from the editorial board, and Wolpe, who had been my mentor in South Africa, and with whom I served on the faculty at Temple University Medical School from 1967–1970, tried to get me fired" (2005, p. 151).

More recently, this eclectic approach is still being criticized and called the "cocktail school" of CBT (David & Szentagotai, 2006). Such professionals make a cocktail of a variety of behavioral and cognitive procedures, without paying due attention to the hypothesized theory of change:

> Although such a cocktail might prove effective, and even be manualized, it is still not informative enough for the science of cognitive-behavioral therapy (CBT). Without a clearly hypothesized theory of change (e.g., precisely which cognitions we want to restructure by using which specific techniques) accompanying each manualized treatment, CBT can hardly be considered a reference scientific therapeutic system. (p. 284)

Empirically Supported Therapies

In recent years, the claim for accountability of psychotherapy has hugely affected the current appraisal of the role of theory underlying effective interventions. In a major part of the field, the emphasis is now on demonstrating efficacy and effectiveness of specific procedures for specific DSM-IV disorders. Rather than brooding on theoretical innovations, a number of practitioners and researchers alike are now in the process of manualizing treatment procedures, often in the form of session-by-session treatment protocols.

In the system proposed by Division 12 of the American Psychological Association Task Force, a treatment method is given the title "possibly efficacious" if it is found to be more effective than no treatment in a single randomized controlled trial (RCT) ("bronze medal"). If this finding is replicated in a second RCT conducted by an independent research team, the treatment method is referred to as "efficacious" ("silver medal"). Treatments found to be superior to conditions that control for nonspecific processes or to another bona fide treatment are even more highly prized ("gold medal") and are said to be efficacious and specific in their mechanisms of action (Chambless & Hollon, 1998; Chambless & Ollendick, 2001).

[handwritten margin notes: bronze, silver, gold]

Renewed Emphasis on Theory

Although the empirically supported treatments approach is currently followed by a majority of CBT researchers, a growing minority argues for a need to put greater emphasis on individual case formulation based on empirically tested theories instead of treatment protocols. Examples are the case formulation approach by Persons (2006) and ACT (Hayes et al., 2006).

Concluding Remarks

Evidently, the once close relationship between theory and practice in behavior therapy and CT has changed considerably over the past decades. Today the dominant paradigm is *evidence-based treatment*. This normative approach emphasizes group means rather than individual cases. In the early days of behavior therapy the emphasis was on a more idiosyncratic approach: the individualized case formulation, firmly based in theory. Of course, throughout the years both the normative and the idiosyncratic approaches have had their proponents, but the relative emphasis has changed considerably over time. In the following, we examine the advantages and disadvantages of the two positions.

ADVANTAGES AND DISADVANTAGES OF THE EVIDENCE-BASED APPROACH

The empirically supported treatment approach of the Division 12 Task Force of the American Psychological Association should be seen in the context of a broader movement: evidence-based medicine. The reasons why certified, evidence-based treatments are proclaimed to be superior include their enhancement of patient care and informing clinicians of recent empirical knowledge. It was felt that therapists in busy clinical practice would find it difficult to keep abreast of the recent literature and would need summaries of the research evidence provided by "expert reviews," such as the National Institute for Clinical Excellence (NICE) guidelines in the United Kingdom and the American Psychological Association "empirically supported treatments" in the United States. In many other countries, similar "expert committees" have now provided guidelines for evidence-based treatment of mental disorders.

Although it is acknowledged that theory may have been important in the development of the various therapeutic approaches, the main criterion for "certifying" a certain treatment for a certain population is its proven efficacy in RCTs. As a consequence, any treatment "that works" without any sound theoretical basis may be accredited in such committees. To enhance the implementation of these guidelines, treatment manuals are developed and validated for specific target populations.

Advantages

There are a number of advantages of the evidence-based approach. First, there are clear, objective criteria for clinical decision making with respect to which treatment would be particularly effective for patients with specific mental disorders. This would make the cumbersome and often problematic idiosyncratic decision making by clinicians superfluous. Although there are many advocates of an individualized clinical approach, hardly any research has actually been conducted to ascertain the validity of this approach. In a study conducted some time ago, we found that the clinical decision making was not so reliable. In a study on the treatment of persons with obsessive–compulsive disorder, therapists held interviews to gather material to make a problem analysis, a functional analysis, and a treatment plan. Based on the interviews, other clinicians came up with their own problem analysis, functional analysis, and treatment plan. Unfortunately, the interrater reliability was low. There appeared to be good consensus on a scale from 0 to 10 between the therapist and other clinicians with respect to the problem areas involved, moderate consensus with respect to the antecedents of the problem behavior and the treatment prescribed, and lowest consensus with respect to the presumed causality in the functional analysis (Emmelkamp, 1992).

A second advantage of the empirically supported treatments (ESTs) movement is that the manualized treatments are easy to disseminate. By definition, each treatment needs to be manualized, and each manual is a convenient vehicle to transport the package to other academic and community settings for training. Third, governing agencies and associations can now develop treatment guidelines based on clearly defined, manualized ESTs. For example, training in CBT is now required for psychiatry residence programs (Beck, 2000). Finally, it is simple to establish new treatments with the clear EST criteria.

Disadvantages

Much criticism that has been raised is emotionally rather than theoretically or empirically driven. For example, some have viewed manuals as "promoting a cookbook mentality" or a therapist as "an improvisational artist, not a manual-driven technician" (Chambless & Ollendick, 2001, p. 701). However, there are also a number of more serious problems related to the evidence-based approach, for example, what to do when individual patients do not fit nicely into target groups for which evidence-based treatments exist. One of the biggest problems for evidence-based psychotherapy is the problem of comorbidity. For example, a substantial number of patients with anxiety disorders have not only concurrent anxiety disorder but may also have a concurrent depressive disorder. Similarly, in patients with substance use disorders, a dual diagnosis is the norm rather than the exception (Emmelkamp & Vedel, 2006). Comorbidity is not limited to Axis I disorders; it also occurs frequently between Axis I and Axis II disorders (Emmelkamp & Kamphuis, 2007). From this perspective, the prescription of evidence-based manualized treatment is not realistic. One can hardly expect practitioners to follow a number of manuals targeting different disorders sequentially. There is a clear need for more theoretically driven decision making in prioritizing treatment targets.

The evidence-based approach is based on disorder-specific thinking; it assumes that qualitatively distinct groups can be defined by shared symptoms. This approach assumes that patients with a certain diagnosis respond in a uniform way to a certain treatment. However, there might be important differences within such patient groups. Take, for example, patients with a borderline personality disorder diagnosis. According to DSM-IV-TR, a patient qualifies for a diagnosis of borderline personality disorder if five out of nine criteria are fulfilled. This means, however, that there is a large variation in how patients with borderline personality disorder present themselves. What if DBT is more effective in patients with borderline personality disorder, who are primarily characterized by impulsivity and parasuicidal behavior, and transference-focused therapy or mentalization-based therapy is more effective for patients who primarily are characterized by problems in interpersonal relationships, distorted self-image, and feelings of emptiness?

Another problem has been negative views regarding treatment manuals (Carroll & Nuro, 2002). Treatments were originally manualized to increase the internal validity of RCTs (Luborsky & DeRubeis, 1984; Waltz, Addis, Koerner, & Jacobson, 1993). It was then assumed that once the manualized treatment was validated in research, practitioners in the community would adopt the manuals for routine care (Torrey et al., 2001). However, in actual practice, very few practitioners are inclined to use treatment manuals (Powers & Emmelkamp, 2009). Only 7% of psychologists report using treatment manuals regularly, and only 20% report being clear on what a treatment manual is (Addis & Krasnow, 2000).

Finally, a criticism pertinent to the theoretical underpinning of CBT involves the lack of any test of the theoretical foundation of the treatment method certified. To establish clear causal links between interventions and outcomes, operationalizations of intervention techniques must be rooted in a solid theoretical foundation. As cogently argued by Rosen and Davison (2003), "any authoritative body representing the science of psychology should work toward the identification of 'empirically supported principles of change' (ESPs); it should not list empirically supported treatments (ESTs); and it certainly should never list proprietary, trademarked methods" (p. 303). Interventions that lack any guiding theory, if proven effective, will generate post hoc speculations regarding possible active components (Strauman & Merrill, 2004).

Concluding Remarks

While the shift in emphasis on empirically effective treatments, with neglect of the empirical theoretical foundations, is understandable from the perspective of the insurance companies, in the end it may turn out to be penny-wise but pound-foolish. Unfortunately, in shifting the emphasis from theory-based therapy to evidence-based therapy, one runs the risk of throwing away the baby with the bathwater. Indeed, current CBT procedures are far from effective for all patients. About 30–40% of patients cannot be successfully treated with current CBT procedures (Emmelkamp, 2004), still leaving room for improvement of the failure rate. This figure has not changed over the past 25 years (Foa & Emmelkamp, 1983); apparently, no significant progress has been made over the last decades. If we want to improve our treatments, we need a better understanding of why treatments work and why they often fail. Progress in psychotherapy in general, and in CBT in particular, is dependent on the synergy between theoretical developments and empirical testing of theories in "lab situations." Of course, the proof of the pudding still is to established evidence in clinical practice: "However interesting, plausible, and appealing a theory may be, it is techniques, not theories that are actually used on people" (London, 1964, p. 33).

ADVANTAGES AND DISADVANTAGES OF INDIVIDUALIZED, THEORY-BASED APPROACHES

An alternative for the evidence-based movement would be to ground treatment more on validated theories of psychopathology and change (see Eifert, 1996; Hayes et al., 2006; Persons, 2006). The main difference between this approach and the evidence-based approach is that treatment decisions are based on not just the application of evidence-based standardized manuals, but on more flexible applications of different strategies derived from the background of a specific model.

There are a number of different individualized treatment approaches, but the common ground is that therapists rely on an empirical hypothesis testing approach to each case. In the individualized treatment approach of Emmelkamp (1982), a distinction is made between a microanalysis and a macroanalysis. A *microanalysis, or functional analysis,* analyzes the behavior within a certain problem domain. The key questions that the therapist attempts to answer are the following: What are the situations in which the behavior occurs? Which responses (emotional, physiological, cognitive, overt behavior) occur? What are the consequences of the behavior? When conducting a macroanalysis, the therapist charts the various problem domains, while seeking possible causal connections between the problems. Based on both of these analyses, the therapist provides an idiographic case formulation to guide treatment planning and intervention (for practical applications see Emmelkamp, Scholing, & Bouman, 1992; Emmelkamp & Vedel, 2006). In the Persons (2006) approach, the therapist uses evidence-based nomothetic formulations and treatment plans as templates for the idiographic formulation and treatment plan. ACT is another approach that includes individualized, theory-driven treatment planning (Hayes, Strosahl, & Wilson, 1999).

There are clear advantages of a more individualized approach. Individual case conceptualization allows targeted treatment for patients with unusual problems for which no evidence-based manuals exist, and for the more difficult cases with more than one disorder. Such a strategy is much more flexible than the application of manualized treatment and allows the therapist to adapt strategies to a range of patient characteristics. Furthermore, such an individualized approach presumably is also more gratifying to the therapist conducting the therapy. In addition, proponents of such an approach suggest that it should lead to faster and more successful innovation in clinical practice (but see below for a critical view on this issue).

On the other hand, there are also disadvantages associated with such an idiosyncratic approach. First of all, the therapy will only be as effective as the therapist's creativity. An individualized treatment approach is certainly much more difficult to learn, teach, and practice than manual-based, standardized, evidence-based treatments. Second, while its flexibility is certainly an advantage, especially in more difficult cases, a weakness of the method is the ease with which it can "slide down a slippery slope and become non evidence-based, in part, because of its very flexibility" (Persons, 2006, p. 168). In addition, it may be naive to assume that theoretical ideas can easily be translated into effective interventions. For example, it turns out that negative appraisals or dysfunctional cognitions can be modified in different ways, including not only traditional cognitive restructuring but also behavior experiments or imagery rescripting (Leahy, 2003). Which technique is most effective for which type negative appraisal is then an empirical question. Finally, there is no robust evidence yet for superior effectiveness of treatment based on a functional analysis over effects achieved with manualized evidence-based treatments. The results of studies conducted so far demonstrate that the individualized treatments are no better than the standardized treatment protocols (Emmelkamp, Bouman, & Blaauw, 1994; Schulte, Kunzel, Pepping, & Schulte-Bahrenberg, 1992). As an aside, it is astonishing how little research effort has gone into what once was considered to be the cornerstone of (cognitive) behavior therapy; the field gets the manualized treatments it deserves!

INTEGRATION OF THEORY-FOCUSED
AND EVIDENCE-BASED TREATMENTS

It is important to note that the dichotomy between evidence-based and theory-based approaches is rather artificial. In fact, extreme views on this issue are rare, and most authors discussing the role of theory versus efficacy of manualized treatments come to the conclusion that both views need to be integrated. However, there are differences in the relative weight assigned to the different components. For example, Persons (2006) puts a clear emphasis on theory-based individual case formulation. Salkovskis (2002), on the other hand, assigns an equally important role to theory and related experimental research, treatment outcome research, and clinical practice in his model on empirically grounded clinical interventions. Finally, researchers from different theoretical orientations have suggested that treatment development would benefit most from a strategy that starts with the development and rigorous testing of a theoretical model that is then translated into manualized treatment protocols that are finally tested in outcome studies (Clark, 2004; Hayes et al., 2006).

A number of current developments may turn out to be fruitful in the future. These include the suggestion to focus more on empirically supported principles of change rather than on whole treatment packages (Rosen & Davison, 2003). In addition, there is the increasing recognition that many processes involved in the development and maintenance of emotional disorders appear to be transdiagnostic rather than disorder specific (Harvey, Watkins, Mansell, & Shafran, 2004). Future treatments may therefore focus more on targeting relevant processes rather than on distinct diagnostic categories. Although it remains to be tested whether these approaches result in more effective interventions, it appears that they may help to overcome some of the dichotomies between theory-based and evidence-based approaches in the current literature.

HOW MUCH EVIDENCE IS THERE
FOR THE PRESUMED THEORETICAL PROCESSES?

In the CBT literature, there has been a surprising lack of interest for studying mediational factors in treatment. However, this type of research can inform the current discussion by testing whether variables derived from theoretical models indeed mediate the effects of psychological treatment on symptom reduction. The theoretical model underlying a specific type of treatment is supported if (1) success is related to change in process variables that are assumed to be crucial for recovery from the disorder (e.g., reduction in dysfunctional appraisals in cognitive therapy), (2) this relationship is *specific* to the type of treatment that is based on the respective theory, and (3) these changes in key processes precede the changes in the targeted complaint (e.g., depression, anxiety). In the following, examples of research in this area are given for anxiety disorders (social phobia and panic disorder), depression, and substance use disorders.

Social Phobia

A recent meta-analysis of 32 RCTs ($N = 1,479$) investigated the effects of cognitive and behavioral therapies in social anxiety disorder (Powers, Sigmarsson, & Emmelkamp, 2008). Whereas treatment outperformed waiting-list ($d = 0.86$) and placebo conditions ($d = 0.38$) across outcome domains and at follow-up, no significant difference was found between exposure therapy and cognitive therapy, or their combination. Interestingly, all types of treatments resulted in significant improvements on both behavioral and cognitive measures with similar effect sizes. Therefore, the hypothesis of differential mechanisms of change in treatments with different theoretical background could not be supported.

A set of additional studies investigated whether treatment effects on symptoms of social phobia are mediated by a reduction in cognitive biases, especially the overestimation of the likelihood/probability of threat, as well as the cost or severity of the threat typically found in social phobics (e.g., Foa, Franklin, Perry, & Herbert, 1996). Results of a first study showed that changes in estimated social cost mediated social phobia improvement in both cognitive therapy and exposure treatment again not showing any specificity in mechanisms of change for different treatment protocols (Hofmann, 2004). In an additional study, Smits, Rosenfield, McDonald, and Telch (2006) examined social cost and probability biases among 53 adults with social phobia undergoing CBT. The found evidence that both biases (cost and probability) mediated social phobia improvement. However, temporal analyses showed that the probability bias resulted in fear reduction, which in turn resulted in a lower cost bias. Taken together, although there is preliminary evidence for a cognitive mediation of treatment effects in social anxiety disorder, there is as yet no evidence for its specificity for cognitively oriented treatments.

Panic Disorder

Somewhat more consistent results come from research into mediators of treatment in panic disorder. From a cognitive perspective, anxiety sensitivity (i.e., a fear of benign bodily sensations [heart rate, sweating, etc.] caused by anxiety; Reiss, Peterson, Gursky, & McNally, 1986), is considered to be a key mechanism in the development and maintenance of the disorder, and has been supported in a large number of studies (see Barlow, 2002). Importantly, results from several studies suggest that anxiety sensitivity mediates improvement in the treatment of panic disorder (Cho, Smits, Powers, & Telch, 2007; Hofmann et al., 2007; Smits, Powers, Cho, & Telch, 2004). For example, Smits et al. randomized 130 patients with panic disorder to CBT or to a waiting list. Anxiety sensitivity fully mediated improvements in disability and partially mediated changes in agoraphobia, general anxiety, and panic frequency. Similar results emerged at a 6-month follow-up (Cho et al., 2007). Furthermore, results of an additional study suggest that the reduction in anxiety sensitivity is specific for CBT treatment. Hofmann et al. (2007) examined changes in panic-related cognitions among 91 patients with panic who were randomized to CBT alone, imipramine alone, CBT plus imipramine, and CBT plus placebo. They found that panic-related cognitions only mediated improvement in patients who received CBT. Importantly, reductions in anxiety sensitivity precede reductions in panic symptoms, thereby showing temporal precedence (Smits et al., 2008). The literature on anxiety sensitivity as a mediator of change in panic disorder treatment therefore provides one of the few examples meeting the criteria outlined at the beginning of this section.

Depression

Behavior therapy, cognitive therapy, and their combination all have been shown to be effective treatments for major depression, and recent reviews and meta-analyses show that no consistent differences in efficacy, among the treatment approaches can be found (Emmelkamp, 2004; Ekers, Richards, & Gilbody, 2008). The same conclusions can be drawn from directly comparing the different treatments in RCTs (e.g., Dimidijian et al., 2006; Gortner, Gollan, Dobson, & Jacobson, 1998). In the treatment of bereavement, however, behavioral exposure was found to be more effective than cognitive therapy (Boelen, de Keijzer, van den Hout, & van den Bout, 2007).

Theoretically, one would expect that cognitive therapy and behavior therapy would have differential effects on cognitive and behavioral variables. Although a number of studies were designed to show that these treatments have specific effects on relevant targets, the results are rather negative. Generally, relevant behavioral and cognitive variables are changed as much by cognitive therapy as by behavior therapy (Emmelkamp, 2004). Thus, effects of behavioral and cognitive programs appear to be "nonspecific," changing both behavioral and cognitive components, thus precluding conclusions with respect to the therapeutic processes responsible for the improvement. To complicate matters further, comparison of cognitive therapy with phar-

macotherapy shows that in most studies cognitions are changed as much by pharmacotherapy as by cognitive therapy (Garratt, Ingram, Rand, & Sawalani, 2007). Thus, it seems that cognitive distortions act as symptoms of depression rather than as mediators of treatment outcome.

Substance Abuse/Dependence

Whereas the first three examples have mainly focused on the role of cognitive factors as mediators of treatment effects, the following example is instead based on a behavioral variable, namely, coping skills in substance use disorders. Training in coping skills to deal with high-risk situations is assumed to be the essential ingredient of effective CBT treatment approaches for substance use disorders (Emmelkamp & Vedel, 2006). Although it is generally held that the results of coping skills training are mediated by a change in coping skills, this has hardly been investigated. In a review by Morgenstern and Longabaugh (2000), support for a mediational role of coping was found in only one study. In a more recent study (Litt, Kadden, Cooney, & Kabela, 2003) with alcohol-dependent patients, researchers investigated whether specific coping skills training was essential for increasing the use of coping skills. Patients received either coping skills training or interactional group treatment, and coping skills were measured at multiple time points. Both treatments yielded very good drinking reduction outcomes throughout the follow-up period, and increased coping skills were indeed a significant predictor of outcome. However, in contrast to what one would expect, coping skills training did not improve coping more than did interactional group treatment. Similarly, in the Marijuana Treatment Project, coping skills-oriented treatment did not result in greater use of coping skills than motivational enhancement therapy (Litt et al., 2005). Thus, although coping skills training has been found to be effective in a number of studies, it is unclear which components in the treatment package are responsible for the results achieved. Further studies are needed to determine which of the various components in the treatment package (e.g., self-monitoring, identification of high-risk situations, strategies for coping with craving, and training in problem solving) are the necessary ingredients for successful therapeutic outcome and prevention of relapse, and which are redundant.

Concluding Remarks

Research so far has not shown unequivocally that the effects of CBT approaches can be attributed to the presumed underlying mechanisms. From our point of view, it is astonishing to see how few efforts have gone into investigating the mediators of treatment outcome. There is a clear need for further studies into the presumed theoretical mechanisms of CBT.

SOME GENERAL REFLECTIONS ON THEORY IN CBT

Up to now, we have referred to *theory* in general, without making any further distinctions. However, when taking a closer look, it appears necessary to distinguish between different levels or domains to which this may refer. In the following, we briefly describe three different types of theory as relevant to CBT research and practice.

Theories Regarding the Development and Maintenance of Emotional Problems

The most commonly used types of theoretical models in CBT research and practice aim at explaining the etiology of emotional problems. Apart from highly eclectic approaches, almost all treatments are based on explicitly formulated theories that often distinguish between factors involved in the development of emotional disorders and those leading to its maintenance. A number of criteria are commonly applied to evaluate psychological theories of this kind (for a detailed description see Westmeyer, 1989). First, they should be logically consistent, parsimonious/simple, and precise; they should allow an operationalization of the theory's key constructs and should be falsifiable. Second, theories are evaluated regarding the amount and quality of their empirical support, as well as their heuristic value for research and practice.

On a broad level, theoretical approaches can be distinguished by their basic ideas and concepts, as exemplified in our historical overview, as well as the structure of this book, wherein each chapter represents one basic theoretical approach. Whereas the same theoretical principles were applied to all emotional problems in early behavior therapy, recent decades have seen a strong trend toward developing and empirically testing disorder-specific models. In practice, it is mainly these disorder-focused theories that are empirically tested rather than the underlying broader theories. However, in recent years, a renewed emphasis on transdiagnostic approaches to emotional disorders has emerged (e.g., Harvey et al., 2004; Hayes, Wilson, Gifford, & Follette, 1996).

Basic Philosophical Assumptions

Psychological theories can be distinguished from basic philosophical ideas with relevance to CBT research and practice. As Hayes et al. (1999) have argued, philosophical assumptions underlying psychological treatment are neither empirically supported nor empirically testable. Instead, they comprise the axioms on which the more specific and testable theoretical constructs are based. The most important philosophical issues with relevance for clinical research and practice fall into two different domains: namely (1) theory of science and (2) basic assumptions about human nature.

Theory of Science

A literature search into the role of theory of science in CBT shows that the field is surprisingly silent about its epistemological assumptions. As a consequence, most introductory textbooks immediately start describing methodological issues, without explicitly presenting CBT's philosophical underpinnings. In the small, specialized literature on philosophy of science and psychology, empiricism, rationalism, idealism, realism, and constructivism are often distinguished as prototypical positions (see Westmeyer, 1989). For example, early behaviorism was rooted in empiricism and aimed at deriving rules from repeated observations. Researchers influenced by basic cognitive psychology typically held more rationalist positions, for example, those derived from critical rationalism (Popper, 1935). However, research practice tends to deviate considerably from the expected relative to the background of these philosophical orientations (see also Kuhn, 1962). Possibly the clearest example is the fact that most psychological research is focused on collecting evidence *supporting* theoretical ideas despite the strong emphasis on the importance of *falsification* in critical rationalism. A number of contemporary positions within philosophy of science, such as social constructionist (Gergen, 1985) or structuralist approaches (Westmeyer, 1992), appear to be potentially fruitful for clinical psychology but have hardly been taken up by theorists and researchers in the field. A number of authors have suggested that the science and practice of CBT may benefit from paying more attention to its epistemological foundations (see Erwin, 2006; Mahoney, 2005; Woolfolk & Richardson, 2008).

Basic Assumptions about Human Nature

Some theoretical traditions within CBT are explicitly linked to specific philosophical traditions. For example, CT (Beck, 1976) and REBT (Ellis, 1975) explicitly refer back to the Greek Stoic philosophers. The resulting emphasis on appraisal and rational thinking clearly distinguished CT from the then-dominating paradigms psychoanalysis and behaviorism. A recent example is ACT, which is explicitly based on functional contextualism (Hayes et al., 2006). In addition to describing their own philosophical foundations explicitly, ACT theorists generally call for greater attention to these issues: "We can ignore philosophy only by mindlessly and implicitly assuming a philosophy, but it seems much better to own up to our assumptions consciously" (Hayes et al., 1999, p. 16). However, this viewpoint is currently an exception in the field. Most theoretical models on the development and maintenance of emotional disorders are silent about the philosophical background. It is open to discussion whether CBT science and practice would indeed benefit from a closer examination of its philosophical foundations. Among others, important issues may include the question of determinism versus individual freedom, and normative questions surrounding the selection of individual and therapeutic goals, as well as ethical issues.

Theories of Change during Psychological Treatment

The third set of theories that can be distinguished from etiological models on the one hand and philosophical foundations on the other concerns the way in which change is thought to take place during psychological treatment. At first sight, one may assume that this can be deducted directly from psychological theories of psychopathology, as these tell us which mechanisms to target during treatment. However, this does not appear to be sufficient for at least two reasons. First, in most cases, there are different ways to target a certain mechanism. For example, to change dysfunctional appraisals in anxiety disorders, purely cognitive strategies may not be the best method. Instead *in vivo* exposure or behavioral experiments may be at least equally effective. Second, there is convincing evidence that theories of change must take into account general factors that are not specific for certain emotional disorders but generally are necessary for change to occur (e.g., motivational processes or therapeutic alliance; see Schulte & Eifert, 2002). Therefore, a stronger emphasis on the development and empirical testing of theories of behavioral and cognitive change appears timely.

SOME CRITICAL THOUGHTS

In this book we intend to promote the view that a stronger emphasis on theory and philosophy can help to strengthen science and practice of CBT. The current chapter has introduced the role of theory in the historical development, as well as current practice of CBT, and highlighted a number of basic issues surrounding the relationship between theory and clinical practice. The historical overview has shown that the emphasis on theory has waxed and waned over the years, and has resulted in a currently strong focus on evidence-based treatments. Although we generally agree with the book's editors that a return to a stronger focus on theory is promising to overcome some of the current problems faced by pure, evidence-based approaches, we would nevertheless like to conclude with a number of critical comments to keep in mind.

First, the structure of each chapter in this book implicitly suggests to the reader that treatment development follows nicely from sound, empirically supported theoretical approaches and their application in treatment. However, from our experience, this is almost never the case. Instead, it appears that development of theory and practice often happen at the same time. This may need to be acknowledged appropriately in order not to run the danger of erroneously disregarding the innovative potential of clinical practice. The jury is still out as to whether successful clinical innovation mainly emerges from theory and basic science or directly from clinical observation and practice. Arguably, a combination of both, as recently described by Clark (2004) and Salkovskis (2002), and generally reflected in the scientist-practitioner model, would be most fruitful.

On a more radical note, looking back at the development of CBT in the past 30 years we might argue that the innovative character of theories may even be a myth. Although systematic desensitization is based on laboratory studies on reciprocal inhibition in cats (Wolpe, 1958), many subsequent innovations in CBT interventions have emerged from clinical practice rather than being the result of theoretically driven experimental work. In addition, many theoretical developments in recent years/decades have not led to any innovation in clinical practice. Take, for example, the considerable efforts by research groups around the world focusing on experimental psychopathology. Hundreds of laboratory studies have been conducted into fine-tuning and testing of theories with respect to learning theory approaches and information processing of psychopathological conditions. While this has certainly improved our theoretical understanding of emotional problems (e.g., Craske, Hermans, & Vansteenwegen, 2006; McNally, 2007), to the best of our knowledge, it has had no real clinical impact on diagnosis, treatment planning, or innovations in treatment of patients with these disorders. One could argue that such research is justified by a slogan popular among pharmacologists: "This type of research is like looking for a needle in the haystack and then ... finding the farmer's daughter." But unfortunately we have not yet come across the farmer's daughter in the field of CBT. An exception may be attentional training in social phobia, which can be considered a direct result of the experimental studies into selective attention in anxiety disorders (but also note the lack of evidence that attentional training is more effective than other CBT interventions for social phobia; Powers et al., 2008). Additional examples are CT for panic disorder, which is related to basic research into misinterpretation of bodily sensations (Clark, 1999), and ACT, which is related to basic research based on relational frame theory (Hayes et al., 2006). Despite these examples, the contribution of basic experimental psychopathology as a whole to clinical practice has been at best modest. We often speak to clinicians who are disappointed with the progress of experimental psychopathology, and who find the studies presented at conferences and published papers hardly relevant to the day-to-day clinical problems with which they are confronted. From this perspective, it is understandable that clinicians "don't care about theories as long as treatment works." This may be one of the reasons why procedures such as eye movement desensitization and reprocessing (EMDR), which, according to Rosen and Davison (2003), "rest on assumptions outside the mainstream of science" (p. 303), are so popular among clinicians. EMDR is as effective as trauma-focused therapies such as prolonged exposure (Bisson et al., 2007), but its theoretical underpinnings have not been validated. There is a clear challenge for scholars working in experimental psychopathology to make their studies more relevant and palatable for the workers in the field. Another example is the considerable research on safety behaviors in anxiety disorders (Powers, Smits, & Telch, 2004; Rachman, Radomsky, & Shafran, 2008; Salkovskis, Clark, Hackmann, Wells, & Gelder, 1999; Sloan & Telch, 2002; Wells et al., 1995). *Safety behaviors* are defined as actions people take to prevent a perceived threat, such as drinking alcohol before giving a speech. Since the beginning of exposure-based treatment (i.e., Wolpe, 1958; Emmelkamp, 1982), clinicians report asking patients to eliminate any kind of avoidance behaviors. However, officially, research on "safety behaviors" only began in the 1990s. During this fruitful time, authors described how engaging in safety behaviors maintained anxiety, whereas fading them improved long-term outcome. Clinicians saw this as a modern-day explanation for what they had been doing all along. It appears important to acknowledge the currently existing gap between basic experimental research and innovative clinical practice to stimulate translational research to connect these two fields. In this context, research programs explicitly acknowledging the importance of interaction between basic science and treatment development are encouraging (Clark, 2004; Hayes et al., 2006).

Finally, a largely neglected but important area appears to be the investigation of treatment processes and mechanisms of change. Treatment process research can provide valuable information for theoretical accounts. One could argue that there are currently a number of empirically well-supported interventions in search of a fitting and empirically supported theory. This is even true for one of the best supported evidence-based treatments, exposure therapy for anxiety disorders: We know that it works, but we do not know exactly why. Bridging the gaps between basic science, treatment development, treatment process research, and everyday clinical practice remains an important challenge for future CBT research.

REFERENCES

Addis, M. E., & Krasnow, A. (2000). A national survey of practicing psychologists' attitudes toward psychotherapy treatment manuals. *Journal of Consulting and Clinical Psychology, 68*, 331–339.

Barlow, D. H. (2002). *Anxiety and its disorders: The nature and treatment of anxiety and panic* (2nd ed.). New York: Guilford Press.

Beck, A. T. (1976). *Cognitive therapy and the emotional disorders.* New York: International Universities Press.

Beck, A. T., Freeman, A., & Associates. (1990). *Cognitive therapy of personality disorders.* New York: Guilford Press.

Beck, A. T., Rush, A. J., Shaw, B. F., & Emery, G. (1979). *Cognitive therapy of depression.* New York: Guilford Press.

Beck, J. S. (2000). *Finally!: Cognitive therapy enters psychiatry training!* Bala Cynwyd, PA: Beck Institute for Cognitive Therapy and Research.

Bisson, J. I., Ehlers, A., Matthews, R., Pilling, S., Richards, D., & Turner, S. (2007). Psychological treatments for chronic post-traumatic stress disorder: Systematic review and meta-analysis. *British Journal of Psychiatry, 190,* 97–104.

Boelen, P. A., de Keijzer, J., van den Hout, M. A., & van den Bout, J. (2007). Treatment of complicated grief: A comparison between cognitive behavioral therapy and supportive counseling. *Journal of Consulting and Clinical Psychology, 75,* 277–284.

Carroll, K. M., & Nuro, K. F. (2002). One size cannot fit all: A stage model for psychotherapy manual development. *Clinical Psychology: Science and Practice, 9,* 396–406.

Chambless, D. L., & Hollon, S. D. (1998). Defining empirically supported therapies. *Journal of Consulting and Clinical Psychology, 66,* 7–18.

Chambless, D. L., & Ollendick, T. H. (2001). Empirically supported psychological interventions: Controversies and evidence. *Annual Review of Psychology, 52,* 685–716.

Cho, Y., Smits, J. A., Powers, M. B., & Telch, M. J. (2007). Do changes in panic appraisal predict improvement in clinical status following cognitive-behavioral treatment of panic disorder? *Cognitive Therapy and Research, 31,* 695–707.

Christensen, A., & Jacobson, N. S. (2000). *Reconcilable differences.* New York: Guilford Press.

Clark, D. M. (1986). A cognitive approach to panic. *Behaviour Research and Therapy, 24,* 461–470.

Clark, D. M. (1999). Anxiety disorders: Why they persist and how to treat them. *Behaviour Research and Therapy, 37,* S5–S27.

Clark, D. M. (2004). Developing new treatments: On the interplay between theories, experimental science, and clinical innovation. *Behavioral Research and Therapy, 42,* 1009–1104.

Craske, M. G., Hermans, D., & Vansteenwegen, D. (Eds.). (2006). *Fear and learning: From basic processes to clinical implications.* Washington, DC: American Psychological Association.

Davey, G. C. L. (1997). A conditioning model of phobias. In *Phobias: A handbook of theory, research and treatment* (pp. 301–318). New York: Wiley.

David, D., & Szentagotai, A. (2006). Cognitions in cognitive-behavioral psychotherapies: Toward an integrative model. *Clinical Psychology Review, 26(3),* 284–298.

Dimidijian, S., Hollon, S. D., Dobson, K. S., Schmaling, K. B., Kohlenberg, R. J., Addis, M. E., et al. (2006). Randomized trial of behavioral activation, cognitive therapy, and antidepressant medication in the acute treatment of adults with major depression. *Journal of Consulting and Clinical Psychology, 74,* 658–670.

Dollard, J., & Miller, N. E. (1950). *Personality and psychotherapy.* New York: McGraw-Hill.

Eifert, G. H. (1996). More theory-driven and less diagnosis-based behavior therapy. *Journal of Behavior Therapy and Experimental Psychiatry, 27,* 75–86.

Ekers, D., Richards, D., & Gilbody, S. (2008). Meta-analysis of randomized trials of behavioural treatment of depression. *Psychological Medicine, 38,* 611–623.

Ellis, A. (1975). *Reason and emotion in psychotherapy.* Secaucus, NJ: Stuart.

Emmelkamp, P. M. G. (1982). *Phobic and obsessive–compulsive disorders: Theory, research and practice.* New York: Plenum Press.

Emmelkamp, P. M. G. (1992). Behaviour therapy in the *fin de siécle.* In J. Cottraux, P. Legeron, & E. Mollard (Eds.), *Which psychotherapies in 2000* (pp. 151–166). Lisse: Swets & Zeitlinger.

Emmelkamp, P. M. G. (2004). Behavior therapy with adults. In M. Lambert (Ed.), *Bergin and Garfield's handbook of psychotherapy and behavior change* (5th ed., pp. 393–446). New York: Wiley.

Emmelkamp, P. M. G., Bouman, T., & Blaauw, E. (1994). Individualized versus standardized therapy: A comparative evaluation with obsessive–compulsive patients. *Clinical Psychology and Psychotherapy, 1,* 95–100

Emmelkamp, P. M. G., & Kamphuis, J. H. (2007). *Personality disorders.* Hove: UK Psychology Press/Taylor & Francis.

Emmelkamp, P. M. G., Scholing, A., & Bouman, T. K. (1992). *Anxiety disorders.* Chichester, UK: Wiley.

Emmelkamp, P. M. G., & Vedel, E. (2006). *Evidence-based treatment of alcohol and drug abuse.* New York: Routledge/Taylor & Francis.

Erwin, E. (2006). Randomized clinical trials in psychotherapy outcome research. *Philosophy of Science, 73,* 135–152.

Eysenck, H. J. (1952). The effects of psychotherapy: An evaluation. *Journal of Consulting Psychology, 16,* 319–324.

Eysenck, H. J. (1970). A mish-mash of theories. *International Journal of Psychiatry, 9,* 140–146.

Foa, E. B., & Emmelkamp, P. M. G. (Eds.). (1983). *Failures in behavior therapy.* New York: Wiley.

Foa, E. B., Franklin, M. E., Perry, K. J., & Herbert, J. D. (1996). Cognitive biases in generalized social phobia. *Journal of Abnormal Psychology, 105,* 433–439.

Forman, E. M., Herbert, J. D., Moitra, E., Yeomans, P. D., & Geller, P. A. (2007). A randomized controlled effectiveness trial of acceptance and commitment therapy and cognitive therapy for anxiety and depression. *Behavior Modification, 31,* 772–799.

Garratt, G., Ingram, R. E., Rand, K. L., & Sawalani, G. (2007). Cognitive processes in cognitive therapy: Evaluation of the mechanism of change in the treatment of depression. *Clinical Psychology: Science and Practice, 14,* 224–239.

Gergen, K. J. (1985). The social constructionist movement in modern psychology. *American Psychologist, 40,* 266–275.

Gortner, E. T., Gollan, J. K., Dobson, K. S., & Jacobson, N. S. (1998). Cognitive behavioral treatment of depression: Relapse prevention. *Journal of Consulting and Clinical Psychology, 66*, 377–384.

Hanley, G. P., Iwata, B. A., & McCord, B. E. (2003). Functional analysis of problem behavior: A review. *Journal of Applied Behavior Analysis, 36*(2), 147–185

Harvey, A. G., Watkins, E., Mansell, W., & Shafran, R. (2004). *Cognitive behavioural processes across psychological disorders.* Oxford, UK: Oxford University Press.

Hayes, S. C. (2004a). Acceptance and commitment therapy and the new behavior therapies: Mindfulness, acceptance and relationship. In S. C. Hayes, V. M. Follette, & M. M. Linehan (Eds.), *Mindfulness and acceptance: Expanding the cognitive-behavioral tradition* (pp. 1–29). New York: Guilford Press.

Hayes, S. C. (2004b). Acceptance and commitment therapy, relational frame theory, and the third wave of behavioral and cognitive therapies. *Behavior Therapy, 35*, 639–665.

Hayes, S. C., Brownstein, A. J., Haas, J. R., & Greenway, D. E. (1986). Instructions, multiple schedules, and extinction: Distinguishing rule-governed from schedule controlled behavior. *Journal of the Experimental Analysis of Behavior, 46*, 137–147.

Hayes, S. C., Luoma, J. B., Bond, F. W., Masuda, A., & Lillis, J. (2006). Acceptance and commitment therapy: Model, processes and outcomes. *Behaviour Research and Therapy, 44*, 1–25.

Hayes, S. C., Strosahl, K. D., & Wilson, K. G. (1999). *Acceptance and commitment therapy: An experiential approach to behavior change.* New York: Guilford Press.

Hayes, S. C., Wilson, K. G., Gifford, E. V., & Follette, V. M. (1996). Experiential avoidance and behavioral disorders: A functional dimensional approach to diagnosis and treatment. *Journal of Consulting and Clinical Psychology, 64*, 1152–1168.

Hofmann, S. G. (2004). Cognitive mediation of treatment change in social phobia. *Journal of Consulting and Clinical Psychology, 72*, 393–399.

Hofmann, S. G., & Asmundson, G. J. G. (2008). Acceptance and mindfulness-based therapy: New wave or old hat. *Clinical Psychology Review, 28*, 1–16.

Hofmann, S. G., Meuret, A. E., Rosenfield, D., Suvak, M. K., Barlow, D. H., Gorman, J. M., et al. (2007). Preliminary evidence for cognitive mediation during cognitive-behavioral therapy of panic disorder. *Journal of Consulting and Clinical Psychology, 75*, 374–379.

Jones, M. C. (1924). A laboratory study of fear: The case of Peter. *Pedagogical Seminary, 31*, 308–315.

Kanfer, L. (1990). History of behavior modification. In A. S. Bellack, M. Hersen, & A. E. Kazdin (Eds.), *International handbook of behavior modification and therapy* (pp. 3–26). New York, Plenum Press.

Kelly, G. (1955). *The psychology of personal constructs.* New York: Norton.

Kohlenberg, R. J., & Tsai, M. (2007). *Functional analytic psychotherapy: Creating intense and curative therapeutic relationships.* New York: Springer.

Kuhn, T. S. (1962). *The structure of scientific revolutions.* Chicago: University of Chicago Press.

Lazarus, A. A. (1967). In support of technical eclecticism. *Psychological Reports,* *21*, 415–416.

Lazarus, A. A. (2005). Is there still a need for psychotherapy integration? *Current Psychology, 24*, 149–152.

Leahy, R. L. (2003). *Cognitive therapy techniques: A practitioner's guide.* New York: Guilford Press.

Linehan, M. M. (1993). *Cognitive-behavioral treatment of borderline personality disorder.* New York: Guilford Press.

Litt, D., Kadden, R. M., Stephens, R. S., & The Marijuana Treatment Project Research Group. (2008). Coping and self-efficacy in marijuana treatment. *Journal of Consulting and Clinical Psychology, 73*, 1015–1025.

Litt, M. D., Kadden, R. M., Cooney, N. L., & Kabela, E. (2003). Coping skills and treatment outcomes in cognitive-behavioral and interactional group therapy for alcoholism. *Journal of Consulting and Clinical Psychology, 71*, 118–128.

London, P. (1964). *The modes and morals of psychotherapy.* New York: Holt, Rinehart, and Winston.

Luborsky, L., & DeRubeis, R. J. (1984). The use of psychotherapy treatment manuals: A small revolution in psychotherapy research style. *Clinical Psychology Review, 4*, 5–14.

Lundgren, T., Dahl, J., & Hayes, S. C. (2008). Evaluation of mediators of change in the treatment of epilepsy with acceptance and commitment therapy. *Journal of Behavioral Medicine, 31*, 225–235.

Mahoney, M. J. (2005). Suffering, philosophy, and psychotherapy. *Journal of Psychotherapy Integration, 15*, 337–352.

McCullough, J. P. (2000). *Treatment for chronic depression: Cognitive behavioral analysis system of psychotherapy.* New York: Guilford Press.

McNally, R. J. (2007). Mechanisms of exposure therapy: How neuroscience can improve psychological treatments for anxiety disorders. *Clinical Psychology Review, 27*, 750–759.

Morganstern, J., & Longabauch, R. (2000). Cognitive-behavioral treatment for alcohol dependence: A review of evidence for its hypothesized mechanisms of action. *Addiction, 95*, 1475–1490.

Muris, P., & Merckelbach, H. (2001). The etiology of childhood specific phobias. In M. W. Vasey & M. R. Dadds (Eds.), *The developmental psychopathology of anxiety* (pp. 355–385). New York: Oxford Press.

Öst, L. G. (2008). Efficacy of the third wave of behavioral therapies: A systematic review and meta-analysis. *Behaviour Research and Therapy, 46*, 296–321.

Persons, J. B. (2006). Case formulation-driven psychotherapy. *Clinical Psychology: Science and Practice, 13*, 167–170.

Popper, K. (1935). *Logik der Forschung* [The logic of scientific discovery]. Vienna: Julius Springer.

Powers, M. B., & Emmelkamp, P. (2009). Dissemination of research findings. In D. Richard & S. Huprich (Eds.), *Clinical psychology: Assessment, treatment, and research.* Burlington, MA: Elsevier.

Powers, M. B., Sigmarsson, R., & Emmelkamp, P. M. G. (2008). A meta-analytic review of psychological treatments for social anxiety disorder. *International Journal of Cognitive Psychotherapy, 1*, 94–113.

Powers, M. B., Zum Vörde Sive Vörding, M. B., & Emmelkamp, P. M. G. (2009). Acceptance and commitment therapy: A meta-analytic review. *Psychotherapy & Psychosomatics, 78*, 73–80.

Powers, M. B., Smits, J. A., & Telch, M. J. (2004). Disentangling the effects of safety-behavior utilization and safety-behavior availability during exposure-based treatment: A placebo-controlled trial. *Journal of Consulting and Clinical Psychology, 72*, 448–454.

Rachman, S., Radomsky, A. S., & Shafran, R. (2008). Safety behaviour: A reconsideration. *Behaviour Research and Therapy, 46*, 163–173.

Reiss, S., Peterson, R. A., Gursky, D. M., & McNally, R. J. (1986). Anxiety sensitivity, anxiety frequency and the prediction of fearfulness. *Behaviour Research and Therapy, 24*, 1–8.

Rosen, G. M., & Davison, G. C. (2003). Psychology should list empirically supported principles of change (ESPs) and not credential trademarked therapies or other treatment packages. *Behavior Modification, 27*, 300–312.

Salkovskis, P. M. (2002). Empirically grounded clinical interventions: Cognitive-behavioural therapy progresses through a multi-dimensional approach to clinical science. *Behavioural and Cognitive Psychotherapy, 30*, 3–9.

Salkovskis, P. M., Clark, D. M., Hackmann, A., Wells, A., & Gelder, M. G. (1999). An experimental investigation of the role of safety-seeking behaviours in the maintenance of panic disorder with agoraphobia. *Behaviour Research and Therapy, 37*, 559–574.

Schulte, D., & Eifert, G. H. (2002). What to do when manuals fail?: The dual model of psychotherapy. *Clinical Psychology: Science and Practice, 9*, 312–328.

Schulte, D., Kunzel, R., Pepping, G., & Schulte-Bahrenberg, T. (1992). Tailor-made versus standardized therapy of phobic patients. *Advances in Behaviour Research and Therapy, 14*, 67–92.

Segal, Z. V., Williams, D., & Teasdale, J. D. (2001). *Mindfulness-based cognitive therapy for depression: A new approach to preventing relapse.* New York: Guilford Press.

Skinner, B. F. (1953). *Science and human behavior.* New York: Macmillan.

Sloan, T., & Telch, M. J. (2002). The effects of safety-seeking behavior and guided threat reappraisal on fear reduction during exposure: an experimental investigation. *Behaviour Research and Therapy, 40*, 235–251.

Smits, J. A., Berry, A. C., Rosenfield, D., Powers, M., Behar, E., & Otto, M. W. (2008). Reducing anxiety sensitivity with exercise. *Depression and Anxiety, 25*, 689–699.

Smits, J. A., Powers, M. B., Cho, Y., & Telch, M. J. (2004). Mechanism of change in cognitive-behavioral treatment of panic disorder: Evidence for the fear of fear mediational hypothesis. *Journal of Consulting and Clinical Psychology, 72*, 646–652.

Smits, J. A., Rosenfield, D., McDonald, R., & Telch, M. J. (2006). Cognitive mechanisms of social anxiety reduction: An examination of specificity and temporality. *Journal of Consulting and Clinical Psychology, 74*, 1203–1212.

Strauman, T. J., & Merrill, K. A. (2004). The basic science/clinical science interface and treatment development. *Clinical Psychology: Science and Practice, 11*, 544–554.

Torrey, W. C., Drake, R. E., Dixon, L., Burns, B. J., Flynn, L., Rush, A. J., et al. (2001). Implementing evidence-based practices for persons with severe mental illnesses. *Psychiatric Services, 52,* 45–50.

Waltz, J., Addis, M. E., Koerner, K., & Jacobson, N. S. (1993). Testing the integrity of a psychotherapy protocol: Assessment of adherence and competence. *Journal of Consulting and Clinical Psychology, 61,* 620–630.

Watson, J. B., & Rayner, R. (1920). Conditioned emotional reactions. *Journal of Experimental Psychology, 3,* 1–14.

Wells, A. (2000). *Emotional disorders and metacognition: Innovative cognitive therapy.* Chichester, UK: Wiley.

Wells, A., Clark, D. M., Salkovskis, P., Ludgate, J., Hackmann, A., & Gelder, M. (1995). Social phobia: The role of in-situation safety behaviors in maintaining anxiety and negative beliefs. *Behavior Therapy, 26,* 153–161.

Westmeyer, H. (1989). *Psychological theories from a structuralist point of view.* Berlin: Springer.

Westmeyer, H. (Ed.). (1992). *The structuralist program in psychology: Foundations and applications.* Toronto: Hogrefe & Huber.

Wolpe, J. (1958). *Psychotherapy by reciprocal inhibition.* Stanford, CA: Stanford University Press.

Woolfolk, R. L., & Richardson, F. C. (2008). Philosophy and Psychotherapy. *Journal of Psychotherapy Integration, 18,* 25–39.

CHAPTER 2

Beck's Cognitive Therapy

Jan Scott
Arthur Freeman

INTRODUCTION AND HISTORICAL BACKGROUND

Cognitive therapy (CT) is probably the most widely researched and practiced short-term psychotherapy worldwide. Prior to its introduction, the two dominant models of psychotherapy were psychoanalysis/psychodynamic psychotherapy and behavior therapy. Although several individuals can be regarded as crucial to the development of CT and closely associated and derivative therapy models, the key figure associated with both theory and therapy research is Aaron T. Beck, MD. Because most proponents of CT can trace their research and academic ancestry back to Beck and Beck's work, he is widely acknowledged as the "founding father" of CT.

Various cognitive or cognitive-behavioral models and the application of these therapies to clinical problems and disorders are detailed in other chapters. This chapter focuses on Beck's work. As noted by Enright (1997), although there are many variants of CT, they share a similar underlying model that suggests psychological problems and mental disorders can be a consequence of cognitively distorted views of events or experiences, or can be maintained by faulty patterns of thinking and behavior, as originally posited by Beck (1967, 1976) and Beck, Rush, Shaw, and Emery (1979). This chapter explores the history of CT and details of the theory and therapy, including empirical support for the approach, followed by comments on some of the issues related to clinical practice and potential future developments, and a case description that illustrates the described model.

The profession of psychotherapy is over 100 years old. Despite the vast expansion that has occurred in the number of different psychotherapies now

28

practiced, most approaches may be categorized as either "insight-oriented" or "action-oriented" (Scott, 1998). In the early years, insight-oriented approaches, such as Freudian psychoanalysis and its multiple offshoots, which emphasized the development of greater insight, self-awareness, or self-understanding, were predominant. The paradigm shift toward action-oriented therapies began in the 1950s and arose because of the development within psychology toward behavioral models of emotional disorders, together with the failure of psychoanalysts to build an empirical basis for the support of their approach. The history of cognitive theory and therapy is best understood within this context of psychoanalysis and behaviorism (Scott, 1998). The focus of cognitive theory on intrapsychic processes that mediate actions and reactions has parallels with psychoanalytic theory. However, the clear definition and selection of targets for therapeutic intervention, the routine inclusion of specific measures of change, and the use of structured therapy sessions make evident the influence of behavior therapy on CT (Weishaar, 1993).

In the early part of the 20th century, psychodynamic psychotherapists created a sophisticated topography of the mind, comprising conscious, preconscious, and unconscious domains, and later incorporating important *structural* concepts, such as the id, ego, and superego. A core element of these models was the notion that the thoughts, feelings, and behaviors that shaped relationships and experiences were the result of unconscious drives and conflicts (Weishaar, 1993). In contrast, the behaviorists viewed such models as lacking empirical support and developed therapies derived from their scientific observations of animal and human behavior (Clark & Beck, 1999). The development of learning theory, in which behaviorists such as Skinner, Eysenck, and Wolpe, proposed that mental disorders are the product of faulty learning, led to the introduction of behavior therapy (BT) as the first brief psychological model of treatment (Scott & Beck, 2008). Followers of Skinner used reinforcement contingencies (reward systems) to try to overcome previous inappropriate conditioning in people with severe mental disorders, while Wolpe focused on systematic desensitization (imaginal graded exposure to a stimulus after the induction of a relaxed state) as a fear-reducing technique in people with "neuroses." However, the early success of BT in treating disorders such as anxiety and agoraphobia was not matched by equivalent results in the treatment of depression—a disorder with an obvious and large cognitive element. A further important prompt in the move away from pure learning theory toward cognitive science was the discontent in some quarters at working exclusively with models developed through animal experiments, when the ultimate goal was to explain human behavior and experience. However, behaviorists continued to support the "environmental determinism" or "conditioning" model, while psychoanalysts continued to support the "motivational model," which proposed that behavior was driven by unconscious beliefs and processes. As such, by the midpoint of the 20th century, the two dominant models of therapy viewed cognitions that may determine feelings and behaviors as either inaccessible to the client (thus requiring a long-term therapeutic relationship to expose these mental events) or regarded them as unimportant to the therapeutic process (which modified overt behavioral responses to stressors).

Beck graduated as a medical doctor at Yale University; his postgraduate training in neurology included placements in psychiatry. He later sought and earned certification in psychoanalysis. Ironically, it was Beck's attempt to convince other researchers, particularly those working in experimental psychology, of the scientific basis of psychoanalytic theories that gave impetus to the development of the cognitive theory of depression. In Philadelphia, Beck had believed that psychoanalysis offered a way of viewing the whole range of human experiences and problems. Like Freud, he began by exploring the links between the environment and the individual, and the individual's emotions and motivations, as well as how disturbances in the balance between and within these factors resulted in emotional problems and disorders. However, Beck's research experiments with depressed patients undermined rather than supported the motivational theory. The results did not suggest that internal determinism was based on unconscious motivations or biological drives, but on how the individual constructed his or her experience (Clark & Beck, 1999). Beck realized that a cognitive or information-processing model offered a far more powerful explanation of both the experimental data and the phenomena he observed in his clinical practice.

During the 1960s, Beck (1963, 1967) wrote his seminal papers on depression, detailing a cognitive model of psychopathology. The core elements of his cognitive model are as follows:

- It is a normalizing model: Cognitive processing in depression is viewed as being on a continuum with unhappiness.
- It is a stress–vulnerability model: The individual's spontaneous interpretations (automatic thoughts) or more considered interpretations of events or experiences are attributed to the activation of underlying cognitive structures (dysfunctional beliefs and schemas).
- The processing of external events or internal stimuli is biased and therefore systematically distorts the individual's construction of his or her experiences, leading to a variety of cognitive errors (e.g., overgeneralization, selective abstraction).
- There are distinct cognitive profiles for different mental disorders, referred to as the cognitive content specificity hypothesis, with different underlying themes (e.g., loss in depression, fear in anxiety).

Interestingly, Albert Ellis in New York had reported a similar hypothesis independently. Ellis (1962) had identified a further implication of cognitive theory that an individual's belief system, which is important in determining the meaning given to events or experiences, could be assumed to be accessible to both the patient and the therapist (see Chapter 4, this volume for details). This suggested that such beliefs could be approached by direct questioning rather than indirectly, through the therapist's interpretations. Ellis contacted Beck to share his ideas, and so began years of lively correspondence that continued until Ellis died in 2006. At about the same time, Beck also noted the parallels between his own ideas and Kelly's "personal construct theory" (1955), which led to the rapidly developing field of cognitive psychology generally and cognitive therapy specifically.

Initially, radical behaviorists, who supported the environmental determinism theory, expressed negative views of CT. Wolpe (1993) was particularly critical of the Beckian hypothesis that the patient could consciously make a choice to change. It was Wolpe's contention that "the cognitive" elements offered nothing additional to behavior therapy. It should be noted, however, that Wolpe made extensive use of imagery in his work, labeling imagery a behavioral tool, whereas cognitivists maintained that imagery was clearly a cognitive tool. However, the rise of cognitive science increasingly led clinicians to explore Beck's approaches. The process of acceptance was helped by the fact that CT also incorporated techniques and adopted the structured therapy session approach typical of BT. CT routinely included specific measures of change and acknowledged the behaviorists' emphasis on empiricism. The gradual move toward cognitive interventions in psychotherapy for common mental disorders in the 1970s and 1980s was driven by clinical need and by the inadequacy of existing models to deal with patients' internal dialogue. Many psychiatrists with a strong track record in pharmacology research have been sympathetic to the use of CT, mainly because it is based on an accessible and understandable theory that is open to empirical testing (e.g., Paykel, 2007). In some ways this also created a climate where exponents of CT were able to pilot interventions for psychoses and other chronic and/or severe mental disorders in which CT is used as an adjunct to medication. Approaches have also been developed for personality disorders and problems of substance misuse. However, the acceptability of CT is not only a function of its scientific foundations, but it also relates to the tenets of good clinical practice, which include the therapeutic alliance and empowerment of the client.

PHILOSOPHICAL AND THEORETICAL UNDERPINNINGS

Beck's model offers a *continuity hypothesis*, since it suggests that syndromes such as clinical depression are exaggerated forms of normal emotional responses, such as sadness. It also views emotional and behavioral responses to events or experiences as being largely determined by the cognitive appraisal that is made of them by the individual (e.g., social avoidance may arise if an individual experiences negative thoughts, such as "Others will find me boring"). The information-processing paradigm has two critical elements: cognitive structures and cognitive mechanisms. The underlying structures are termed *schemas*. These are defined as containing a network of core beliefs, but there is also a more accessible yet involuntary level of cognition that Beck termed *automatic thoughts*. These occur at the same time as, or immediately prior to, an emotional response to an event or experience. Such thoughts are particularly important in therapy, as they encapsulate the individual's response to a specific situation in an "event–thought–feeling–behavior" link. The analysis of automatic thoughts across different situations allows underlying themes to be identified, thereby giving clues to the content of the underlying schema. The automatic thoughts serve as guides or directional signals to the schema.

The term *cognitive mechanisms* refers to the faulty information processing that may occur when individuals selectively include or screen out information from their environment that either supports or refutes their view of themselves, their world, and their future.

The diathesis–stress component of the cognitive model postulates that some individuals are at greater risk of developing depression in response to certain events because, as a result of early learning experiences, they have developed constellations of dysfunctional core beliefs. For example, individuals who experience physical or emotional abuse or neglect as a child may develop a collection of negative beliefs (e.g., "I am unlovable," "I am damaged or defective and no one will ever want me," "I am only good for one thing," or "I will always be a victim"). Such beliefs may be latent for long periods but become activated or reactivated by events that carry a specific meaning for that person (e.g., the experience of personal rejection for an individual who already believes he or she is unlovable). J. Beck (1995) suggests that the underlying beliefs that render an individual vulnerable to depression may be broadly categorized into beliefs about being helpless or unlovable. Thus, events that are deemed uncontrollable or that involve relationship difficulties may be important in the genesis of depressive symptoms (Scott, 2001). Cognitions about the self, the world, and the future—termed the *cognitive triad*—are concomitants of depression when these views are negative but serve to reinforce the core underlying dysfunctional beliefs. These thoughts dominate the thinking of many depressed patients and are sustained through systematic distortions of information (e.g., focusing only on negative aspects of an interpersonal interaction) and contribute to further depression of affect (Hollon, Kendall, & Lumry, 1986). Beck states that while the vicious cycle of low-mood-enhancing negative thinking, which then leads to further lowering in mood, may represent a causal theory in some cases, it acts as a perpetuating factor in other forms of depression.

Beliefs about the self seem especially important in the onset or maintenance of depression and these beliefs, particularly when connected with low or variable self-esteem, are frequent targets for change in CT (Haaga, Dyck, & Ernst, 1991).

Beck's cognitive theory of anxiety disorders suggests that underlying danger-oriented beliefs (1) predispose individuals to restrict their attention to perceived threats in their environment, (2) to make catastrophic interpretations of ambiguous stimuli, (3) to underestimate their own coping resources (or the likelihood that others can help them if a dangerous situation arises), and (4) to engage in dysfunctional "safety behaviors" such as avoidance (Beck, 2005). The latter (e.g., leaving a crowded environment for fear of collapsing) means that individuals are restricted in their activities and also never collect the evidence to counter their original belief that they were in danger (e.g., at risk of collapse). There are, of course, some variations, depending on the perceived nature of the threat or danger. For example, in panic disorder, ambiguous stimuli or subjective experiences are given catastrophic interpretations that are often focused on the presumed pathological significance of what is happening. Normal or quite benign experiences, such as a brief period of tachycardia, may be interpreted as a potentially fatal event, such as a heart attack (Beck & Emery with Greenberg, 1985; Clark et al., 1997). Cognitive theory and therapy have been important in helping clinicians understand that guiding clients through a detailed examination of the evidence that supports or refutes their individual catastrophic automatic thoughts is a more important element in overcoming anxiety than the repeated use of reassurance (which leads to rebound anxiety). Furthermore, behavioral experiments to collect data can help the individual to challenge actively and overcome safety behaviors.

It is hypothesized that in social anxiety disorders, maladaptive beliefs focus on individuals' perceptions of their potential social performance and the potential reaction of others. They then conclude that others will make negative evaluations and reject them as they have already done to themselves (Clark & Wells, 1995). This assumption is often associated with a failure to register objective social clues and exaggerated negatively biased interpretations of the situation.

In posttraumatic stress disorder (PTSD), Clark and Ehlers (2004). suggest that the two core components of the cognitive model are (1) negative appraisal of actual events and exaggerated negative appraisal of the symptoms produced by the trauma, and (2) inadequate integration of the traumatic experience into the individual's autobiographical memory. Common cognitions that maintain the symptoms and distress, which can be tackled through sensitive intervention, are "The world is a dangerous place," "I am not in control," and "Things will never be the same again." The CT of PTSD has been important in demonstrating that the consequences of real life traumatic events can be understood and treated (Gillespie, Duffy, Hack-mann, & Clark, 2002).

The previously discussed models evolved from not only the template laid down initially in the experimental and observational studies of Beck and his colleagues and students, but also all the key figures who developed cognitive models for other disorders, worked alongside, spent time with, or were encouraged by Beck in their research. It is no surprise that he has been honored for his contributions to science and clinical practice by international organizations representing psychologists and psychiatrists. Beck has continued to contribute original research for over 50 years. His later publications on cognitive models highlight the importance of cognitive distortions as factors that maintain psychotic or affective symptoms in schizophrenia, chronic and severe depressions, and bipolar disorders (Beck, 1996, 2005; Beck & Rector, 2002). In psychosis research, work on attributional style has established that individuals who experience delusions "jump to conclusions" when drawing inferences, underutilize disconfirming data, and tend to attribute negative events to external causes. The classical cognitive characteristics of a delusion are that it is a culturally unacceptable explanation of an experience that attributes the cause of the experience to factors outside of the individual (Morrison, 2002). Because, according to this hypothesis, delusions could be amenable to structured reasoning and behavioral approaches, a model of CT was developed that allowed exploration of delusions in the same way that techniques to modify core beliefs in common mental disorders had been adapted and modified for working with individuals with personality disorders (Beck et al., 2004; Scott et al., 1992; Kingdon & Turkington, 1994).

Most CT interventions share a common core: Because psychological distress is a function of disturbed cognitive processes, the focus of therapy is on modifying cognitions. Beck's model is the most widely practiced; it differs from Ellis's approach in important ways. Ellis proposes that individuals have a common set of assumptions; Beck maintains that an individual's underlying beliefs are idiosyncratic. The practice of Beckian CT also differs from Ellis's rational-emotive behavior therapy in other important aspects, notably that Beck employs a "guided discovery" (see Table 2.1) approach to help the individual explore ideas and cognitions, whereas Ellis uses rational disputation to challenge openly an individual's assumptions. For instance, Ellis may say to a client who is affected by an adverse event, "Why should you assume that everything which happens in the world is designed to increase your happiness?" Beck's model provides a template of questions that the individual applies initially with the help of the therapist but can then utilize independently when dealing with any maladaptive or unhelpful thoughts or ideas in the future, after he or she has left therapy. One of the best descriptions of the process of "guided discovery" is provided by Padesky (1993).

TABLE 2.1. Guided Discovery

Socratic Questioning

- This involves asking questions that:
- The client has the knowledge to answer.
- Draw the client's attention to information that is relevant to the issue being discussed but which may be outside the client's current focus.
- Generally move from the concrete to the more abstract so that ...
- The client can, in the end, apply the new information either to reevaluate a previous conclusion or to construct a new idea.

For example, to help a client identify useful information about a topic being discussed in therapy, the therapist might ask:

- Have you ever been in similar circumstances before?
- What did you do? How did that turn out?
- What do you know now that you didn't know then?
- What would you advise a friend who told you something similar?

The Four Stages of Guided Discovery

- *Stage 1: Asking informational questions.* Socratic questions are used to delineate the client's concerns in a concrete (e.g., specific example) and understandable way for the client and therapist.
- *Stage 2: Listening.* To be exactly clear about the issues, but also to listen for idiosyncratic words and emotional reactions.
- *Stage 3: Summarizing.* The therapist should summarize the discussion or ask the client to provide a brief summary every few minutes.
- *Stage 4: Synthesizing or analytical questions.* The therapist completes the guided discovery process by asking a synthesizing or analytical question that applies to the client's original concern and the new information that has been discussed and summarized, along with idiosyncratic meanings that have been explored (e.g., "How do all of the information and data we have reviewed fit with your idea that you are unlovable?")

Note. Data from Padesky (1993).

Beck's model of therapy is regarded as a collaborative "hypothesis-testing" approach; it uses deductive reasoning (also referred to as Socratic questioning or guided discovery), to help individuals identify and challenge their distorted cognitions and dysfunctional beliefs for themselves. As well as devising techniques to educate individuals about their problems and to explore their automatic thoughts, CT integrates interventions targeting definable modes of behavior that can be readily monitored and addressed (Scott & Beck, 2008). Although Beck acknowledges the use and importance of the behavioral technique in CT, he emphasizes that it is only one of several mechanisms for producing change. Furthermore, the therapy is not simply technique-driven; the therapeutic relationship is a crucial aspect of the approach, as described below.

In the course of therapy, interventions that are proposed to help a particular individual are selected on the basis of a cognitive conceptualization. This draws together key information about the individual; it identifies the individual's likely core negative beliefs, the critical incidents that have occurred in his or her life that uniquely explain the onset and maintenance of distress. If an individual with depression shows a low level of functioning, then behavioral techniques may be used initially to improve activity levels and enhance problem-solving and coping skills. This can help to improve mood by providing the individual with an early "success" experience. However, a further goal of behavioral intervention is to identify negative cognitions and underlying beliefs. Verbal interventions are initially employed to teach the individual to recognize and challenge negative cognitions. This usually leads to further improved mood, positive changes in behavior, and a reduction in acute symptoms. Between-session experiments, frequently focused on interpersonal functioning, are used to reevaluate ideas. Negative automatic thoughts are characteristically situation-specific interpretations, but as well as reviewing these cognitions and the processing errors that may be manifest, the patient and therapist analyze the patterns or recurring themes in the recorded automatic thoughts as this helps identify the probable underlying beliefs (Beck, 1976). The therapist helps the client to explore his or her perceptions of events and experiences, and facilitates self-discovery of evidence to support or refute client's hypotheses. This collaborative–empirical approach is crucial to the success of the therapy. Later, when the client has developed his or her independent use of cognitive and behavioral skills and can employ the techniques to reduce depressive symptoms, the therapist and client apply similar cognitive interventions and behavioral experiments to try to modify underlying dysfunctional beliefs (which operate across situations). Events that hold specific meaning for the individual, and that may make him or her vulnerable to distress in the future, are also identified and discussed. The aim of this part of the therapy is to identify high-risk situations for the future and to reduce the individual's underlying vulnerability to relapse. It is noteworthy that this latter element of CT may differentiate effective from ineffective applications of the therapy (Salkovskis, 1996). In general, counseling and therapy approaches that begin and end with interventions targeted at change in symptoms, generic problem solving, or nonspecific support, without any consideration of underlying mechanisms and formulation, can produce temporary symptomatic improvements but usually fail to deliver any durable posttherapy change in vulnerability to relapse (Hollon, Shelton, & Davis, 1993; Scott, 2001).

While cognitive theory provides plausible and clinically applicable models of common mental disorders in which CT may be used as an alternative to medication (or in combination, in certain instances), there has been greater ambivalence about trying to apply "continuity hypotheses" to individuals with severe mental disorders that also have biological triggers. However, from an early stage, Beck noted that the principles of CT could be applied to certain phenomenological features (e.g., delusional beliefs) or to factors maintaining the biological processes (e.g., maladaptive use of alcohol by individuals with bipolar disorders to contain mood swings). As such, as early as 1952, Beck published the first case description of the use of reasoning techniques with an individual with systematized paranoid delusions (today, this case would probably be classified as schizophrenia) prior to the advent of antipsychotics. Beck described some of the key elements of a new structured psychotherapy of schizophrenia, which, at least in this case, was extremely successful. He engaged with the client and established a working therapeutic alliance in which trust developed. Together they worked on the sequence of events that had preceded the emergence of the client's systematized paranoid delusion. A phase of systematic, graded reality testing followed, in which the client was guided to examine the evidence in relation to the behavior of his presumed persecutors. Having done this with the help of the therapist in session, he reviewed all the evidence at his disposal from his homework exercises and gradually started to eliminate false beliefs about his presumed persecutors. In this case, there was no emergence of depression or anxiety as the delusion receded, and the effect appeared to be durable, with the client remaining well at follow-up. In their CT manual, Kingdon and Turkington (1994) highlight that differences in CT with clients with psychosis are generally a matter of emphasis, in addition to some specific techniques to supplement those used for anxiety and depression. For example, agenda setting may need to be more flexible and simple, and sometimes less explicit; the length and frequency of sessions may also need to vary. If an individual is experiencing severe symptoms, then the length of sessions can be attenuated to take into account reduced attention and concentration, or if the individual is suspicious of others, then early sessions can focus more on building a trusting therapeutic alliance to ensure that later attempts to explore delusional beliefs are not viewed by the client as threatening. The skill of the therapist is obviously important in such circumstances and can be a major factor in predicting the degree of benefit from adjunctive CT.

EMPIRICAL EVIDENCE

Support for Cognitive Models

This section initially explores evidence supporting cognitive theories, followed by a limited overview of randomized controlled treatment trials of CT across the range of emotional and mental disorders; we comment on moderators and mediators of the effects of CT, using mood disorders as an example.

Theory Research

An overview (Beck, 2005) highlighted the breadth of research on different cognitive models of psychopathology and noted a substantial body of supportive evidence for the model of depression, with somewhat less evidence for the other disorders for which CT has been applied as a treatment. Although empirical support for the different theoretical formulations may vary, it is clear that research by advocates of these models follows a well-established systematic process, namely, that the development of a coherent conceptual framework always precedes the introduction of therapeutic strategies. Thus, there is more research on depression, followed by anxiety disorders, with less empirical data for psychoses, personality disorders, and bipolar disorders.

Key elements of the cognitive theory that have been investigated empirically are the concept of cognitive vulnerability and the notion that unhelpful, negative cognitions arising under stress are critical in the onset, maintenance, and relapse of emotional disorders (Segal & Ingram, 1994; Scher, Ingram, & Segal, 2005). There are a number of different conceptualizations of cognitive diathesis: the cognitive reactivity model, the cognitive risk model, and the personality style perspective. Research supports the notion of cognitive reactivity in adults, and a growing literature suggests that this concept has validity in children and adolescents. This model identifies the presence of negative self-schemas as necessary but not sufficient precipitating factors for depression. The critical additional element that dictate whether transient unhappiness may become a clinical depressive episode is a stimulus that "matches" the themes within the schemas, thus reactivating them. Some early research did not include this aspect and therefore was not able to demonstrate the presence of high levels of dysfunctional beliefs in individuals remitted from but at risk of future depressive relapse. To demonstrate underlying schemas in euthymic clients often requires "priming" designs, such as mood induction to increase the accessibility of underlying beliefs (Segal et al., 1994).

Other models of cognitive risk explored self-report measures, such as levels of dysfunctional attitudes, self-esteem level and stability, and recall of self-descriptions (Alloy & Abramson, 1999; Teasdale & Dent, 1987). Some studies adopted longitudinal prospective designs to try to delineate characteristics of those at risk of later depression. For example, Lewinsohn, Joiner, and Rohde (2001) reported on more than 1,500 adolescents; their findings were suggestive of a threshold view of vulnerability to depression. Adolescents who experienced negative life events had depressive onset related to dysfunctional attitudes if their initial level of dysfunctional attitudes exceeded a certain level (low = intermediate < high). The Temple–Wisconsin Cognitive Vulnerability to Depression Project (Alloy & Abramson, 1999) was a large-scale prospective cohort study of young adults who were followed up to determine whether cognitive styles measured at baseline could help to predict later development of depression. Cognitive high-risk participants experienced more episodes of depression, more severe episodes, and more chronic courses than did low-risk participants. However, no group differences were observed for age of onset or duration of episodes.

A frequently asked question is how cognitive vulnerability may relate to personality characteristics. An interesting conceptual framework was proposed by Beck (1996), who suggested that predisposing "depressogenic" beliefs could be differentiated according to whether the patient's personality was primarily autonomous or sociotropic. Although the findings were mixed, the predominant evidence indicated that autonomous individuals were more likely to become depressed following an autonomous event (e.g., a failure) than following a sociotropic event (e.g., loss of a relationship), and the reverse was true of sociotropic individuals. Meanwhile, Teasdale (1988) demonstrated that dysfunctional beliefs can be state and trait markers; he especially drew attention to the often discredited concept of "neuroticism," demonstrating that it identifies individuals with high levels of dysfunctional beliefs as a trait characteristic, and that this may in part explain the predisposition of this personality style to depressive episodes.

It is worth noting that in Beck's (2005) review, he identified the number of supportive–unsupportive studies for the three key components of the cognitive theory: the negative cognitive triad in depression (150 supportive and 14 nonsupportive), negatively biased cognitive processing of stimuli (19 supportive and 0 nonsupportive), and identifiable dysfunctional beliefs (31 supportive and 6 nonsupportive). Studies of the content specificity hypothesis indicate that in homogeneous samples of clients with depressive or anxiety disorders, it is possible to differentiate between the cognitive themes of depression (loss and self-devaluation; high levels of hopelessness and negative expectancies) and anxiety (threat and vulnerability).

This research should not be taken to indicate a robust, universally accepted cognitive model for depression and/or anxiety. Ongoing debate focuses on the fact that many dysfunctional beliefs are not disorder specific (Hollon, Kendall, & Lumry, 1986; Jones et al., 2006) and that there are transdiagnostic abnormalities in cognitive content and processing (Harvey, Watkins, Mansell, & Shafran, 2004). Furthermore, the cognitive biases and content reported during depressive or anxiety episodes may be epiphenomena rather than critical factors in dictating the evolution of an episode. Matthews (2006) suggests that to progress, relevant cognitive operations contributing toward the maintenance of psychological disorders need to be specified more precisely with the use of objective means rather than subjective reports of cognitive content. He notes that while clients' reports of their conscious cognitions are a critically important source of hypotheses about cognitive factors in etiology, the underlying processes are not always amenable to conscious introspection. One of the best examples of such operations is *rumination* (repetitive, self-related ideation), which is now clearly regarded as an important maintaining factor in depression (Nolen-Hoeksema, 1991; Miranda & Nolen-Hoeksema, 2007). However, research has shown that the content of rumination can be conceptualized as brooding and reflection (which can involve problem solving); furthermore, the former is more toxic than the latter for depression-prone individuals. Matthews (2006) points out that the adverse effect of brooding is likely to arise because it reactivates existing negative thought patterns and makes personal interpretations of new ambiguous events more likely. Such issues are not just of academic interest. Work on how rumination may operate to maintain depression suggests that one way to prevent these consequences is to focus more therapy time on the detail of this processing bias rather than simply using thought records to explore cognitive content. Clients can be taught to strengthen habits of thought that are incompatible (i.e., less self-related) with brooding. A pilot study of rumination-focused CT indeed produced impressive results. However, as noted previously by Foa and Kozak (1997), as well as embracing the concepts of cognitive psychology, clinicians need to draw on experimental cognitive psychology more often if they are to develop the scientific underpinnings for new treatment strategies.

Treatment Research

The majority of the treatment trials employ a CT model that fulfills the criteria for "well-established" empirically supported treatments (ESTs; Chambless & Hollon, 1998). Recognition as an EST means that the efficacy of the therapy has been established in two or more carefully designed, methodologically reliable randomized controlled trials that evaluate the treatment of a specific disorder (Task Force on Promotion and Dissemination of Psychological Procedures, 1995). The criteria require that trial samples be well-defined and of adequate size to establish statistical significance of the findings, and use reliable and valid outcome measures. Therapists involved in the trial should use treatment manuals and their adherence to the therapy protocol and competency in delivering the interventions should be monitored (see Table 2.2). There are concerns among some psychotherapy researchers about the criteria that are usually employed to judge the value of pharmacotherapies; indeed, opponents of EST argue that such approaches to the assessment of the benefits of psychotherapy are fundamentally flawed. However, this evidence-based approach is invariably employed in the development of clinical practice treatment guidelines, and psychological therapies that have been evaluated through randomized trials and are the subject of meta-analytic review are more likely to be considered as either an alternative or an adjunct to pharmacotherapy (Roth & Fonagy, 1996; Thase et al., 1997). There may be some issues in evaluating therapies whose approaches primarily assess the benefits of new medications, but the reality is that the adoption of this research framework has clearly raised the CT profile and increased its acceptability to nonpsychotherapists working in general psychiatry and general medical settings. As such, treatment guidelines in the United States, many countries across Europe, and Australia and New Zealand have incorporated CT into several of its key guidelines (e.g., in the United Kingdom, it is a recommended treatment of depression, schizophrenia, and anxiety disorders).

A recent review by Butler, Chapman, Foreman, and Beck (2006) identified over 300 published outcome studies on CT and over 16 meta-analyses. These authors used data on mean effect sizes (ES) to try to answer key questions about the utility of CT: (1) the effectiveness of CT, and the disorders for which is it most effective and (2) the durability of therapy gains. These findings are summarized in Table 2.3. This meta-analysis and other reviews suggest that compared to waiting-list or placebo treatments, CT is highly effective (CT vs. control condition: grand mean ES = 0.95; SD = 0.08) for unipolar depression, childhood anxiety and depressive disorders, and a number of specific anxiety disorders, especially generalized anxiety disorder (GAD), panic and social phobia disorders, and obsessive–compulsive disorder (OCD). Although the heterogeneity of studies incorporated in other meta-analyses make the findings less robust, CT is also associated with large improvements (mean ES = 1.27; SD = 0.11) in symptoms of bulimia nervosa that exceed the gains from medication alone, and CT shows additional benefits over treatment as usual for persistent medication refractory delusions in schizophrenia (ES for CT varied from 0.54 to 1.20 compared to an ES of 0.17 for treatment as usual). However, when compared to an active treatment condition, CT for depressive disorders shows equivalent or

---

TABLE 2.2. Empirically Supported Treatments: Requirements for a Well-Established Treatment

Criteria for a "Well-Established" Therapy

I. At least two good between-group design experiments demonstrating efficacy in one or more of the following ways:

    A. Superiority to pill or psychological placebo or alternative treatment

    B. Equivalence to an already established treatment in experiments with adequate statistical power

II. Experiments must be conducted with treatment manuals.

III. Characteristics of the client samples must be clearly specified.

IV. Effects must have been demonstrated by at least two different investigators or investigatory teams.

only marginal superiority. In other disorders, such as OCD, in a comparison of BT, and the treatments appeared to be equally effective. Moderate ES (0.50–0.80) are reported for CT compared to control conditions for marital distress, pain syndromes, anger management, and childhood somatic disorders.

The other key issue is whether the benefits of CT extend after completion of therapy (i.e., has the individual learned to apply CT techniques independently and have underlying beliefs been modified to reduce relapse risk?) A major methodological problem is that few therapy trials have adequate statistical power to assess reliably the durability of the treatment benefits, and many follow-ups involve a "treatment sieve" that focuses only on a

TABLE 2.3. Summary of Findings from Meta-Analyses of Acute and Longer-Term (6 Months to 8 Years) Benefits of CT

Evidence from one or more meta-analyses of CT > control condition and/or CT = Active Treatment (Number of studies in analysis)	Consistent Evidence of Durable CT Benefit
Adult Unipolar Depression ($n = 75$)	Adult Unipolar Depression (acute and chronic disorders)
Bulimia Nervosa ($n = 24$)	
Childhood Depressive and Anxiety Disorders ($n = 22$)	
Panic Disorder with or without Agoraphobia ($n = 20$)	Panic Disorder
PTSD ($n = 14$)	
Adolescent Depression ($n = 13$)	
Generalized Anxiety Disorder ($n = 8$)	Generalized Anxiety Disorder
Social Phobia ($n = 7$)	Social Phobia
Schizophrenia ($n = 7$)	Medication-refractory psychotic symptoms
OCD ($n = 4$)	OCD

Note. Data from Butler, Chapman, Foreman, and Beck (2006).

selected subsample of the original trial population (Paykel et al., 1999). However, bearing these limitations in mind, Butler et al. (2006) concluded that there is evidence of persistent benefit and reduced relapse rates in unipolar depression and a range of adult anxiety disorders. Grant, Young, and DeRubeis (2005) note that CTs are quite versatile, and that the absolute limits have yet to be empirically defined. Like any treatment, however, a number of factors may impede engagement with CT, and certain client or therapist characteristics mean that many individuals do not benefit from CT. In this context it is important to note that large-scale effectiveness trials, especially of CT combined with medication, do not always show across-the-board benefit (DeRubeis et al., 2005; Scott et al., 2006; Garety et al., 2008). Although these studies have consistently identified subgroups of clients who benefit from this approach, there is a need to avoid overstating the case for CT, as this may lose rather than win support for increasing its availability in general psychiatry (Parker, Roy, & Eyers, 2003; Scott, 2008).

Moderators and Mediators

Beyond determining the efficacy and effectiveness of CT, it is important to determine the mechanisms, moderators, and predictors of response to this therapy. Finding the answers to questions (e.g., "How does therapy work?"; "What determines/predicts the effectiveness of therapy?"; "How do we target therapy more effectively?") is essential to developing better therapy and matching therapy to clients systematically rather than by trial and error. Moderators of therapy response are often similar to the individual client factors that predict poor outcome with a variety of treatment approaches (Scott, 2001). There is evidence that nonspecific mediators and predictors (e.g., factors common across psychotherapies), as well as specific processes (e.g., cognitive mechanisms) may be important in CT.

A number of client variables have been found to predict poor outcome with CT (Hamilton & Dobson, 2002). Perfectionistic beliefs adversely influence outcome for medications and a number of therapies, including CT, as well as placebo, even when researchers control for features of personality disorder (Shahar, Blatt, Zuroff, & Pilkonis, 2003). This effect is partially mediated by perfectionists' difficulties in developing strong therapeutic alliances (Zuroff et al., 2000). Shahar et al. (2003) also found that odd–eccentric and depressive personality features independently predicted poor outcome for all the brief treatments for depression. In bipolar disorders, multiple comorbidities, lifetime substance misuse, and multiple previous episodes predicted poor response from CT; in contrast, those with fewer than 12 prior relapses (and especially more than six) at the time CT was added to their medication regimen, did extremely well, with longer relapse-free periods (Scott, Paykel, Morriss, Bentall, Kinderman, et al., 2006). This suggests that earlier introduction of CT in treatment of bipolar disorders may improve longer-term outcomes before maladaptive coping strategies become ingrained. It is also clear that therapist expertise, especially adherence to the therapy model, and competent and skillful use of therapy techniques, impact on client outcomes (Crits-Cristoph et al., 1991; Davidson et al., 2004). The relationship between the therapist and client is also an important determinant of the process and outcome of CT. Previous research has shown that both the patient's contribution to the alliance (e.g., the patient's openness, honesty, active engagement and agreement with therapist, as rated on videotapes of therapy sessions), and the quality of therapeutic relationship, as reported by the patient, independently predict outcome for CT (Blatt, Zuroff, Quinlan, & Pilkonis, 1996; Krupnick, Sotsky, Simmens, Moyer, Elkin, et al., 1996). Later, Meyer, Pilkonis, Krupnick, Egan, Simmens, et al. (2002) reanalyzed these data and found that clients' pretreatment expectations of therapeutic effectiveness predicted their active engagement in therapy, which then led to greater improvement with CT. It is also notable that some research indicates that patient's expectancies after some experience of therapy (e.g., ratings of the therapeutic alliance after session 3 to 4) may be an even stronger predictor of outcome.

Work on mediators of change in depression is of great interest. Despite evidence clearly demonstrating that CT can be an effective treatment of acute or chronic depressive disorders, how CT achieves these effects is not well understood. For example, Tang and DeRubeis (1999) found that a significant minority of depressed clients undergoing CT showed substantial symptom improvement in one between-session interval rather than gradual and steady improvement over time. This rapid improvement, called sudden gains, accounted for over half of the total symptom improvement, usually occurred early in therapy, and was associated with better long-term outcomes. Clients who experienced sudden gains were significantly less depressed than other clients at 18-month follow-up. In CT, sudden gains seemed to be preceded by critical sessions in which substantial cognitive changes occurred. Hayes et al. (2007) investigated an additional pattern of change: a transient period of apparent worsening that they called a *depression spike*. Statistical modeling revealed that spike patterns also predict lower posttreatment depression, but weekly diary records suggest that clients with depression spikes show more cognitive–emotional processing during this period of arousal than those without a spike. This is of interest because clinicians have previously reported the presence of depression spikes (e.g., in the treatment of chronic depression) and observed that it is not necessarily associated with poor outcome.

Prevention of relapse is a key focus of CT. Segal, Gemar, and Williams (1999) found that individuals who become euthymic during CT might still be at risk of early relapse. They undertook a study that showed that following mood induction, those individuals who still maintained high scores on measures of dysfunctional attitudes were at significantly higher risk of relapse than those whose scores had normalized and did not show reactivity in negative mood states. However, Persons (1993) noted that the changes in *depressogenic attributional style* (a tendency to attribute negative events to internal, stable, global causes) produced by CT are equivocal. This led her to propose that a key therapeutic process may not be simply modification of underlying beliefs but the acquisition of compensatory skills that allow the individual to cope with isolated depressive symptoms and prevent the symptoms from evolving into a depressive episode.

In recent years, a number of studies have indicated that changes in the way clients process information rather than changes in thought content may be important in the mechanism of action of CT. For example, Teasdale et al. (2000) found that CT helps clients with residual depression by changing not the content of their thinking but the form of their thinking. In particular, CT reduced absolutist, dichotomous thinking that in turn was found to mediate the effects of CT on preventing relapse. Individuals with persistent extreme response styles to depression-related material were more than 2.5 times as likely to experience early relapse compared with individuals without this extreme style (relapse rate = 44 vs. 17%). Teasdale and colleagues' examination of metacognitive awareness suggests that shifting the mode of processing adopted by patients is a critical factor. Taking this idea forward, Watkins et al. (2007) developed a model of CT that targeted ruminative response style and found that this led to significant improvements in individuals with chronic, often comorbid, depressive disorders. Fresco, Segal, Buis, and Kennedy (2007) found that CT responders exhibited significantly greater gains in decentering when compared with antidepressant responders. In addition, high postacute treatment levels of decentering and low cognitive reactivity were associated with the lowest rates of relapse in the 18-month follow-up period. An experimental study by Singer and Dobson (2007) sheds some light on these observations: 80 remitted depressed participants were randomized to training in the metacognitive style of rumination, distraction, acceptance or to a "no-training control" condition prior to a negative mood induction. Rumination prolonged the intensity of the negative mood, consistent with no training. Both distraction and acceptance reduced the intensity of the negative mood, but attitudinal changes were only found in the acceptance condition, as these participants reduced negative attitudes toward negative experiences. These results imply that preventive interventions may operate by both reducing the intensity of sad moods and altering one's attitudes toward temporary moments of sadness.

CLINICAL PRACTICE

The following session excerpt is an attempt to demonstrate what can be done in the shortest possible therapy, a single session with a woman with borderline personality disorder (BPD). The context of the session was a workshop on the treatment of BPD. Debbie was aware that the session was being recorded and that the written text would be reported in a professional chapter.

The annotations to the session highlight the therapist's development of hypotheses and the treatment conceptualization, and include the strategies that led to the implementation of that CT conceptual model through specific therapeutic techniques.

Patient Data

Debbie[1] was a 43-year-old white woman employed as an elementary school teacher in a public school. She had completed both undergraduate and master's degrees at a state teachers college. Debbie had never married and lived alone. She had no close friends and a few distant friends that she saw very occasionally on holidays. She had no social contact with her teaching colleagues. While relating well to the children, she had interpersonal problems with teacher colleagues, administrators, and parents of the children in her class.

For the last 10 years she has had no contact with her mother and a younger sister. Her father died when Debbie was 3 years old, and her mother remarried when Debbie was 5. The stepfather's mother lived with them. Debbie was sexually abused from ages 6 through 12 by her stepfather. He would come into her room three or four times a week and have her touch his genitals, then rape or sodomize her. On several occasions she had told her mother and stepgrandmother about the sexual abuse, but they did not believe her. They criticized and insulted her for even commenting on such a thing, and punished her for her comments. Ultimately, nothing was done. Her stepfather gloated and told Debbie that no one would ever believe her, that she was worthless, and that she deserved what happened to her. At other times he would cry after raping Debbie and tell her what a horrible child she was for making him do these sexual things. The abuse stopped when Debbie was 12. She brought a steak knife to bed and when her stepfather came into her bed she threatened him and told him that she

---

1. The patient's name, the name of her therapist, her geographic location, and other identifying data have been changed to maintain privacy and confidentiality. While there was a vast amount of data available about Debbie, it is not included here. What is included is the barest outline, but enough to conceptualize, plan, and enact the single-session therapy.

would castrate and then kill him if he ever touched her again. He called her "crazy" and never touched her again.

Debbie met six criteria for BPD (DSM-IV-TR). Debbie had been in therapy with several different therapists over the last 18 years. She had been seeing her present therapist for 1½ years. She reported anxiety, depressive symptoms, and seemingly inexplicable expressions of anger in which she verbally "exploded" at people at work. Finally, she engaged in frequent self-damaging behavior.

Case Conceptualization

The specific criteria-focused data were gathered from her therapist Dr. John Smith, and from elucidation by Debbie in a presession meeting. The criteria she met were as follows:

1. *Unstable interpersonal relationships.* Debbie had difficulty with coworkers that often led her to avoid them and to be excluded from social functions and even to be ignored during the work day. The problems took the form of Debbie insulting, being sarcastic, or being angry with others, who saw no reason for her verbal assaults.

2. *Self-mutilating behavior.* Debbie had for many years practiced self-mutilation.

3. *Affective instability.* Debbie reported that she experienced her moods shifting almost instantly. She could go from calm to anger in what she described as "a flash." She also described having experienced going through many "moods" in the course of the day.

4. *Inappropriate, intense anger.* Debbie reported that her anger responses to others appeared to "come out of the blue." The level, content, focus, extent, and duration of the anger often surprised Debbie.

5. *Chronic feelings of emptiness.* By her own report, Debbie described herself as "a nothing," "without value," "like an empty shell."

6. *Dissociative symptoms.* When Debbie was "upset," she had for many years used the technique of holding her breath until she became what she called "dizzy." She reported being able to see herself from a distance, sometimes looking down from the ceiling of the room. (This was what she learned to do during the childhood abuse.)

Given this information, Debbie likely had developed the following schemas: (1) The world was a dangerous place; (2) people, especially people in power, not to be trusted; (3) her value was based on sex; (4) her value was negative; (5) sex was negative; (6) she was to blame for what had happened to her; (7) she hoped for, and was disappointed when she could not find, support from others; (8) displays of emotion were to be hidden; (9) she was helpless; and (10) she was hopeless about changing.

Therapeutic goals were as follows:

1. Identify problem areas.
2. Reduce those areas to a small-enough piece for the single-session therapy.
3. Develop a conceptualization of the patient's problems.
4. Decide which parts of the conceptualization can be worked on in the single session.
5. Decide what specific techniques would be most useful.
6. Implement the technical therapy.
7. Evaluate the success of the interventions.
8. Make midcourse changes, as needed.
9. Get frequent feedback from the patient.
10. Be sure to leave time for appropriate closure and debriefing after the session.

Of specific note is the use of Socratic questioning throughout the session. To enhance the rapport in this brief time, many of the questions are closed-ended and elicit an affirmative response. This assisted in overcoming the negative set Debbie had about men, therapy, and so forth.

Several questions and issues that had to be kept in mind included the following:

• *Issue 1: Did Debbie have the potential for violence, either verbal or physical?* It would not have been helpful to Debbie and might have been seen by her as a failure and an embarrassment. Given her history, the therapist's response, and my own estimation, there was little chance of this potential for violence.

• *Issue 2: Were Debbie's social skills adequate and appropriate for her appearance in front of a group?* The goal was to demonstrate a particular set of interventions, not to put Debbie on display as an example of a diagnostic category. Again, based on her history, Debbie had social skills but often had trouble using them.

• *Issue 3: Were Debbie's intelligence and verbal ability adequate for the task?* History and interviews confirmed no problem in this area. Furthermore, her intelligence and verbal ability were strengths to be used.

• *Issue 4: What would be the effect of the audience?* Debbie's reaction to the therapist and to the audience would be crucial. Although she had agreed to participate after several discussions with her therapist, it was not clear what effect the audience would have. Would she use it as an opportunity to try to embarrass and humiliate me (an authority figure and a male)? Would she use it as an opportunity to get the audience to feel sorry for her as a way to justify her anger and upset?

- Ideally, the setting for this would be a consultation room with video capability. This way, the audience could see and hear the session without being present in the room. However, as in life, the ideal is not always available. The second choice was to have Debbie sit in front of the audience, with her back to the group. This allowed the therapist to face the audience and to keep his session notes on an overhead projector. In this way both the audience and Debbie could see what notes were being written in the session. The lights in the room were dimmed, and the only bright lights were on the stage. Aside from some coughing, there were few sounds from the audience. On several occasions Debbie's responses evoked supportive laughter from the group.

- *Issue 5: What was Debbie's frustration tolerance level?* This would be the key to the single session and to the treatment as a whole. It would be essential to establish how much flexibility and strength of boundaries Debbie had. If her boundaries were crossed, she would likely (and reasonably) retreat. If Debbie's boundaries or safety zone were not expanded, there would be minimal growth. If Debbie perceived a threat, she would withdraw. The best way to establish her boundaries (or how far and fast she could be pushed) would be to test the boundaries gingerly and gently. The therapist had to be prepared to back off immediately and, if needed, apologize quickly for the intrusion.

Schemas about intrusion, boundary violations, lack of remorse by the offender, lack of support, and victimization were all part of Debbie's life and had to be considered throughout the session. Overall, concerns included any motivational or compliance problems, and her ability to maintain control. Having been satisfied in an extensive discussion with her therapist and also with Debbie prior to the on screen interview, I was assured that there would not likely be any major problems.

Session Transcript

T1: Hi Debbie. I really appreciate your willingness to do this. We'll talk for about forty minutes, is that all right?

P1: Yes.

T2: How are you feeling about doing this?

P2: I'll be fine in about 40 minutes.

T3: It feels OK now, but you'll feel better later?

P3: Yeah.

T4: Again, I'd like to thank you for doing this. I think that it's interesting that you volunteered to do this because it says something about a level of courage. It takes an awful lot of courage to come into a room of strangers, to talk to a stranger about some very personal things. Given that we're going to talk for about 40 minutes, are there particular things that you would like to try to address in the time we have?

In addition to establishing rapport, the therapist is testing hypotheses regarding Debbie's view of self. If she is offered a positive statement (e.g., "You have courage") how does Debbie deal with it? It is likely dissonant with her negative self-view and will probably evoke a "Yes, but" response, or it may be ignored, as if she did not hear it at all.

P4: What seems to keep me stuck is how bad I feel about myself.

T5: That's pretty general. Can you be more specific, what does that mean?

What is the patient's idiosyncratic meaning for her often used terms, such as "bad"? The therapist can never assume idiosyncratic meanings.

P5: I'm not mad at the appropriate people. I take everything out on myself, even if it's not my fault.

T6   So, if someone does something, you'll take responsibility for it?

P6: I tend to take a lot and then it starts oozing out in inappropriate ways.

T7: Can you give me an example, Debbie, of how this would show itself? What would be a typical example?

P7: If a situation occurs at work, and it might have happened for the fifth time that week, I would blow up at whatever person is in front of me, even if it had nothing to do with that person. It was something underneath and they just happened to get in the way.

T8: OK, so things have been happening, the anger builds up, and then there's a trigger and then you explode?

P8: Right.

This summary of the chain of events does two things. First, it indicates to the patient that the therapist is listening. Second, it establishes a basis for further clarification.

T9: The other person is saying what to themselves?

P9: "Where did that come from?"

T10: He is saying, "Where did that come from?"

This reflective statement also encourages perspective taking by asking what Debbie guesses the other person might be thinking.

P10: And then I feel so guilty about laying somebody out, but it's too much to deal with.

T11: Do you feel guilty because you got angry, or do you feel guilty that you got angry to such a high degree?

Guilty is too broad a concept. It is important to delineate not only Debbie's meaning but also the nature of the "guilt" problem and any second-order problems attached to it.

P11: The degree.

T12: The degree? Is getting angry OK?

P12: No. Periodically, yes, it's good. I mean I know that I'm angry, but it's not OK for any long time.

T13: Why not? Why isn't anger OK?

P13: I haven't had much experience seeing appropriate anger and I'm afraid that I end up looking like what I grew up with.

This is a very broad invitation to explore issues of childhood experience, early learning, parental interactions and reactions, and a general theme of the past. Given the parameter of the setting and the single-session format, this will be left aside. The basic schema regarding anger will have to be addressed as a "here-and-now" issue.

T14: OK, so one thing we might be able to focus on in the time we have is this issue of appropriate anger or inappropriate anger, just kind of looking at that.

P14: Right.

T15: Anything else you might what to look at in the time we have, and then we can see what would be reasonable for the limited time that we have?

P15: I think anger pretty much covers everything that I do.

As in the overall therapy, this sets out an early problem list that ideally would be broad enough to fill the available time, and focused enough to allow the most effective use of the time.

T16: So anger is really something with a big capital "A"?

P16: Yeah.

T17: And it's with you pretty much all the time?

P17: I feel like I'm just boiling mad and I take it out on myself, and I'm trying to find other ways ...

T18: Are you boiling mad right now?

P18: No, I'm scared to death right now.

T19: Is that an alternative, either you're angry or you're scared?

P19: Yeah.

T20: So we have two possibilities. You can be angry or scared. Is scared a way of not dealing with your anger?

Is this one method of coping? If it is, then it can be used as the start of a list of coping strategies. For many patients, the predominant idea is that they have no coping strategies and are driven by the winds of chance or fate. By identifying any strategies they may attempt, we can introduce the idea that control is already part of their repertoire and the therapeutic goal is to enhance and build that list. What we know of Debbie's childhood is that until she got angry, she was scared of the abuse. For Debbie, anger was a useful way of coping.

P20: Well, I think I become angry when I'm really scared, because I don't know how to deal with being afraid, but at least anger leads me someplace. I feel paralyzed by the fear.

T21: So being scared, you're stuck?

This is another summary statement that elicits a positive response. Debbie knows the therapist is listening.

P21: Yeah.

T22: Anger gives you what?

P22: I don't want anybody to see me when I'm mad. I end up cleaning the house.

T23: Lot's of cleaning?

P23: Yeah.

T24: So anger gets you moving, anger gets you mobilized, so it's a good part of anger, you get your house clean. . . . very clean.

P24: Yeah.

This is the beginning of a cost–benefit analysis. The idea of this type of analysis is introduced here and expanded over the session. Just what is the function and value of anger in Debbie's life?

T25: But the anger's also upsetting, is that what you're saying?

P25: Because it's unpredictable and it oozes out, and I don't always see it until it's pointed out.

T26: You say it's unpredictable. Let me use an extreme example. Let's suppose someone from the audience comes up to you and kicks you in the ankle. Would that make you angry?

By constructing and introducing an extreme example, the therapist can see how Debbie responds to a scenario that is "here-and-now" rather than to situations that are outside of the therapy situation.

P26: Yes.

T27: Would you express your anger?

P27: Probably in an instant.

T28: So if someone comes up and kicks you in the ankle, you'd say, "You know you have a helluva nerve doing that. Who do you think you are? You shouldn't do that?" You'd get pretty angry?

P28: I probably wouldn't be that wordy.

T29: Is that right? Would that be appropriate anger?

P29: Off the top of my head, yes.

T30: So if someone comes up to you and kicks you in the ankle and you got angry at them, would you feel guilty afterwards for being angry?

P30: Yeah.

T31: Why? What would get you from being angry at what they did to you and then feeling bad about being angry? Can you describe the process?

How does Debbie construct and process the event? By asking her to explicate and describe the process in detail, possibly the thought–feeling–action connection can be elicited.

P31: It would be because of my response. It's like I would have to have a reason why I did that. Obviously I did something to them. Its because I'm the kind of person that I am that they did that. This is what I deserved, and on and on and on.

T32: So if you were a better person, a nicer person, a sweeter person, a gentler person, they wouldn't have kicked you in the ankle?

P32: That's right.

T33: What if I told you that I knew the person who kicked you, and that they were a mean, nasty individual.

There is an obvious segue to move to the likelihood of Debbie's response in this example being similar to her response as a child when she was abused and hurt. It was then that she likely developed the idea that if she were a better person, the abuse would not have occurred. As before, this avenue is too much of a jump for the context or this brief contact. This avenue is likely a rich one for further and future therapy work.

P33: I would be more angry that, if you knew that about him, why you wouldn't you try to warn me or to defend me.

T34: So you'd then get angry at me?

P34: And then I'd be angry at you.

T35: So that the anger is with you all the time?

P35: Pretty much.

T36: There are two ways to look at anger in my view. One is that people carry around with them a kind of basket filled with anger, and they keep pulling from the basket and spreading the anger around the world, but if that were true, then at some point the basket might be empty and you'd say, "Whew I finally got rid of that last piece of anger." What you're describing, though, is kind of a well that keeps being replenished from underneath, so that you always have this anger that keeps being there. Is that right?

P36: Yeah.

T37: Is that an accurate view on my part?

P37: Yeah.

T38: Have you thought about—either by yourself or with your therapist—what generates the anger, what keeps filling the well?

P38: A lot of times it's situational. If something happens and there's like, someone who could have spoken up for me or in some ways defended me and didn't. (*Patient's voice breaks and she gets teary.*)

Here are the data to support the hypothesis of the anger, the lack of control, and the early abuse. This lead is very compelling, but the therapist has decided that it is not be in the patient's best interest to explore it in this context.

T39: Let me just stop. You're getting really upset right now. Can you tell me, if you're comfortable in this setting, what is getting you upset right now? As you start talking about "why haven't I been warned or defended," the tears come. What's going on right now that's generating those tears?

By immediately focusing on the emotional response, we can access the disturbing cognitions (automatic thoughts). Once again, the focus has the effect of bringing the therapy work into the here and now.

P39: That so many things happened, and that there was no one there for me . . .

T40: So what really gets upsetting is the idea that "I should have been defended or helped or supported."

P40: Yes.

T41: But I wonder. Maybe the upsetting part is not just that. What it sounds like is not simply that "I should have been defended or helped or supported," but the last part of what you haven't said—"and you weren't." When you have that idea, "I should have been defended and I wasn't," how does that make you feel?

This addresses the patient's rules about how others should have acted. Her rules or expectations are, of course, entirely reasonable. The connection between the thoughts and feelings is important here. The therapist has chosen not to explore the broad or specific parts of the abuse in the context of being in front of an audience. The operative piece for Debbie is that she was not defended. This is also the clue as to how to focus the therapy. Her issue was not being defended, either externally or internally. Does she, for example, defend herself against her negative cognitions?

T42: Does the thought that you were not defended make you happy?

P42: No.

T43: Does it make you sad?

P43: It's just the way it was.

T44: Does it make you angry?

P44: It's just the way it was.

T45: That's true, but as you look back on it, does it make you angry?

P45: I suppose. To be safe, to be protected, to be helped to survive.

T48: Right, and that wasn't your experience?

P48: No, it wasn't.

T49: But that was a while ago, wasn't it? You still carry it in your head?

P49: Like it was yesterday.

T50: Like it was yesterday. But physically it wasn't yesterday, was it?

P50: No.

T51: But in your head it could have been this morning?

P51: Right.

T52: What goes on in your head for you that keeps you upset all this time?

The thought–feeling connection is very important. This is basic in the cognitive-behavioral therapy (CBT) model. Debbie has been in CBT with an experienced CBT therapist, so there is no need to offer a formal description of the therapy. To emphasize the therapy, I chose to demonstrate throughout the session the connections between thoughts, feelings, and behavior.

P52: The noise in my head that's very loud and critical. I can't do anything right.

T53: The noise in your head. What does that noise sound like?

P53: Sometimes it's a loud critical voice, and sometimes there are so many of them that its like having airplanes fly over your head, one after another.

T54: When you hear the critical voices, what do the critical voices say to you?

P54: That I'm really bad, I'll never amount to anything. This is a joke. I'm kidding myself if I think that things are going to be any better.

This is likely only a small sample of the internal negative dialogue. The initial hypothesis of difficulty in accepting positives is clearer here. How can Debbie see things as positive when there are all of these negative voices? A goal of therapy to work to quiet the negative voices and allow some room for the positive seems a better bet.

T55: As you hear the voice say those things, how does that make you feel?

P55: Like I don't stand a chance.

T56: You don't stand a chance?

P56: No.

T57: If anyone of us had a bunch of people following us, saying, "You'll never amount to anything, you're worthless, you're a waste," what effect do you think it would have on any one of us?

P57: After a while, you'll begin to believe it.

This was an attempt at normalizing her experience.

T58: Right, have you ever tried to argue with those voices?

P58: I must have at some point.

T59: You must have ...

P59: I'm sure ...

T60: How about in the last 6 months? Have you tried to argue with those voices recently?

My choice is to choose a proximal point; 6 months is long ago but still recent. To focus on the more likely time frame of the last 40 years would be far too upsetting. This introduces the therapeutic notion of countering the automatic thoughts.

P60: I argue with my therapist instead.

T61: Maybe we can do it for here for free.

P61: OK.

T62: OK, there are some advantages, for example, tell me again what those voices say. I want to write them down. What are some typical things those voices say?

P62: "You're no good, you don't deserve good things."

T63: Wait a minute, slow down, "You're no good, you don't deserve good things." I want to write them down. What else?

The thoughts run through Debbie's head like a runaway train. By directly slowing her down and writing each thought down, the therapist can highlight each and every thought.

P63: "You'll never amount to anything."

T64: "You'll never amount to anything."

P64: "You are kidding yourself if you believe that things could be better."

T65: "You're kidding yourself to think that things will ever be better." : If we took anybody in this room and we attached a tape recorder to their waist, and there was a constant tape that ran "You're no good, you don't deserve good things. You'll never amount to anything. You're kidding yourself to think you deserve any better," what effect do you think it would have, say, on your therapist? John's a pretty strong guy. I've known him for a long time. What effect do you think it would have on him?

Before challenging the negative thoughts, the goal was to explicate the thoughts. Debbie could see that having the thoughts is normal, reasonable, and expected. Given her life experience, it should not be a surprise to Debbie that there were many negative self-referential thoughts. The problem for Debbie is that she never stopped to question the thoughts.

P66: After a while it weighs you down.

T67: Yeah, after a while you start saying, yeah, it's true.

P67: Uh huh.

T68: Is that what you're saying now? "Yeah, it's true."

P68: Uh huh.

T69: You're agreeing with it.

P69: Uh huh.

T70: What do you think would happen, Debbie, if you challenged those voices ... challenged those ideas? What effect do you think it would have on you?

P70: Hopefully it would change.

T71: OK, hopefully it would change? What would be your guess if you could answer these voices back? If you could, what would happen to the voices? What's your prediction?

P71: I'd ... it would get louder and then go away.

T72: You think it may get louder and shout you down?

P72: Initially.

T73: Initially? I'd agree with that, I think initially the voices will get louder, but then they'd probably . ideally, go away. When you hear these voices, is there a particular person or voice attached to them?

Here is the family-of-origin connection. It is a great lead that we let pass for now.

P73: Sometimes it's my own, sometimes its my stepfather's, sometimes its my grandmother's.

T74: So there are specific people that you can hear saying these things?

P74: Uh huh.

T75: Let me just explore something with you in terms of this, because what you're saying is that by believing these things, you then say, "I should have been defended and not have heard these things, and I wasn't and that makes me really sad and angry."

P75: Uh huh.

T76: Is it true that you're no good?

Can she examine the evidence for goodness or badness?

P76: I've had a good day now.

T77: So you have a good day. What would be a good day?

P77: I don't really know. It's kind of ... like I guess ... I haven't had one in a very long time, so that I don't remember what it's like.

T78: But if you were to have one of these infrequent good days, you wouldn't easily say you're no good. You would say, what, maybe you're not so bad?

P78 : No, it would probably have more to do with the environment, with the sun being out and going for a walk.

Debbie externalizes her good days. She has no control. This is a basic schematic element. Rather than confronting and disputing the schema, I try to collect data to have her challenge the absolutistic nature of this idea.

T79: OK. Do you believe you don't deserve good things?

P79: Most of the time.

T80: So you only deserve bad things?

P80: Yeah, basically.

T91: OK, if you could quiet these voices there's a chance that you might feel better, all right. Do you ever try to argue with the voices, to challenge these ideas?

P91: Yeah.

T92: And the result of that?

P92: The noise gets louder and I begin to hurt myself.

T93: I'm not clear. If you try to answer the voices the noise gets louder and then you hurt yourself.

P93: It's part of a chain of events; it's just so loud, it wins.

T94: And when it wins, its reward is that you hurt yourself?

P94: Yes, I know it doesn't make sense, but ...

T95: Help me understand it, Debbie. I'm trying to understand the sequence. The voice says, for example, "Debbie, you're no good," and you say, "Yes I am," then the voice says, "Forget it. No you're not," and you say, "OK, you're right, no I'm not" and then you do what? You hurt yourself?

P95: I start getting more and more agitated, and it pretty much plays into the noise, but, yeah, you're right. I say, "This is the truth. You are a worthless piece of crap."

T96: ... and, and what? You're a worthless piece of crap and ...

P96: Yeah.

T97: If the result is that you hurt yourself, then you say you're a worthless piece of crap and you want to do something to prove it?

P97: No, I just know. It just happens.

T98: What just happens, you hurting yourself?

P98: Yeah, sometimes the pressure feels so big, its like sometimes it eases ...

P104 : When I'm experiencing a lot of emotional pain I tend to hold my breath and sort of black out. I have to go to someplace else that eases the pain, so what I'm working on is trying to bring it out, so that it won't stay stuck inside.

T105: And then you don't dissociate?

P105: I do, but I can come down from being up in the ceiling, and I can hear the voices and be able to work it through.

T106: OK. What do you think would happen, Debbie, if you could answer these voices back as soon as you hear them? What do you think the result of that would be?

P106: The way to go is that I could talk back to the voices. I could be louder and make myself heard.

T106: And what do you think would be the result of that?

P106: That I could feel better.

T107: And what would be the result of that?

P107: That I wouldn't have to hurt myself anymore.

T108: And what would be the result of that?

P108: I wouldn't see my therapist anymore.

T109: And what would be the result of that?

P109: I would be very sad.

T110: That you wouldn't see him?

P110: Yeah, even though it would hurt sometimes ...

The downward arrow technique has Debbie looking at each successive level of belief.

T111: Sometimes. If you're able to not hurt yourself, if you're able to feel better about yourself, if you can answer all of these negative voices, then you wouldn't need therapy and you would lose John as a support.

P111: By that time I wouldn't need it.

T112: You're not so sure about that?

P112: Well, definitely no. I've really taken a long time to be able to talk with him.

T115: So if you do something really positive, really in effect very powerful, you dismiss it how?

P115: I don't know it's that I'm doing this and just keep on doing it.

P117: It's a very negative thing right now and I'd beat myself up, because it's just too much.

T121: So you kind of dismiss the positive?

P121: Uh huh.

T122: And emphasize what you don't do or what you see as a negative? Would you be willing to try a little experiment with me? I'll tell you what it is. Don't agree to it until I tell you what it is.

P122: OK.

T123: You've gone to school. Have you ever been in a debate at school?

P123: No.

T125: Have you ever seen a debate?

P125: Yeah.

T126: What's your understanding of a debate?

P126: You do your best to be the most convincing.

T127: Right. What if you and I were to have a debate? I would like to be this really negative voice and what I want you to do is debate with me. I want to see if you can quiet me down. Would you be willing to try that?

The session is about half over. I have made a clinical decision. By external-izing the negative voices I think that several points can be made. First, I can demonstrate the technique to the audience. Second, we can see exactly how Debbie copes with the negative voices. Third, Debbie can see just how she copes. Finally, we can use the data from the experience to try to help her to respond in a more adaptive fashion.

P127: Yeah.

T128: OK, so I'm going to be the negative voice and you're going to debate with me. You're going to try to quiet me. Got it?

P128: Yeah.

T129: OK. In fact one of the things we can do here that we can't otherwise do, I'd like to stack the deck in your favor, of course. John, I'd like to invite you to join us. I would like you to sit next to Debbie, and if she starts having trouble I would like you to help her out. OK? Would that be all right with you?

P129: Yeah.

T130: *(to John)* You don't have to say a word until she gets into trouble. *(to Debbie)* You in trouble yet?

P130: No.

T131: No? OK. So this is you and me.

P131: You know, you're really no good, you're really a worthless person.

P132: You're right.

That was fast. Debbie immediately agreed with the negative voice.

T133: Wait a minute, wait a minute. What kind of a debate is that?

(John says something to her. She moves back into the role.)

P133: Why would you say that?

T134: Oh, no reason. I just think it.

P134: Of course, you need a reason.

T135: No, I just think you're a worthless person, you're just a bad person.

P135: Nobody's worthless.

T136: Except you. You're no good and you don't deserve anything good happening to you.

P136: That's not true.

T137: It is true. *(stopping)* What's happening?

P137: All I hear are negative voices. It's like I'm lying to you.

T138: That's right. So we have a problem with this debate, because you hear the negative idea and the voice inside you says "True, you're right." If you could say the things that would quiet me, that would be a beginning. You don't have to believe it. At first you have to practice saying it. You OK? What I'd like to do is switch roles. OK?

P138: Uh huh.

T139: I would like for you to be the negative voice, and I want to see if I can model for you a way of responding. OK? Can you be the negative voice that beats you up?

P139: No problem.

Certainly Debbie has no problem being the negative voice. I want to model a strong and assertive adaptive voice that is not afraid of the negative voice, but is assertive and reasonable. To try to be too unreasonable will be rejected by Debbie. If I try to be too positive, then it will be rejected as "cheerleading." I have to model some level of adaptive response that Debbie can copy.

T140: No problem? Do it.

P140: You really aren't worth a piece of crap.

T141: Says who?

P141: Says me.

T142: Who the hell are you to tell me that I'm no good?

P142: I know it all.

T143: I think you know very little. You have no right to make judgments on anyone.

P143: It's not just anyone. I'm talking to you.

T144: Oh, it's me, and you have no right to make judgments about me. I'm not worthless and I don't have to listen to this garbage from you. If you weren't so damn stupid you wouldn't even say something like that. Just who in the hell do you think you are talking to me like that? I'm sick and tired of hearing it. (*Debbie sits back in her seat, shakes her head, and smiles.*) Where's that negative voice, Debbie? Where is it?

P144: You're being a pain in the butt.

T145: I may be a pain in the butt, but I'm tired of feeling bad. I'm tired of hurting myself, I'm tired of blaming myself for everything, and it's your fault and I want to hear no more of it. Where's the negative voice?

P145: I don't hear it.

T146: Wait, let's back up. Where did the negative voice go?

P146: It went away.

T150: Does it feel better or worse when that negative voice is quiet?

P150: Better.

T151: When I was really doing a job on that negative voice you were smiling. Why?

I wanted to do two things here: first, to understand why Debbie was smiling, and second, to give her some breathing space.

P151: Well, you're quite powerful.

T152: Yeah. Why were you smiling?

P152: 'Cause it was kind of funny.

T153: It's funny? You weren't laughing, you were smiling.

P153: Well, I guess I never stood up to myself in that way.

T154: And you were smiling because of what?

P154: Because of how you were saying it.

T155: Are those things you could say?

P155: Today? Yeah. Only one thing ...

T156: I have a hunch. Let me share my hunch with you, Debbie. My experience over the years has been that very often people carry voices that they give great power to. That the voices are kind of like..... .Did you ever see the film *The Wizard of Oz*? The part where they are in the wizard's castle and want to talk to the wizard, and they see this fearsome image on a screen saying, "I'm the great and powerful Oz." Remember that scene?

P156: Uh huh.

I decide to use a metaphor that has great power. If the image had no meaning for Debbie, it would not be worth explaining. I would try to find another image.

T157: What was he? Was he a great wizard? What was he?

P157: A sorry old man.

T158: Using all kinds of tricks to make himself look bigger and sound bigger. I wonder ... and I'd just like to present that for your consideration ... is it possible that this negative voice is like the Wizard of Oz? Because if we could shut that voice up so easily, then it's a lot of bluster and a lot of noise, and a lot of smoke, but it's not as powerful as it makes out to be. Is that possible?

At this point I am addressing her beliefs that people in power are indeed as powerful as they make themselves out to be. I am fully aware that the image of the "pathetic old man" may well be the stepfather who was viewed as very powerful. Again, given the context and the limit of our contact, I will plant the seed for John to harvest.

P158: It feels like it.

T159: Right now it feels like it? OK. So what I'd like to do, if that's true, I'm going to be the negative voice again and I'd like you to really be tough. No messing around, and John's there to help you. I want you ... don't just be gentle. I want you to really quiet me 'cause I'm not doing you any good. I'm not your friend. I make you feel bad, you get angry, you hurt yourself. OK?

Having offered the metaphor that the voice may not be that powerful after all, we need to try the debate again. Can Debbie be helped to feel powerful?

You know Debbie, you're no good. You're worthless.

P159: That's not true.

T160: Yeah it is. Yeah it's true. You're no good, you'll never amount to anything. (*I encouraging her ... "Come on, that's it."*)

P160: (*John offers her a response. Debbie gulps and then repeats it.*) Who the hell are you?

T161: I'm the negative voice. I've been here a long time. And don't you talk to me that way.

P161: OK.

T162: Oh boy! In that one time when you said what John did, how did you feel?

P162: It was great.

I wanted Debbie to identify what she was feeling at that moment, and to offer her feedback about her response.

T163: Again, I wish you could see yourself. If we had a mirror to see you weren't smiling, you were grinning, you gulped once and then said, "Who the hell do you think you are anyway?" But it felt good?

P163: Uh huh.

T164: Let's do it again. You're a worthless individual, you don't deserve anything good to happen to you.

P164: That's not true.

T165: It's been true for years, Debbie. Let's just face it, you're a worthless piece of crap.

P165: Who the hell are you?

T166: I am just your voice. I've been with you along time. That gives me great longevity and seniority, and I know you're worthless.

P166: Things can change.

T167: Oh yeah, sure, the oceans can all dry up. You know you're worthless and you'll be that way forever. (*Whispers to Debbie.*)

P167: You're just like the character in *The Wizard of Oz.*

T168: You know you're just kidding yourself if you think that things will ever get better. You'll always be … you know … no good, worthless, a loser, a piece of crap.

P168: You don't know that.

T169: Well I'm inside your head. I know everything. I'm the smartest thing going.

P169: Who says so? You don't know everything.

T170: Well, I know I may not know everything, but I know you're no good.

P170: You're a disturbed, pathetic old man. Now. (*Covers her mouth and starts giggling.*)

T171: Let me stop. You've gone from smiling to grinning to being almost giggly. Why?

The here-and-now focus invites Debbie's response.

P171: I guess it's all the things he's (*pointing to John*) saying about you.

T172: He's not saying it. You're saying it. I'm running out of things to say.

P172: It's the same stuff. You'll run out of them.

T173: Exactly. But … "Yeah, says you." How does it feel for you right here, right now to say those things?

P173: It's like you're talking about somebody else.

T174: So if you practice and then they get to be yours. How does it make you feel when you start getting giddy and start giggling? What are you feeling?

Here we can focus on the need for practice via homework.

P174: A lot lighter.

T175: Lighter? Does it make you want to go out and hurt yourself?

P175: No, not at the moment.

T176: So when you're able to answer that voice back, to be really tough, do you feel guilty for quieting that voice down?

P176: Not yet.

T177: But you might.

P177: Uh huh.

T178: OK. And that's something else that you're going to work on with John. Right here, right now, you've gone from smiling to grinning, to giggly just answering this negative voice back. Debbie, what's been going on inside your head?

P178: Well, I haven't been thinking about the voice.

T179: OK. Having someone nearby is real helpful.

P179: Yeah.

T180: OK. Well, let me recommend something that might be a good exercise, some good homework for you. Was this little exercise painful?

P180: In the beginning, I was afraid I wouldn't have the right answer.

T181: And then?

P181: I would fail.

T182: And then what happened?

P182: I get really nervous in front of all these people.

T183: That's right, but what happened instead of that

P183: I'm still here, I didn't move.

T184: Are you embarrassed in front of all these people?

P184: Not yet.

T185: Not yet? OK. let me suggest something that can be helpful. Do you have a cassette recorder at home?

P185: Yes.

T186: OK. I would like to recommend something, and again, this is something I'll recommend for John and you to work on. I don't think your negative voice is that terribly clever. OK? I don't think it's terribly smart. I think it's kind of a Johnny One Note. It says just the same things—"You're no good"—you know, the same kind of crap over and over again. First thing that I'd like to recommend is that you write those thoughts down. Try to identify all of the thoughts, those negative thoughts that this really insistent negative voice annoys you with. Then what I'd recommend you do is to record them on a tape recorder in the following way: "You're no good. You're a worthless piece of crap." Give yourself about 10 seconds between each negative statement: "You'll never amount to anything in your life," 10 seconds, "You're just a piece of crap. No one even cares about you." And then I'd like to recommend.... Do you understand what I'm asking so far, to work with John, 'cause John's a good helper on this. You just saw what he did ... to come up with responses that you can write down. So what I'd like for you to do is that you're going to go home and you're going to put on your cassette recorder and a voice is going to say "You're no good." And you're going to practice, "You know you're full of shit. I don't have to take that from you. You're a worthless jerk, you're a stupid,

stupid voice. I don't have to agree with you any longer. The voice will say "Nothing's going to ever work out for you." And you'll say "Well, that's not true, something is working out right now, I'm shutting you up." Write those down and practice them a couple of times a week. So you're going to become your own negative voice on the tape and John's going to help you respond. Does that make sense?

P186: Yup.

T187: What do you hear me asking you to do?

I want to be sure that Debbie and I are talking about the same thing. By having her repeat the homework, I can monitor and change, if necessary.

P187: Change the way it is.

T188: Is this something you think you'd be able to manage to do?

P188: Yeah.

T189: You can practice it in the office, and then you can work on it at home. John, is that something you'd be willing to work with Debbie on? (*John says, "Oh yeah."*) OK. If you could quiet that negative voice, what would the result be?

P189: I wouldn't need to hurt myself.

T190: Would that be good or bad?

P191: Good.

T192: OK. We're running close on our time. Let me ask you, as our time is almost up, what are you going to take home from today's session? What have you learned?

I wanted to have Debbie review the session work for herself, for me, and also to have the audience hear what she was taking home.

P192: What I did.

T193: With what?

P193: Change.

T194: Yeah and ...

P194: Quieting the voice.

T195: Yeah, what else?

P195: That I have a way now of trying to use the mechanisms I have ...

T196: OK. How likely do you think it is you'll be able to do this?

P196: Well, I want to be realistic, because you suggested and it seemed like a pretty good idea. It's not like its going to change right away like today.

T197: You're right. You know, maybe it wouldn't change your behavior at all. Maybe it won't change things one bit. How are you going to find out?

P197: I'd have to try it.

T198: OK. Sounds like a good idea. In closing, Debbie, how do you feel about what we've done in the last 45 minutes?

P198: I'm more relaxed than in the beginning.

T199: More relaxed than in the beginning?

P199: Uh huh.

T200: Did I say anything that upset you or hurt you?

P200: No.

T201: Did I say anything that you found obnoxious or difficult to deal with?

P201: No.

T202: OK. What's your overall impression of the 45 minutes we spent?

P202: I was on the hot seat.

T203: You certainly were. OK. How do you think you did on the hot seat?

P203: Well, I'm still talking.

T204: You survived?

P204: Yeah.

T205: On a scale of 0 to 100, where 0 is total failure and 100 is really positive, how do you think you did today?

P205: 60.

T206: Better than half. You know I'm going to ask them [the audience] the same question. They're listening to us, of course, and I'm going to see what their view is. Once again, if what you said is accurate, that you underestimate your value, you're giving yourself a 60, which is still pretty good, then would you be interested in hearing what they think? Or would you rather not hear it?

P206: OK.

T207: OK, we're going to stop and what we're going to do, they're going to have a chance to ask me questions. Would you like to stay and maybe they'll have a some questions for you? And if you feel comfortable maybe you can answer them.

P207: OK.

Summary

On follow-up, Debbie was able to do the homework with the therapist's assistance and found that it was helpful in countering the negative thoughts. This led to a lifting of the depression and a diminution in the self-injurious behavior.

SUMMARY AND CONCLUSIONS

CT has been applied successfully to a number of problems and disorders for nearly half a century. The philosophy of CT entirely reflects the scientist-practitioner approach that is widely advocated as a model for clinical practice for mental health professionals. Ongoing research continues to establish whether the notion of cognitive vulnerability is a robust and plausible hypothesis. It is important to note that most of the evidence linking selective processing with emotional vulnerability is correlational, and the cognitive biases shown by clients compared to healthy controls are usually reduced or reversed with recovery (Matthews, 2006). Furthermore, reversal of cognitive abnormalities occurs whether individuals are treated with CT or other approaches, including pharmacotherapy. Thus, we are still seeking predictors of differential benefit from CT, so that we may target the intervention more effectively (Scott, 2001). Cognitive therapy trials for different disorders commenced as much as 30 years apart, so it is not surprising that research on the efficacy of CT, and explorations of its adaptation and range of applications are at different stages for disorders. Examples of the breadth of this research are studies of the utility of extended courses of individual CT that encompass acute treatment and maintenance sessions to reduce relapse rates in highly recurrent depressive disorders, which are often treated in specialist affective disorders clinics (Jarrett et al., 2001); at the other end of the spectrum, brief computerized and guided self-help versions of CT have been used successfully in the treatment of common mental disorders and eating disorders, and may be applied in primary care settings (Bara-Carril et al., 2004; Wright et al., 2002). There is a scientific rationale for the former approach but the latter may be driven by convenience, as we are still unable to specify the active ingredients of CT and it is not yet clear whether techniques unique to CT specifically benefit certain emotional disorders and distinguish CT from other therapies.

An important area of developing research is the process of change in CT (DeRubeis & Feeley, 1990). This is important when trying to differentiate between the general characteristics of effective therapies, such as the strength of the therapeutic alliance compared to any unique effects. A snapshot of some of the exciting research on CT process is provided in this chapter, and Kraemer, Wilson, Fairburn, and Agras (2002) suggest that treatment trials should now routinely include an evaluation of the mediators and moderators of outcomes. This is an attractive proposition for studies of CT in depressive disorders, but it is premature for studies of bipolar disorders, which require more detailed theoretical work and coherent modeling to produce a robust cognitive explanation of the ascent into mania that would then allow the introduction of CT interventions with greater specificity and durability. It is important to heed the warnings of leading CT researchers, such as Hollon (Hollon, Stewart, & Strunk, 2006), who comments that it remains unclear whether the durable benefits of CT are a consequence of the amelioration of the causal processes that generate risk or the introduction of compensatory strategies that offset them. Furthermore, we are still not certain whether these effects reflect the mobilization of cognitive or of other mechanisms.

Last, an exciting field of research is the exploration of the mind–brain interface by using scanning technology, such as functional magnetic resonance imaging (fMRI) and positron emission tomography (PET) and looking at changes before and after CT and comparing these with changes observed with pharmacological treatments, such as antidepressants. Two recent publications on response to CT provide examples of this evolving area of research. First, Goldapple et al. (2004) undertook before-and-after PET scans on 17 unmedicated, unipolar depressed outpatients, 14 of whom responded to 15–20 sessions of CT. Scan results were compared with an independent group of 13 paroxetine-treated responders. Treatment response with CT was associated with significant metabolic changes, notably, increases in hippocampus and dorsal cingulate cortical activity and decreases in dorsal ventral and medial frontal cortical activity. Furthermore, this pattern was distinct from that with paroxetine-facilitated clinical recovery, where prefrontal increases and hippocampal and subgenual cingulate decreases in activity were found. The researchers concluded that, as with antidepressants, clinical recovery with CT is associated with modulation in the functioning of specific sites in limbic and cortical regions. However, the differences in the directional changes in frontal cortex, cingulate, and hippocampus with CBT relative to paroxetine may reflect modality-specific effects.

In a separate study, Siegle and colleagues (2006) used fMRI scans to monitor areas of the brain that are activated or deactivated in response to emotional stimuli. Fourteen unmedicated depressed clients and 21 never-depressed controls were asked to rate as quickly and accurately as possible the relevance to them of positive, negative, and neutral emotionally valenced cue words. Following the scans, the depressed participants received 16 sessions of CBT. It was reported that seven out of nine depressed clients in whom pretherapy had shown low sustained reactivity in the subgenual cingulate cortex after they read and rated negative words responded to CBT. Furthermore, increased activity in a region of the right amygdala was associated with improved response to CBT even when initial severity of symptoms was taken into account. However, amygdala activity was only marginally predictive of recovery status. The researchers concluded that CBT was most useful to those who demonstrated increased emotional reactivity and who could not engage regulatory structures.

These studies represent an important area of research in psychotherapy, but it should be noted that they are but early attempts to use these approaches with small samples of selected clients, and there are many methodological hurdles to overcome. The fact that more such studies and the beginnings of some consistency in differential observed patterns of changes with CT and medication are under way opens up exciting opportunities for future empirical research on the neuroscientific underpinnings of CT (Miterschiffthaler, Williams, Scott, & Fu, 2008).

REFERENCES

Alloy, L., & Abrahamson, L. (1999). The Temple–Wisconsin Cognitive Vulnerability to Depression Project: Conceptual background, design, and methods. *Journal of Cognitive Psychotherapy, 13*, 227–262.

Bara-Carril, N., Williams, C. J., Pombo-Carril, M. G., Reid, Y., Murray, K., Aubin, S., et al. (2004). A preliminary investigation into the feasibility and efficacy of a CD-ROM-based cognitive-behavioral self-help intervention for bulimia nervosa. *International Journal of Eating Disorders, 35*, 538–548.

Beck, A. T. (1952). Successful outpatient psychotherapy of a chronic schizophrenic with a delusion based on borrowed guilt. *Psychiatry, 15*, 305–312.

Beck, A. T. (1963). Thinking and depression: Idiosyncratic content and cognitive distortions. *Archives of General Psychiatry, 9*, 324–333.

Beck, A. T. (1967). *Depression: Clinical, experimental, and theoretical aspects*. New York: Harper & Row.

Beck, A. T. (1976). *Cognitive therapy and the emotional disorders*. New York: International Universities Press.

Beck, A. T. (1996). Beyond belief: A theory of modes, personality, and psychopathology. In P. Salkovskis (Ed.), *Frontiers of cognitive therapy* (pp. 1–25). New York: Guilford Press.

Beck, A. T. (2005). The current state of cognitive therapy: A 40-year retrospective. *Archives of General Psychiatry, 62*, 953–959.

Beck, A. T., & Emery, G., with Greenberg, R. L. (1985). *Anxiety disorders and phobias: A cognitive perspective*. New York: Basic Books.

Beck, A. T., Freeman, A., Davis, D. D., Pretzer, J., Fleming, B., Arntz, A., et al. (2004). *Cognitive therapy of personality disorders* (2nd ed.). New York: Guilford Press.

Beck, A. T., & Rector, N. A. (2002). Delusions: A cognitive perspective. *Journal of Cognitive Psychotherapy: An International Quarterly, 16*(4), 455–468.

Beck, A. T., Rush, A. J., Shaw, B. F., & Emery, G. (1979). *Cognitive therapy of depression*. New York: Guilford Press.

Beck, J. (1995). *Cognitive therapy: Basics and beyond*. New York: Guilford Press.

Blatt, S. J., Zuroff, D. C., Quinlan, D. M., & Pilkonis, P. A. (1996). Interpersonal factors in brief treatment of depression: Further analyses of NIMH TDCRP. *Journal of Consulting and Clinical Psychology, 64*, 162–171.

Butler, A. C., Chapman, J. E., Foreman, E. M., & Beck, A. T. (2006). The empirical status of cognitive behavioural therapy: A review of meta-analyses. *Clinical Psychology Review, 26,* 17–31.

Chambless, D. L., & Hollon, S. D. (1998). Defining empirically supported therapies. *Journal of Consulting and Clinical Psychology, 66,* 7–18.

Clark, D. A., & Beck, A. T. (1999). *Scientific foundations of cognitive theory and therapy of depression.* New York: Wiley.

Clark, D. M., & Ehlers, A. (2004). Posttraumatic stress disorder: From cognitive theory to therapy. In R. L. Leahy (Ed.), *Contemporary cognitive therapy: Theory, research, and practice* (pp. 43–71). New York: Guilford Press.

Clark, D. M., Salkovskis, P. M., Öst, G. L., Westling, B., Loehler, K. A., Jeavons, A., et al. (1997). Misinterpretation of body sensations in panic disorder. *Journal of Consulting and Clinical Psychology, 65,* 203–213.

Clark, D. M., & Wells, A. (1995). A cognitive model of social phobia. In R. G. Heimberg, M. Liebowitz, D. A. Hope, & F. Schneier (Eds.), *Social phobia: Diagnosis, assessment, and treatment* (pp. 15–37). New York: Guilford Press.

Crits-Christoph, P., Baranackie, K., Kurcias, J. S., Greenberg, R., Conte, H., et al. (1991). Meta-analysis of therapist effects in psychotherapy outcome studies. *Psychotherapy Research, 1,* 81–91.

Davidson, K., Scott, J., Schmidt, U., Tata, P., Thornton, S., & Tyrer, P. (2004). Therapist competence and clinical outcome in the POPMACT trial. *Psychological Medicine, 34,* 855–863.

DeRubeis, R. J., & Feeley, M. (1990). Determinants of change in cognitive therapy for depression. *Cognitive Therapy and Research, 14,* 469–482.

DeRubeis, R. J., Hollon, S. D., Amsterdam, J. D., Shelton, R. C., Young, P. R., Salomon, R. M., et al. (2005). Cognitive therapy vs medications in the treatment of moderate to severe depression. *Archives of General Psychiatry, 62*(4), 409–416.

Ellis, A. (1962) *Reason and emotion in psychotherapy.* New York: Lyle Stuart.

Enright, S. J. (1997). Cognitive behaviour therapy: Clinical applications. *British Medical Journal, 314,* 1811–1816.

Foa, E., & Kozak, M. (1997). Beyond the efficacy ceiling: Cognitive behavior therapy in search of theory. *Behavior Therapy, 28,* 601–611.

Fresco, D., Segal, Z., Buis, T., & Kennedy, S. (2007). Relationship of post-treatment decentring and cognitive reactivity to relapse in major depression. *Journal of Consulting and Clinical Psychology, 75,* 447–455.

Garety, P. A., Fowler, D. G., Freeman, D., Bebbington, P., Dunn, G., & Kuipers, E. (2008). Cognitive-behavioural therapy and family intervention for relapse prevention and symptom reduction in psychosis: Randomised controlled trial. *British Journal of Psychiatry, 192,* 412–423.

Goldapple, K., Segal, Z., Garson, C., Lau, M., Beiling, P., Kennedy, S., et al. (2005). Modulation of cortical–limbic pathways in major depression: Treatment-specific effects of cognitive behavior therapy. *Archives of General Psychiatry, 61,* 34–41.

Gillespie, K., Duffy, M., Hackmann, A., & Clark, D. M. (2004). Community based cognitive therapy in the treatment of posttraumatic stress disorder following the Omagh bomb. *Behaviour Research and Therapy, 40,* 345–357.

Grant, P., Young, P., & DeRubeis, R. (2005). Cognitive and behavioural therapies.

In G. Gabbard, J. Beck, & J. Holmes (Eds.), *Oxford textbook of psychotherapy* (pp. 79–107). Oxford, UK: Oxford University Press.

Haaga, D. A., Dyck, M. J., & Ernst, D. (1991). Empirical status of cognitive theory of depression. *Psychological Bulletin, 110,* 215–236.

Hamilton, K., & Dobson, K. (2002). Cognitive therapy of depression: Pretreatment patient predictors of outcome. *Clinical Psychology Review, 22,* 875–893.

Harvey, A., Watkins, E., Mansell, W., & Shafran, R. (2004). *Cognitive behavioural processes across psychological disorders.* Oxford, UK: Oxford University Press.

Hayes, A. M., Feldman, G. C., Beevers, C. G., Laurenceau, J. P., Cardaciotto, L. A., & Lewis-Smith, K. (2007). Discontinuities and cognitive changes in an exposure-based cognitive therapy for depression. *Journal of Consulting and Clinical Psychology, 75,* 409–421.

Hollon, S. D., Kendall, P. C., & Lumry, A. (1986). Specificity of depressotypic cognitions in clinical depression. *Journal of Abnormal Psychology, 95,* 52–59.

Hollon, S. D., Shelton, R. C., & Davis, D. D. (1993). Cognitive therapy for depression: conceptual issues and clinical efficiency. *Journal of Consulting and Clinical Psychology, 62,* 270–275.

Hollon, S. D., Stewart, M. D., & Strunk, D. (2006). Enduring effects for cognitive behavior therapy in the treatment of depression and anxiety. *Annual Review of Psychology, 57,* 285–315.

Jarrett, R. B., Kraft, D., Doyle, J., Foster, B. M., Eaves, G., & Silver, P. C. (2001). Preventing recurrent depression using cognitive therapy with and without a continuation phase: A randomized clinical trial. *Archives of General Psychiatry, 58,* 381–388.

Jones, L., Scott, J., Haque, S., Gordon-Smith, K., Heron, J., Caesar, S., et al. (2005). Cognitive styles in bipolar disorder. *British Journal of Psychiatry, 187,* 431–437.

Kelly, G. (1955). *The psychology of personal constructs.* New York: Norton.

Kingdon, D. G., & Turkington, D. (1994). *Cognitive-behavior therapy of schizophrenia.* New York: Guilford Press.

Kraemer, H. C., Wilson, T., Fairburn, C. G., & Agras, W. S. (2001). Mediators and moderators of treatment effects in randomized clinical trials. *Archives of General Psychiatry, 59,* 877–883.

Krupnick, J. L., Sotsky, S. M., Simmens, S., Moyer, Elkin, et al. (1996). The role of the therapeutic alliance in psychotherapy and pharmacotherapy outcome: Findings in the NIMH TDCRP. *Journal of Consulting and Clinical Psychology, 64*(3), 532–539.

Lewinsohn, P. M., Joiner, T. E., Jr., & Rohde, P. (2001). Evaluation of cognitive diathesis–stress models in predicting major depressive disorder in adolescents. *Journal of Abnormal Psychology, 110*(2), 203–215.

Mathews, A. (2006). Towards an experimental cognitive science of CBT. *Behavioral Therapy, 37*(3), 314–318.

Meyer, B., Krupnick, J. L., Simmens, S. J., Pilkonis, P., Egan, M., & Sotsky, S. (2002). Treatment expectancies, patient alliance, and outcome: Further analyses from the NIMH TDCRP. *Journal of Consulting and Clinical Psychology,* 70, 1051–1055.

Meyer, B., Pilkonis, P. A., Krupnick, J. L., Egan, M. K., Simmens, S. J., & Sotsky, S. M. (2002). Treatment expectancies, patient alliance, and outcome: Further analyses from the National Institute of Mental Health Treatment of Depression Collaborative Research Program. *Journal of Consulting and Clinical Psychology,* 70(4), 1051–1055.

Miranda, R., & Nolen-Hoeksema, S. (2007). Brooding and reflection: rumination predicts suicidal ideation at 1-year follow-up in a community sample. *Behaviour Research and Therapy,* 45(12), 3088–3095.

Mittersciffhaler, M. T., Williams, S. C., Scott, J., & Fu, C. (2008). Neural basis of the emotional Stroop interference effect in major depression. *Psychological Medicine,* 38, 247–256.

Morrison, A. (Ed.). (2002). *A casebook of cognitive therapy for psychosis.* Hove, UK: Brunner/Routledge.

Nolen-Hoeksema, S. (1991). Responses to depression and their effects on the duration of depressive episodes. *Journal of Abnormal Psychology,* 100(4), 569–582.

Padesky, C. (1993, September 24). *Socratic questioning: Changing minds or guiding discovery?* Keynote Address at the European Congress of Behavioural and Cognitive Therapies, London.

Parker, G., Roy, K., & Eyers, K. (2003). Cognitive behavior therapy for depression?: Choose horses for courses. *American Journal of Psychiatry,* 160, 825–834.

Paykel, E. S. (2007). Cognitive therapy in relapse prevention in depression. *International Journal of Neuropsychopharmacology,* 10(1), 131–136.

Paykel, E., Scott, J., Teasdale, J., Johnson, A., Garland, A., Moore, R., et al. (1999). Prevention of relapse in residual depression by cognitive therapy: A controlled trial. *Archives of General Psychiatry,* 56, 829–835.

Persons, J. B. (1993). The process of change in cognitive therapy: Schema change or acquisition of compensatory skills? *Cognitive Therapy and Research,* 17, 123–137.

Roth, A., & Fonagy, P. (1996). *What works for whom?: A critical review of psychotherapy research.* New York: Guilford Press.

Salkovskis, P. (1996). *Frontiers of cognitive therapy.* New York: Guilford Press.

Scher, C. D., Ingram, R. E., & Segal, Z. V. (2005). Cognitive reactivity and vulnerability: Empirical evaluation of construct activation and cognitive diatheses in unipolar depression. *Clinical Psychology Review,* 25(4), 487–510.

Scott, J. (1998). Cognitive therapy. In H. Freeman (Ed.), *Century of psychiatry* (pp. 61–72). London: Mosby Wolfe Medical Communications.

Scott, J. (2001). Cognitive therapy for depression. *British Medical Bulletin,* 57, 101–113.

Scott, J. (2008). Cognitive-behavioural therapy for severe mental disorders: Back to the future? *British Journal of Psychiatry,* 192(6), 401–403.

Scott, J., & Beck, A. T. (2008). Cognitive therapy. *In essentials of postgraduate psychiatry* (3rd ed.). Cambridge, UK: Cambridge University Press.

Scott, J., Byers, S., & Turkington, D. (1992). Cognitive therapy with chronic inpatients. In J. Wright, M. Thase, J. Ludgate, & A. T. Beck (Eds.), *Cognitive therapy with inpatients: Developing a cognitive milieu* (pp. 357–390). New York: Guilford Press.

Scott, J., Kingdon, D., & Turkington, D. (2004). CBT for schizophrenia. In J. Wright (Ed.), *APA review psychiatry*. Washington, DC: American Psychiatric Association Press.

Scott, J., Paykel, E., Morriss, R., Bentall, R., Kinderman, P., Johnson, T., et al. (2006). Cognitive-behavioural therapy for severe and recurrent bipolar disorders: Randomised controlled trial. *British Journal of Psychiatry, 188,* 313–320.

Segal, Z., Gemar, M., & Williams, S. (1999). Differential cognitive response to a mood challenge following successful cognitive therapy or pharmacotherapy for unipolar depression. *Journal of Abnormal Psychology, 108,* 3–10.

Segal, Z., & Ingram, R. (1994). Mood priming and construct activation in tests of cognitive vulnerability to unipolar depression. *Clinical Psychology Review, 14,* 663–695.

Shahar, G., Blatt, S. J., Zuroff, D. C., & Pilkonis, P. A. (2003). Role of perfectionism and personality disorder features in response to brief treatment for depression. *Journal of Consulting and Clinical Psychology, 71,* 629–633.

Siegle, G., Carter, C. S., & Thase, M. E. (2006). Use of fMRI to predict recovery from unipolar depression with cognitive behavior therapy. *American Journal of Psychiatry, 163,* 735–738.

Singer, A. R., & Dobson, K. S. (2007). An experimental investigation of the cognitive vulnerability to depression. *Behaviour Research and Therapy, 45,* 563–575.

Tang, T. Z., & DeRubeis, R. J. (1999). Sudden gains and critical sessions in cognitive-behavioural therapy for depression. *Journal of Consulting and Clinical Psychology, 67,* 894–904.

Task Force on Promotion and Dissemination of Psychological Procedures. (1995). Training in and dissemination of empirically validated psychological treatments: Report and recommendations. *Clinical Psychologist, 48,* 3–23.

Teasdale, J. (1988). Cognitive vulnerability to persistent depression. *Cognition and Emotion, 2,* 247–274.

Teasdale, J., & Dent, J. (1987). Cognitive vulnerability to depression: An investigation of two hypotheses. *British Journal of Clinical Psychology, 26,* 113–126.

Teasdale, J., Scott, J., Moore, R., Hayhurst, H., Pope, M., & Paykel, E. S. (2000). How does cognitive therapy for depression reduce relapse? *Journal of Consulting and Clinical Psychology, 69,* 347–357.

Thase, M. E., Greenhouse, J. B., Frank, E., Reynolds, C. F., Pilkonis P. A., et al. (1997). Treatment of major depression with psychotherapy or psychotherapy–pharmacotherapy combinations. *Archives of General Psychiatry, 54*(11), 989–991.

Watkins, E., Scott, J., Wingrove, J., Rimes, K., Bathurst, N., Steiner, H., et al. (2007). Rumination-focused cognitive behaviour therapy for residual depression: A case series. *Behavior Research Therapy, 45*(9), 2144–2154.

Weishaar, M. E. (1993). *Aaron T. Beck.* Thousand Oaks, CA: Sage.

Wolpe, J. (1993). Commentary: The cognitivist oversell and comments on symposium contributions. *Journal of Behavior Therapy and Experimental Psychiatry, 24*(2), 141–147.

Wright, J. H., Wright, A. S., Salmon, P., Beck, A. T., Kuykendall, J., Goldsmith, L. J., et al. (2002). Development and initial testing of a multimedia program for computer-assisted cognitive therapy. *American Journal of Psychotherapy, 56,* 76–86.

Zuroff, D. C., Blatt, S. J., Sotsky, S. M., Krupnick, J. L., Martin, D. J., Sanislow, C. A., et al. (2000). Relation of therapeutic alliance and perfectionism to outcome in brief outpatient treatment of depression. *Journal of Consulting and Clinical Psychology, 68*(1), 114–124.

CHAPTER 3

Problem-Solving Therapy

Arthur M. Nezu
Christine Maguth Nezu
Thomas J. D'Zurilla

INTRODUCTION AND HISTORICAL BACKGROUND

Problem-solving therapy (PST) is a cognitive-behavioral intervention that focuses on training in the adoption and effective application of adaptive problem-solving attitudes and skills. The general aim of this positive approach to clinical intervention is not only to reduce psychopathology but also to enhance psychological and behavioral functioning in a positive direction to prevent relapse and the development of new clinical problems, in addition to maximizing one's overall quality of life. Originally outlined by Thomas D'Zurilla and Marvin Goldfried (1971), the theory and practice of PST has been refined and revised over the years by D'Zurilla, Nezu, and their associates, as noted in the next section. Based on scores of randomized controlled trials by researchers around the world over the past several decades, PST has proven to be an appropriate and effective treatment for a highly diverse population of adolescents and adults with a wide range of psychological, behavioral, and health disorders (see reviews in Chang, D'Zurilla, & Sanna, 2004; D'Zurilla & Nezu, 2007; Nezu, 2004).

Two important trends in clinical psychology and psychiatry during the late 1960s and early 1970s served as the major impetus for the development of PST. The first trend was the growing emphasis in the nascent field of behavior modification on cognitive processes that facilitate self-control and maximize the generalization and maintenance of behavior changes (Kendall & Hollon, 1979). The second trend was the growing recognition that

76

the efficacy of clinical interventions might be facilitated by focusing more on developing positive skills and abilities that enhance social competence, including problem solving (Gladwin, 1967).

In 1971, D'Zurilla and Goldfried conducted a comprehensive review of the relevant theory and research related to real-life problem solving (later termed *social problem solving*; SPS; D'Zurilla, 1986; D'Zurilla & Nezu, 1982) from the fields of experimental psychology, education, and industry. Based on this review, these investigators constructed a prescriptive model of SPS that comprises two different, albeit related, components: (1) general orientation (later relabeled *problem orientation*; D'Zurilla & Nezu, 1982), and (2) problem-solving skills. *General orientation* is viewed as a metacognitive process that primarily serves a motivational function in SPS. This process involves the operation of a set of relatively stable cognitive–emotional schemas that reflect a person's general awareness and appraisals of problems in living, as well as his or her own problem-solving ability (e.g., challenge appraisals, self-efficacy beliefs, positive outcome expectancies). *Problem-solving skills*, on the other hand, refers to the set of cognitive and behavioral activities by which a person attempts to understand problems in everyday living and discovers effective "solutions" or ways of coping with such difficulties. In this model, four major problem-solving skills are identified: (1) problem definition and formulation, (2) generation of alternatives, (3) decision making, and (4) verification (i.e., evaluation of solution outcomes following solution implementation). In addition to describing the components of this model, D'Zurilla and Goldfried (1971) also presented preliminary guidelines and procedures for the clinical application of problem-solving training with patients who present with significant deficits in the ability to cope effectively with stressful problems in living.

In 1974, Arthur Nezu became a graduate student in clinical psychology under the mentorship of D'Zurilla at the State University of New York at Stony Brook, which began a lifelong research collaboration (and friendship). Their initial efforts led to confirmation of several of the theoretical tenets of the then-conceptual model of PST, including the benefits of training individuals to define problems better (Nezu & D'Zurilla, 1981a, 1981b), generate alternatives (D'Zurilla & Nezu, 1980), and make effective decisions (Nezu & D'Zurilla, 1979). Conducting research on the stress-buffering properties of effective problem-solving coping, together and individually, they later developed the relational/problem-solving model of stress described later in this chapter (D'Zurilla & Nezu, 1999; Nezu & D'Zurilla, 1989). Particularly instrumental in this research was George Ronan, a graduate student working with Nezu (e.g., Nezu & Ronan, 1985, 1988).

D'Zurilla and Nezu continued their collaboration by developing the Social Problem-Solving Inventory (D'Zurilla & Nezu, 1990), a self-report measure of real-life problem solving. This measure was subsequently revised, based on a series of exploratory and confirmatory factor analyses, with the help of statistician Albert Maydeu-Olivares. The new version, known as the Social Problem-Solving Inventory—Revised (D'Zurilla, Nezu, & Maydeu-Olivares, 2002), has become the most widely used measure of this construct in the field. Based in part on such changes, the overall model of PST was also revised to include the following five dimensions: positive problem orientation, negative problem orientation, rational problem solving, impulsivity/carelessness style, and avoidance style (D'Zurilla, Nezu, & Maydeu-Olivares, 2004).

In the 1980s, Nezu and his colleagues, particularly Christine Maguth Nezu, focused their research activities on the relationship between problem solving and clinical depression, an effort resulting in the development of both a conceptual model of depression and an adapted version of PST for depression (Nezu, 1987; Nezu, Nezu, & Perri, 1989). Since Nezu's earlier outcome studies evaluating the efficacy of PST for major depressive disorder (e.g., Nezu, 1986c; Nezu & Perri, 1989), PST has come to be viewed as an efficacious, evidenced-based psychosocial treatment alternative for depression, as supported, for example, by recent meta-analyses of this literature (e.g., Bell & D'Zurilla, 2009; Cuijpers, van Straten, & Warmerdam, 2007). Another graduate student working with Nezu, Patricia Aréan, further adopted the basic PST for depression protocol for older adults, eventually demonstrating its efficacy for this population as well (e.g., Aréan et al., 1993).

Because depression and psychological distress are pervasive among individuals experiencing chronic medical illness, Nezu and Nezu, together with social psychologist, Peter Houts and other colleagues, developed a variety of PST treatment programs to help adults with cancer, as well as their families (e.g., Allen et al., 2002; Nezu, Nezu, Friedman, Faddis, & Houts, 1998; Houts, Nezu, Nezu, & Bucher, 1996). More recently, Nezu and Nezu have become interested in the potential efficacy of PST for the treatment of depression in patients with various cardiovascular diseases (e.g., Nezu, Nezu, & Jain, 2005), particularly heart failure (Nezu et al., 2006), as well as the treatment of personality disorders in collaboration with colleagues in the United Kingdom at the Universities of Nottingham and Liverpool (e.g., Mary McMurran, Conor Duggan, and James McGuire).

C. M. Nezu has also been instrumental in creatively adapting the basic PST protocol to treat special populations, including adults with mental retardation and concomitant psychopathology (e.g., C. M. Nezu, Nezu, & Aréan, 1991), sex offenders (C. M. Nezu, 2003), and sex offenders with intellectual disabilities (C. M. Nezu, Fiore, & Nezu, 2006). Additional applications by D'Zurilla, Nezu, and their colleagues include PST for weight loss (Perri, Nezu, & Viegener, 1992), PST as a means of improving adherence (e.g., Nezu, Nezu, & Perri, 2006), and PST as a means of enhancing positive psychology goals (Chang & D'Zurilla, 1996).

Finally, one major outcome that has evolved from our work regarding the major theoretical underpinnings of PST, that is, human problem solving, is the application of problem-solving principles to the task of a therapist's case formulation and treatment planning in cognitive-behavioral therapy (Nezu, Nezu, & Lombardo, 2004; Nezu, Nezu, & Cos, 2007). Specifically, we have developed a structured method by which cognitive-behavioral therapists can improve their clinical decision-making skills with specific regard to better developing an accurate case formulation of a client's problems, and based on such a conceptualization, to develop a better overall individualized treatment plan.

PHILOSOPHICAL AND THEORETICAL UNDERPINNINGS

The goal of PST is to reduce and prevent psychopathology and enhance positive well-being by helping individuals cope more effectively with stressful problems in living. Depending on the nature of the problematic situation (e.g., controllability, aversiveness), effective coping may involve (1) changing the situation for the better (e.g., achieving a desired goal, removing an aversive condition, resolving a conflict) and/or (2) reducing the emotional distress generated by the situation (e.g., acceptance, tolerance, physical relaxation, helping others with similar problems). The theory upon which PST is based comprises two interrelated conceptual models: (1) the SPS model, and (2) the relational/problem-solving model of stress, which integrates SPS theory with Lazarus's relational model of stress (Lazarus & Folkman, 1984).

The Social Problem-Solving Model

As described earlier, the term *social problem solving* refers to problem solving as it occurs in the natural social environment (D'Zurilla & Nezu, 1982). As conceived here, SPS is a learning process, a general coping strategy, and a self-control method. Because solving a problem results in a change in performance in specific situations, SPS qualifies as a learning process (Gagné, 1966). Because effective problem solving increases the likelihood of adaptive coping outcomes across a wide range of problematic situations, it is also a general, versatile coping strategy. Finally, because SPS is a *self-directed* learning process and coping strategy, it is also a self-control method that has important implications for the maintenance and generalization of treatment effects (D'Zurilla & Goldfried, 1971; Mahoney, 1974; Nezu, 1987).

Definitions of Major Concepts

The three major concepts in SPS theory include (1) SPS, (2) problem, and (3) solution. *SPS* is defined as the self-directed cognitive-behavioral process by which an individual, couple, or group attempts to identify or discover effective solutions for specific problems encountered in daily living. As this definition implies, SPS is conceived as a conscious, rational, and purposeful coping activity. As we suggested earlier, the goals of problem solving may include changing the problematic situation for the better, reducing or modifying the negative emotions generated by the situation, or both of these outcomes. As conceived here, SPS can be used to cope with all types of problems in living, including impersonal problems (e.g., insufficient finances, transportation problems), personal/intrapersonal problems (cognitive, emotional, behavioral, health difficulties), as well as interpersonal problems (e.g., relationship conflicts and disputes). Moreover, rather than describing a singular type of coping behavior or activity, SPS represents the multidimensional metaprocess of idiographically identifying and selecting various coping responses to adequately address the unique features of a given stressful situation at a given time (Nezu & Nezu, in press).

A problem (or problematic situation) is represented by the imbalance or discrepancy between adaptive demands and the availability of effective coping responses. Specifically, a *problem* may be defined as any life situation or task (present or anticipated) that requires an effective response to achieve a goal or resolve a conflict, but wherein no effective response is immediately apparent or available to the person due to various obstacles. The demands in a problematic situation may originate in the environment (e.g., job demands, behavioral expectations of significant others) or within the person (e.g., a personal goal, need, or commitment). The obstacles might include novelty, ambiguity, unpredictability, conflicting demands or goals, performance skills deficits, or lack of resources. A problem might be a single, time-limited event (e.g., coming late to work, an acute illness), a series of similar or related events (e.g., repeated unreasonable demands from one's spouse or partner, repeated violations of curfew by an adolescent daughter), or a chronic, ongoing situation (e.g., continuous pain, loneliness, or chronic illness).

A *solution* is a situation-specific coping response (cognitive and/or behavioral) that is the product of the SPS process when applied to a specific stressful situation. An *effective* solution is one that achieves the problem-solving goal (e.g., changing the situation for the better, reducing the distress generated by the situation), and at the same time maximizes positive consequences and minimizes negative ones. The relevant consequences include personal and social outcomes, and both long- and short-term outcomes.

As defined here, SPS should be distinguished from *solution implemen-*

tation (D'Zurilla & Goldfried, 1971). These two processes are conceptually different and require different sets of skills. *Problem solving* refers to the process of *discovering* solutions to specific problems, whereas *solution implementation* refers to the process of *carrying out* those solutions in the actual problematic situations. Problem-solving skills are assumed to be generally applicable across situations, whereas solution-implementation skills are expected to vary across different situations depending on the nature of the problem and the specific solution. Because they are different, problem-solving skills and solution-implementation skills are not always correlated. Hence, some individuals might possess poor problem-solving skills but good solution-implementation skills, or vice versa. Because both sets of skills are required for adaptive functioning, it is often necessary in PST to combine training in problem-solving skills and solution implementation skills (e.g., social skills, parenting skills) to maximize positive outcomes (D'Zurilla & Nezu, 2007; Nezu, Nezu, & D'Zurilla, 2007).

Major Problem-Solving Dimensions

As we noted earlier, the original version of the present SPS model (D'Zurilla & Goldfried, 1971; D'Zurilla & Nezu, 1990) assumed that SPS ability comprises two major, partially independent components: (1) problem orientation, and (2) problem-solving skills (later referred to as "problem-solving proper" [e.g., D'Zurilla & Nezu, 1999] and more recently as "problem-solving style" [e.g., D'Zurilla & Nezu, 2007; D'Zurilla et al., 2002]). Based on this theoretical hypothesis, D'Zurilla and Nezu (1990) developed the Social Problem-Solving Inventory (SPSI), which comprises two major scales: the Problem Orientation Scale (POS) and the Problem-Solving Skills Scale (PSSS). Each scale includes positive items that are assumed to reflect "good" problem-solving ability, as well as negative items, which were assumed to reflect "poor" problem-solving ability. The assumption that problem orientation and problem-solving skills are different, albeit related, components of SPS is supported by data showing that the POS item correlation is high with the total POS score and relatively low with the total PSSS score, whereas the reverse is true for the PSSS items (D'Zurilla & Nezu, 1990).

Based on an integration of the original SPS model and subsequent empirical data generated by factor analyses of the SPSI, D'Zurilla et al. (2002; Maydeu-Olivares & D'Zurilla, 1995, 1996) developed a revised, five-dimensional model of SPS that comprises two different, albeit related, problem orientation dimensions and three different problem-solving styles. The two problem orientation dimensions include positive problem orientation and negative problem orientation, whereas the three problem-solving styles include rational problem solving (i.e., effective problem-solving skills), impulsivity/carelessness style, and avoidance style. Positive problem orientation and rational problem solving are constructive dimensions that increase the probability of positive outcomes, whereas negative problem orientation, impulsivity/carelessness style, and avoidance style are dysfunctional dimensions that are likely to disrupt or inhibit effective problem solving, resulting in negative personal and social outcomes.

Positive problem orientation is the constructive problem-solving cognitive set that involves the general disposition to (1) appraise a problem as a "challenge" (i.e., opportunity for benefit or gain); (2) believe that problems are solvable (positive outcome expectancies, or "optimism"); (3) believe in one's personal ability to solve problems successfully ("problem-solving self-efficacy"); (4) believe that successful problem solving takes time, effort, and persistence; and (5) commit oneself to solving problems with dispatch rather than avoiding them. In contrast, *negative problem orientation* is the dysfunctional or inhibitive cognitive–emotional set that involves the general tendency to (1) view a problem as a significant threat to well-being (psychological, social, behavioral, health), (2) doubt one's personal ability to solve problems successfully ("low self-efficacy"), and (3) easily become emotionally upset when confronted with stressful problems (i.e., low tolerance for frustration and uncertainty).

Rational problem solving is a constructive problem-solving style that is defined as the rational, deliberate, and systematic application of four major problem-solving skills: (1) problem definition and formulation, (2) generation of alternative solutions, (3) decision making, and (4) solution verification (D'Zurilla & Goldfried, 1971). Specifically, the rational problem solver carefully and systematically gathers facts and information about a problem, identifies demands and obstacles, sets realistic problem-solving goals, generates a variety of possible solutions, anticipates the consequences of the different solutions, judges and compares the alternatives, chooses the "best" solution, implements the solution, and carefully monitors and evaluates the outcome. Note that this dimension does *not* include the solution implementation skills that are also necessary for successful problem-solving performance in specific situations.

Impulsivity/carelessness style is a dysfunctional problem-solving pattern characterized by active attempts to apply problem-solving activities, but such attempts are narrow, impulsive, careless, hurried, and incomplete. A person with this problem-solving style typically considers only a few solution alternatives, often impulsively going with the first idea that comes to mind. In addition, he or she scans alternative solutions and consequences quickly, carelessly, and unsystematically, and monitors solution outcomes carelessly and inadequately.

Avoidance style is another dysfunctional problem-solving pattern characterized by procrastination, passivity or inaction, and dependency. The avoidant problem solver prefers to avoid or to put off problem solving, waiting for problems to resolve themselves, or attempts to shift the responsibility for solving his or her problems to other people.

The five problem-solving dimensions we just described are measured by the Social Problem-Solving Inventory—Revised (SPSI-R; D'Zurilla et al., 2002). With this instrument, "good" SPS is indicated by high scores on positive problem orientation and rational problem solving, and low scores on negative problem orientation, impulsivity/carelessness style, and avoidance style, whereas "poor" SPS is indicated by low scores on positive problem orientation and rational problem solving, and high scores on negative problem orientation, impulsivity/carelessness style, and avoidance style. The five-dimensional model measured by the SPSI-R has been cross-validated in young adults (D'Zurilla et al., 2002), adolescents (Sadowski, Moore, & Kelley, 1994), and in a population of incarcerated sex offenders in the United Kingdom (Wakeling, 2007). Using translated versions of the SPSI-R, the model has also been cross-validated in samples of Spanish adults (Maydeu-Olivares, Rodríquez-Fornells, Gómez-Benito, & D'Zurilla, 2000), German adults (Graf, 2003), Chinese adults (Siu & Shek, 2005), and Japanese college students, community adults, and psychiatric patients (Sato et al., 2006).

A Relational/Problem-Solving Model of Stress and Well-Being

A major assumption underlying the use of PST is that symptoms of psychopathology (emotional, cognitive, behavioral, and interpersonal) can often be understood and effectively treated or prevented by viewing them as ineffective, maladaptive, and self-defeating coping behaviors (e.g., aggression, substance abuse), with negative personal and social consequences (e.g., anxiety, depression, low self-esteem, and impaired behavioral and interpersonal functioning; D'Zurilla & Goldfried, 1971). Following from this assumption, the theory of PST is also based on a relational/problem-solving model of stress and well-being in which the concept of SPS is given a central role as a general and versatile coping strategy that increases adaptive functioning and positive well-being, which in turn reduces and prevents the negative impact of stress on well-being and adjustment (D'Zurilla, 1990; D'Zurilla & Nezu, 1999, 2007; Nezu, 1987; Nezu & D'Zurilla, 1989).

The relational/problem-solving model integrates Lazarus's relational model of stress (Lazarus, 1999; Lazarus & Folkman, 1984) with the SPS model presented earlier. In that model, *stress* is defined as a type of person–environment relationship in which demands are appraised by the person as exceeding coping resources and threatening his or her well-being (Lazarus & Folkman, 1984). This relational definition of *stress* is very similar to the definition of a *problem* in SPS theory. Hence, it is reasonable to conclude that a problem is also a "stressor," if it is at all difficult and significant for well-being. In the relational/problem-solving model, stress is viewed as a function of the reciprocal relations among three major variables: (1) stressful life events, (2) emotional stress/well-being, and (3) problem-solving coping.

Stressful life events are life experiences that present a person with strong demands for personal, social, or biological readjustment (Bloom, 1985). Two major types of stressful life events are major negative events and daily problems. A *major negative event* is a broad life experience, such as a major negative life change, that often requires sweeping readjustments in a person's life (e.g., job loss, death of a loved one, major illness or surgery). In contrast, a *daily problem* is a more narrow and specific stressful life event. Although major negative events and daily problems may develop independently in a person's life, they are often causally related (Nezu & D'Zurilla, 1989; Nezu & Ronan, 1985, 1988). For example, a major negative event, such as major heart surgery, usually creates many new daily problems for a person (e.g., pain, self-care problems, financial problems, diet changes). Conversely, an accumulation of unresolved daily problems (e.g., marital conflicts, job problems, excessive alcohol use, poor diet, lack of exercise) may eventually cause or contribute to heart disease and major surgery.

In this model, the concept of *emotional stress* refers to the immediate emotional responses of a person to stressful life events, as modified or modulated by cognitive appraisal and coping processes (Lazarus, 1999). Depending on the nature of stressful life events (e.g., aversiveness, controllability), cognitive appraisals, and coping behavior, emotional stress responses may be negative (e.g., anxiety, anger, depression) or positive (e.g., hope, relief, exhilaration, joy). Negative emotions are likely to predominate when the person (1) appraises a stressful event as threatening or harmful to well-being, (2) doubts his or her ability to cope effectively, and (3) performs coping responses that are ineffective, maladaptive, or self-defeating. On the other hand, positive emotions may compete with negative emotions and sometimes dominate when the person (1) appraises a stressful event as a significant "challenge" or opportunity for benefit, (2) believes that he or she is capable of coping with the problem effectively, and (3) performs coping responses that are effective, adaptive, and self-enhancing.

Emotional stress is an important part of a broader construct of *well-being* that also includes cognitive, behavioral, social, and physical functioning (Lazarus & Folkman, 1984). Hence, the relational/problem-solving model assumes that stressful life events, cognitive appraisals, and coping processes are likely to have a significant impact on well-being *in general* and, ultimately, on the person's adjustment status (e.g., psychological or health disorder vs. positive mental and physical health).

The most important concept in our model is *problem-solving coping*, a process that integrates all cognitive appraisal and coping activities within a general SPS framework. A person who applies the problem-solving coping strategy effectively (1) perceives a stressful life event as a challenge or "problem to be solved," (2) believes that he or she is capable of solving the problem successfully, (3) carefully defines the problem and sets a realistic goal, (4) generates a variety of alternative "solutions" or coping options, (5) chooses the "best" or most effective solution, (6) implements the solution effectively, and (7) carefully observes and evaluates the outcome. Unlike Lazarus's relational model of stress (Lazarus & Folkman, 1984), which views problem solving as a form of *problem-focused coping* (i.e., aimed at changing the problematic situation for the better), problem solving is conceived in this model as a broader, more versatile coping strategy that may also function as a form of *emotion-focused coping* (i.e., aimed at reducing emotional distress and/or increasing positive emotions). The goals set for any particular problematic situation depend on the nature of the situation and how it is defined and appraised. If a situation is appraised as changeable or controllable, then problem-focused goals would be emphasized. On the other hand, if the situation is appraised as largely unchangeable or uncontrollable, then emotion-focused goals should be articulated.

The hypothesized relationships among the major variables in the relational/problem solving model of stress and well-being are summarized in Figure 3.1. As the figure shows, the two types of stressful life events in the model (major negative events and daily problems) are assumed to influence each other. For example a major negative event, such as a divorce, is likely to result in many new daily problems for an individual (e.g., reduced income, conflicts involving children, difficulty meeting new people). Conversely, an accumulation of unresolved daily problems in a marriage (e.g., conflicts or disagreements, differences in sexual needs) may eventually result in a divorce. Figure 3.1 also shows that in addition to influencing each other, both types of stressful life events are assumed to have a direct impact on well-being, as well as an indirect effect via problem solving. In general, stressful life events are assumed to have a *negative* impact on well-being. This negative relationship between stressful life events and well-being is well established (Bloom, 1985; Monroe & Hadjiyannakis, 2002). Moreover, a number of studies have suggested that an accumulation of unresolved daily problems may have a greater negative impact on well-being than the number of major negative events (e.g., Burks & Martin, 1985; DeLongis, Coyne, Dakof, Folkman, & Lazarus, 1982; Nezu, 1986b; Nezu & Ronan, 1985, 1988; Weinberger, Hiner, & Tierney, 1987). These findings suggest that it is important in PST to identify those problems that might be created by major negative events and to focus on solving these daily problems rather than coping with the major negative event itself.

In addition, our model assumes that problem solving influences the

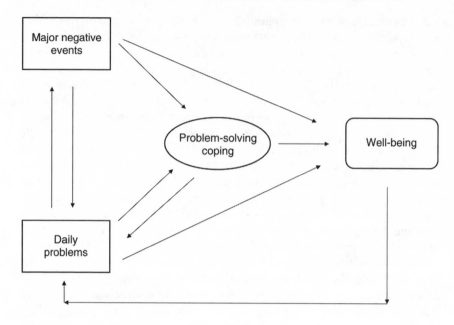

FIGURE 3.1. Relational/problem-solving model of stress and well-being. From D'Zurilla and Nezu (2007). Copyright 2007 by Springer Publishing Company, LLC, New York, NY 10036. Reprinted by permission.

relationship between stressful life events and well-being by functioning as both a mediator and a moderator. The model recognizes two different mediational hypotheses. The first hypothesis is based on the popular A-B-C behavioral model, where stressful life events (A) are assumed to set the occasion for problem-solving behavior (B), which in turn results in personal and social consequences (C) that affect well-being. If problem solving is ineffective, then the consequences for well-being are expected to be negative (e.g., anxiety, depression). On the other hand, if problem solving is effective, then the consequences are expected to be positive (e.g., less negative emotions, more positive emotions). The second mediational hypothesis assumes that SPS is an intervening variable in a causal chain in which stressful life events have a negative impact on problem-solving ability and performance, which in turn has a negative effect on well-being. In contrast with this A-B-C hypothesis, the arrows from stressful life events to problem solving are interpreted as negative causal relationships rather than prompting effects.

With regard to the moderator hypothesis, the major assumption is that stressful life events interact with problem-solving ability to influence well-being. Specifically, the negative relationship between stress and well-being is expected to be stronger when problem-solving ability is low rather than high. In other words, poor problem-solving ability is assumed to increase the negative impact of stressful life events on well-being, whereas effective problem-solving ability is assumed to function as a "buffer" and reduce the negative impact of stress on adjustment. In this hypothesis, the assumption of a causal relationship between stressful life events and problem-solving ability is not necessary. In this respect, the moderator hypothesis is consistent with the first mediational hypothesis described earlier.

As Figure 3.1 depicts, the model also hypothesizes that a *reciprocal* relationship exists between problems and SPS. Specifically, in addition to the assumption that stressful events may have a negative impact on problem solving, the model also assumes that problem solving is likely to influence the frequency of daily problems. Ineffective problem solving is expected to result in an increase in daily problems, whereas effective problem solving is expected is to reduce the frequency of daily problems. Finally, the relationship between stressful events and well-being is also assumed to be reciprocal. Specifically, in addition to the direct and indirect impact of stressful events on well-being, the model also assumes that well-being is likely to have an impact on future stressful events. Specifically, negative adjustment outcomes (e.g., anxiety, depression, impaired social and behavioral functioning) are likely to result in an increase in daily problems and major negative events, whereas positive adjustment outcomes (e.g., hope, self-esteem, happiness, competence) are likely to reduce the frequency of these stressful events.

In addition to providing a theoretical rationale for PST, our model of stress and well-being also provides a useful framework for clinical assessment prior to PST. During assessment, the therapist identifies and pinpoints major negative life events, current daily problems, emotional stress responses, problem-orientation deficits and distortions, problem solving style deficits, and solution implementation skills deficits. Based on this assessment, PST is then applied to (1) increase one's positive problem orientation, (2) reduce one's negative problem orientation, (3) improve rational problem-solving skills, (4) reduce or prevent impulsive/careless problem solving, and (5) minimize the tendency to avoid problem solving. If necessary, other cognitive-behavioral methods (e.g., social skills training, exposure methods) are used to teach effective solution implementation skills and/or reduce anxiety that might be inhibiting effective solution implementation. The successful achievement of these goals is expected to increase adaptive situational coping and positive psychological, social, and physical well-being, while reducing and preventing the negative effects of stress on well-being and adjustment.

EMPIRICAL EVIDENCE

In this section, we review the empirical support for both the relational/problem-solving model of stress and well-being, and problem-solving therapy itself.

Empirical Support for the Relational/Problem-Solving Model of Stress

Over the past two decades, a large number of studies evaluating the correlation between various dimensions of problem solving and psychological distress and adjustment (e.g., depression, anxiety, well-being, optimism), using both behavioral outcome and self-report measures, have provided strong support for this aspect of the relational/problem-solving model. For example, ineffective SPS, particularly the negative problem orientation dimension (Nezu, 2004), has been found to be highly related to depression, anxiety, suicidal ideation, pain, and addictive behaviors (Nezu, 1986a; Nezu, Wilkins, & Nezu, 2004), whereas effective SPS is related to optimism, positive subjective well-being, and positive trait affectivity (Chang, Downey, & Salata, 2004). Although such studies support the view that SPS plays an important role in adjustment, the strongest support for the relational/problem-solving model comes from investigations specifically demonstrating that problem solving both mediates the relationship between stressful life events and personal–social functioning, and moderates the negative impact of stress on psychological well-being and adaptive functioning. Representative studies are described below.

Problem Solving as a Mediator

Folkman and Lazarus (1988) studied coping as a mediator of emotion in two samples of community residents—a middle-aged sample and an older adult sample. They interviewed these residents once each month for 6 months about how they coped with the most stressful situations that occurred during the previous week. Emotions were assessed at the beginning of a stressful encounter, during the encounter, and at the end of the encounter. Results in both samples showed that planful problem solving was the only coping strategy that was consistently associated with less negative emotions and more positive emotions. In their interpretation of these results, these investigators speculated that problem solving may have both a direct and an indirect effect on emotions in stress situations. The direct effect is that people are likely to feel better when they make an attempt to solve the problem that is causing distress. The indirect effect is that problem solving, when effective, can change the problematic situation for the better, which in turn has positive emotional outcomes.

Nezu and Ronan (1985), using path analysis, in a college student sample, tested a model that incorporated major negative life events, daily problems, SPS, and depressive symptoms. The results provided support for the following causal hypothesized relations: (1) Major negative life events increase the number of daily problems; (2) more daily problems result in more depression; and (3) problem solving mediates the relation between daily problems and depression; in other words, the magnitude of the relation between daily problems and depression is at least partly accounted for by problem-solving ability. These results were replicated in a similar study by Nezu, Perri, and Nezu (1987), which included clinically depressed subjects.

Kant, D'Zurilla, and Maydeu-Olivares (1997) examined the role of SPS as a mediator of the relations between daily problems and depression and anxiety among middle-aged and older adult community residents. A significant mediating effect was found in both samples, indicating that problem solving reduced the relation between daily problems and both forms of emotional distress. Further analyses indicated that negative problem orientation contributed most to this mediational effect. SPS was found to account for approximately 20% of the relation between problems and depression and about 34% of the variance between problems and anxiety. Overall, the prediction model that comprised daily problems and SPS accounted for 50% of the variance in depression and 50% in anxiety in both age samples.

Problem Solving as a Moderator

Nezu and his associates conducted several studies designed to evaluate the role of SPS as a moderator or buffer of the negative effects of major negative life events on psychological well-being. In one study that employed a college student sample, with depression as the dependent variable, Nezu, Nezu, Saraydarian, Kalmar, and Ronan (1986) found a significant interaction between major negative life events and problem-solving ability, which indicated that the relationship between such stressors and depression varied with the level of problem-solving ability. Specifically, the relationship was significantly weaker for individuals with effective problem-solving ability than for those with poor problem-solving ability. These findings were replicated by Nezu, Perri, Nezu, and Mahoney (1987) in a sample of individuals diagnosed with major depression. In another study focusing on college students, Nezu (1986d) found that SPS also moderated the impact of major negative events on state and trait anxiety. In a study focusing on cancer patients, SPS was found to moderate the negative effects of cancer-related stress (Nezu, Nezu, Faddis, DelliCarpini, & Houts, 1995). Specifically, under similar levels of cancer-related stress, individuals with poor problem-solving ability reported higher levels of depression and anxiety than those with better problem-solving ability.

Because these studies are all cross-sectional in nature, rival hypotheses regarding the possible influence of emotional distress on problem-solving ability cannot be ruled out. Therefore, Nezu and Ronan (1988), in a prospective study with college students, attempted to predict depressive symptoms 3 months postbaseline, while statistically controlling for the level of depression at baseline. Their results confirmed that problem-solving ability moderates the impact of major negative events on later depressive symptoms even after they controlled for the prior level of depression.

In a more recent study, Londahl, Tverskoy, and D'Zurilla (2005) examined the role of interpersonal problem solving as a moderator of the relationship between interpersonal conflicts and anxiety in college students. The measure of interpersonal problem solving was a modified form of the SPSI-R (D'Zurilla et al., 2002) that focused specifically on interpersonal conflicts (i.e., disagreements or disputes between two people in a relationship) rather than problems in general. The results showed that negative problem orientation was a highly significant moderator of the relationship between romantic partner conflicts and anxiety symptoms. Specifically, the relationship between conflicts and anxiety was weaker when negative problem orientation was low rather than high.

Empirical Support for PST

Since the initial publication of the D'Zurilla and Goldfried (1971) model, clinical researchers around the world have effectively applied PST, both as the sole intervention strategy and as part of a larger treatment package, to a wide variety of problems and patient populations. These include major depression, dysthymia, schizophrenia, suicidal ideation and behaviors, social phobia, generalized anxiety disorders, posttraumatic stress disorder, caregiving problems, substance abuse, sexual offending, AIDS/HIV prevention, obesity, back pain, hypertension, distressed couples, primary care patients, persons with mental retardation, distressed cancer patients, recurrent headaches, personality disorders, and diabetes (D'Zurilla & Nezu, 2007). Recent meta-analyses of this literature basically support this perspective. Specifically, Malouff, Thorsteinsson, and Schutte (2007) conducted a meta-analysis of 32 studies, encompassing 2,895 participants, that evaluated the efficacy of PST across a variety of mental and physical health problems. In essence, PST was found to be as effective as other psychosocial treatments, although not significantly more so (effect size =

0.22). However, it was found to be significantly more effective than either no treatment (effect size = 1.37) or attention control placebo conditions (effect size = 0.54). This strongly suggests that PST is an efficacious clinical intervention. Parenthetically, these authors found that significant moderators of treatment outcome included whether the evaluated PST protocol included training in problem orientation (see Nezu, 2004; Nezu & Perri, 1989), whether homework was assigned, or whether a developer of PST helped conduct the investigation.

Cuijpers et al. (2007) conducted a meta-analysis of 13 randomized controlled studies evaluating PST for depression (total N = 1,133 participants). Based on their results (i.e., mean effect size for a fixed effects model was 0.34, and 0.83 for a random effects model), these authors concluded that although additional research is needed, "there is no doubt that PST can be an effective treatment for depression" (p. 9). However, they also noted substantial heterogeneity of results across investigations. Another meta-analysis, one that also focused exclusively on PST for depression but included seven more studies than the pool in the Cuijpers et al. meta-analysis, came to the same conclusion for both posttreatment and follow-up results (Bell & D'Zurilla, 2009). Moreover, although PST was not found to be more effective than alternative psychosocial therapies or psychiatric medication, it was found to be more effective than supportive therapy and attention control groups. Moreover, significant moderators of treatment effectiveness included whether the PST program included problem orientation training, whether all four problem-solving skills were included, and whether all five components were included (i.e., problem orientation and the four rational problem-solving skills). Another moderator that approached significance was whether the SPSI-R (D'Zurilla et al., 2002) was administered before treatment to assess strengths and weaknesses in SPS abilities.

Due to limited space in this chapter, we are unable to describe this literature in depth; therefore, we refer the reader to other sources (Chang, D'Zurilla, et al., 2004; D'Zurilla & Nezu, 2007; Gellis & Kenaly, 2008; Nezu, 2004) for descriptive reviews of these studies. However, we do wish to highlight the *flexibility* of PST regarding the types of patient populations addressed and methods of service delivery employed (Nezu, 2004). More specifically, not only does PST appear to be an effective cognitive-behavioral intervention, but it is also quite flexible and can be applied in a variety of ways—in a group format, on an individual basis, over the telephone, as the sole treatment modality, as part of a larger "treatment package," as a method to target caregiver populations in addition to the patients themselves, and as a means to enhance the efficacy of other intervention strategies when applied as an adjunct. The following are examples of these types of applications.

Group PST

An example of PST applied in a group format is an outcome study that evaluated the efficacy of PST for adults reliably diagnosed with unipolar depression (Nezu, 1986c). Specifically, depressed individuals in an outpatient setting were randomly assigned to one of three conditions: (1) PST; (2) problem-focused therapy (PFT); or (3) waiting-list control (WLC). Both therapy conditions were conducted in a group setting over eight weekly sessions, each lasting from 1.5 to 2 hours. The PFT protocol involved therapeutic discussions of patients' current life problems but did not include systematic training in problem-solving skills. Both traditional statistical analyses and an analysis of the clinical significance of the results indicated substantial reductions in depression in the PST group compared to both the PFT and WLC conditions. These results were maintained over the 6-month follow-up period. Further analyses revealed that PST participants increased significantly more than the other two groups in problem-solving effectiveness and in locus-of-control orientation (i.e., from external to internal). These improvements were also maintained at the 6-month follow-up. Overall, these results provide support for the basic assumption that PST produces its effects by increasing problem-solving ability and strengthening personal control expectations.

PST for Individuals and Significant Others

Conceptualizing the stress associated with adjusting to cancer and its treatment as a series of "problems" (Nezu, Nezu, Houts, Friedman, & Faddis, 1999), PST has been applied as a means of improving adult cancer patients' quality of life (Nezu, Nezu, Felgoise, McClure, & Houts, 2003). As with most chronic medical conditions, the diagnosis and treatment of cancer can serve as a major stressor and, consequently, can increase the likelihood that such patients will experience heightened levels of psychological distress (Nezu, Nezu, Felgoise, & Zwick, 2003). This study, known as Project Genesis, represents how PST can be applied on an individual and on a couple basis. In this project, adult cancer patients with clinically meaningful elevated scores on measures of depression and psychological distress were randomly assigned to one of three conditions: (1) PST (10 individual sessions); (2) PST-plus (10 sessions of PST provided to both the patient and a patient-selected "significant other" in order to evaluate the effects of including a caregiver as a "problem-solving coach"); and (3) a WLC. Results of pre–post analyses across multiple measures that included self-reports, clinician evaluations, and collateral ratings, provide strong evidence underscoring the efficacy of PST in general for this population. Moreover, these results were maintained at 6-month and 1-year follow-ups. Additional analyses provided evidence that including a significant other in treatment serves to enhance positive treatment effects beyond those attributable to receiving PST by one-self. More specifically, at the two follow-up assessment points, on several of the outcome measures, patients in the PST-plus condition were found to continue to experience significant improvement compared to individuals in the PST condition.

PST as Part of a Larger Treatment Package

PST has also often been included as an important component of a larger cognitive-behavioral treatment package. As an example, García-Vera, Labrador, and Sanz (1997) combined PST with education and relaxation training for the treatment of essential hypertension. Overall, compared to participants comprising a WLC, treated patients were found at posttreatment to have significantly lowered blood pressure. These positive results were further found to be maintained at a 4-month follow-up assessment. Whereas studies evaluating the efficacy of a treatment package cannot provide data specific to any of the included intervention components, a subsequent analysis of their outcome data (García-Vera, Sanz, & Labrador, 1998) revealed that reductions in both systolic and diastolic blood pressure were significantly correlated with improvements in problem solving, as measured by the SPSI-R (D'Zurilla et al., 2002). Moreover, problem solving was found to mediate the antihypertensive effects of their overall stress management protocol, suggesting that PST was at the very least an important and active treatment ingredient.

PST for Caregivers

PST has not always been geared to help patient populations in a direct fashion. In addition to the effects on patients themselves, chronic illness and its treatment can have a significant impact on the lives of a patient's family members, in particular, a primary caregiver (Houts et al., 1996). The impact of the role of caregiver involves increased distress, physical symptoms, and feelings of burden. In this context, several researchers have applied PST as a means of improving the quality of life of caregivers across a range of medical patient problems (C. M. Nezu, Palmatier, & Nezu, 2004). For example, Sahler et al. (2002) evaluated the efficacy of PST for mothers of newly diagnosed pediatric cancer patients. After an 8-week intervention, mothers in the treatment condition were found to have significantly enhanced problem-solving skills associated with significant decreases in negative affectivity. Similarly, Grant, Elliott, Weaver, Bartolucci, and Giger (2002) found PST, provided to caregivers of stoke patients, to be effective in both decreasing caregiver depression and enhancing their problem-solving ability and caregiver preparedness.

PST as a Means to Foster Adherence and Compliance

Beyond application as the major treatment modality to decrease psychological distress and to improve functioning, PST has also been used as an adjunct to foster the effectiveness of other behavioral intervention strategies. For example, Perri et al. (2001) hypothesized that PST would be an effective means to foster improved adherence to a behavioral weight loss intervention by helping subjects to overcome various barriers to adherence, such as scheduling difficulties, completing homework assignments, or the interference of psychological distress. More specifically, after completing 20 weekly group sessions of standard behavioral treatment for obesity, 80 women were randomly assigned to one of three conditions: (1) no further contact (behavior therapy [BT] only); (2) relapse prevention training; and (3) PST. At the end of 17 months, no differences in overall weight loss were observed between relapse prevention and BT only conditions or between relapse prevention and PST. However, PST participants had significantly greater long-term weight reductions than BT only participants, and a significantly larger percentage of PST participants achieved "clinically significant" losses of 10% or more in body weight that did BT only members (approximately 35 vs. 6%). As such, these findings further highlight the flexible applicability of PST for a variety of clinical goals.

PST as a Secondary Prevention Strategy

Recent research has identified a strong association between problem orientation variables and levels of functional disability among persons experiencing low back pain (LBP). For example, van den Hout, Vlaeyen, Heuts, Stillen, and Willen (2001) found that a negative orientation toward problems was associated with higher levels of functional disability in persons with LBP. In addition, Shaw, Feuerstein, Haufler, Berkowoitz, and Lopez (2001), using the SPSI-R, found low scores on the positive orientation scale and high scores on impulsivity/carelessness and avoidant style scales to be correlated with functional loss in LBP patients. Based on such findings, van den Hout, Vlaeyen, Heuts, Zijlema, and Wijen (2003) evaluated whether PST provided a significant supplemental value to a behavioral graded activity protocol in treating patients with nonspecific LBP with regard to work-related disability. Their results indicated that in the second half-year after the intervention, patients receiving both graded activity and problem solving (GAPS) had significantly fewer days of sick leave than their counterparts who received graded activity plus group education. Furthermore, work status was more favorable for the GAPS participants, in that more employees had a 100% return to work, and fewer patients received disability pensions 1-year posttreatment. These results point to the potential efficacy of PST as a *secondary* prevention strategy.

PST and Telephone Counseling

At times, access to university or hospital-based intervention programs can be limited for people living in rural or sparsely populated areas. In addition, due to other responsibilities and commitments such as child care, many medical patients may not have the ability to travel to a university or major medical center where such research is taking place. As such, we need to be able to identify additional means by which to reach such individuals and increase the clinical applicability of such interventions. One approach has been the use of the telephone to administer psychosocial protocols. Allen et al. (2002) conducted a study in which PST was delivered over the telephone as a means of empowering women with breast carcinoma to cope with a range of difficulties when diagnosed in midlife. Specifically, six PST sessions were provided to 87 women with breast cancer: The first and last sessions were in person, and the middle four were provided by a nurse over the phone. Whereas PST was found generally to be an effective approach, results were not as supportive of the efficacy of this method of providing PST *across all subjects*. More specifically, relative to the control group, patients receiving PST who were characterized as "poor problem solvers" at baseline experienced no changes in the number and severity of cancer-related difficulties. However, patients with average or "good" problem-solving skills at baseline compared to controls were found to have improved mental health as a function of the intervention. Collectively, these results provide partial support for this method of PST but suggest that a more intensive form of this intervention (e.g., more sessions, more face-to-face contact) may be required for individuals with premorbid ineffective coping ability. The Grant et al. (2002) study involving PST for caregivers of stroke patients noted previously also used a telephone counseling approach, providing further support for this mode of PST implementation.

Nonsupport of PST

Collectively, the majority of the outcome literature evaluating PST supports the notion that it is an efficacious clinical intervention for a wide range of patient populations and problems. A major exception to these findings is a multisite study by Barrett et al. (2001) that found problem-solving therapy for primary care patients (PST-PC) to be no more effective than a drug placebo condition regarding the treatment of adults diagnosed with minor depression or dysthymia. However, a closer look at PST-PC indicates that this model of PST does not include a treatment component focused on problem orientation variables; rather, it provides training exclusively in the four rational problem-solving skills (cf. Barrett et al., 1999). As mentioned earlier, the link between problem solving and depression lies particularly in the association between depression and negative problem orientation (Nezu, 2004). Coupling this notion with the results from a study by Nezu and Perri (1989) that demonstrated the superior effects of PST when training was included in problem orientation, it is possible that PST-PC represents a truncated version relative to the Nezu (1987; Nezu et al., 1989) model of PST for depression and may not address a significant reason why a problem solving–depression association exists. As such, PST-PC may be clinically less potent, thus explaining the lack of a treatment effect compared to a placebo condition in the Barrett et al. (2001) investigation. A more definitive conclusion awaits additional research; however, two of the meta-analyses described previously (i.e., Bell & D'Zurilla, 2009; Malouff et al., 2007) found that inclusion–exclusion of a major focus on problem orientation moderated the effect sizes regarding outcome (i.e., absence of problem orientation training led to poorer outcome).

CLINICAL PRACTICE

In this section, we provide a brief, step-by-step guide to conducting PST. It should be noted that although PST involves teaching individuals specific skills, similar to other cognitive-behavioral therapy approaches, it should be conducted within a *therapeutic context*. Because PST does focus on skills building, it can easily be misunderstood by the novice therapist as entailing only a "teaching" process. However, it is important for the problem-solving therapist to be careful not to (1) conduct PST in a mechanistic manner; (2) focus only on skills training and not on the patient's emotional experiences; (3) deliver a "canned" treatment that does not address the unique strengths, weaknesses, and experiences of a given patient; and (4) assume that PST focuses only on superficial problems rather than on more complex interpersonal, psychological, existential, and spiritual issues (if warranted). Thus, in addition to requiring the therapist to teach the patient certain techniques to cope better with problems, effective PST requires the therapist to be competent in a variety of other assessment and intervention strategies, such as fostering a positive therapeutic relationship, assessing for complex clinical problems, modeling, behavioral rehearsal, assigning homework tasks, and appropriately providing corrective feedback.

Structurally, PST training can be broken into three major foci: (1) training in problem orientation; (2) training in the four specific rational problem-solving skills (i.e., problem definition and formulation, generation of alternatives, decision making, solution verification); and (3) practice of these skills across a variety of real-life problems. However, as noted in D'Zurilla and Nezu (2007), PST can be implemented in a variety of ways. For example, the guidelines provided in the next section actually depicts how PST might be conducted in a sequential fashion, such as that implemented in various treatment outcome studies (e.g., Nezu, Felgoise, McClure, & Houts, 2003; Nezu & Perri, 1989). In clinical settings, however, application of PST should be based on a comprehensive assessment of a given individual's (couple's, family's) problem-solving strengths and weaknesses. As such, not all training components may be necessary to include across all patients (for a more comprehensive discussion, see D'Zurilla & Nezu, 2007).

Training in Problem Orientation

The goal of training in this problem-solving component is to foster adoption or facilitation of a positive problem orientation. Clinically, we suggest that obstacles to adopting such a perspective include (1) poor self-efficacy beliefs, (2) negative thinking, and (3) negative emotions (i.e., a strong negative problem orientation).

Visualization is a clinical strategy included in PST to enhance a patient's optimism or sense of self-efficacy as a means of creating the experience of successful problem resolution in the "mind's eye" and vicariously experiencing the reinforcement to be gained. Visualization in this context requires individuals to close their eyes and imagine that they have successfully solved a current problem. The focus is on the end point—not on "how one got to the goal," but on "focusing on the feelings of having reached the goal." The central goal of this strategy is to have patients create and "experience" their own positive consequences related to solving a problem as a motivational step toward enhanced self-efficacy. In essence, it helps to create a visual image of "the light at the end of the tunnel."

To help overcome *negative thinking*, various cognitive restructuring strategies can be used, including those advocated in more formal cognitive therapy (e.g., Beck, 1995). For example, we often prescribe use of the A-B-C method of constructive thinking. With this technique, patients are taught to view emotional reactions from the A-B-C perspective, where A is the activating event (e.g., a problem), B is beliefs about the event (including what people say to themselves), and C is emotional and behavioral consequences. In other words, how individuals *feel and act* is often the product of how they *think*. Using a current problem, the PST therapist can use this procedure to diagnose negative self-talk and thoughts that are likely to lead to distressing emotions for a given patient. Such cognitions often include highly evaluative words, such as *should* and *must*, "catastrophic" words to describe non-life-threatening events, and phrases that tend to be overgeneralizations (e.g., "*Nobody* understands me!"). By examining self-talk, the patient can learn to separate realistic statements (e.g., "I wish ... ") from maladaptive ones (e.g., "I must have ... ") as they pertain to problems in living. The patient can also be given a list of positive self-statements to substitute for or to help dispute the negative self-talk (as in the reverse advocacy role-play strategy).

We also suggest applying the *reverse advocacy role-play* strategy. According to this approach, the PST therapist pretends to adopt a particular belief about problems and asks the patient to provide reasons why that belief is irrational, illogical, incorrect, or maladaptive. Such beliefs might include the following statements: "Problems are not common to everyone. If I have a problem, that means I'm crazy," "There must be a perfect solution to this problem," or "I'll never be the same again." At times when the patient has difficulty generating arguments against the therapist's position, the counselor then adopts a more extreme form of the belief, such as "No matter how long it takes, I will continue to try and find the perfect solution to my problem." This procedure is intended to help patients identify alternative ways of thinking, then to dispute or contradict previously held negative beliefs with more adaptive perspectives.

To help overcome negative emotions, patients are taught to interpret such negative feelings as *cues* that a problem exists. In other words, rather than labeling their negative emotions as "the problem," they are helped to conceptualize such an emotion as a "signal" that a problem exists, then observe what is occurring in their environment to recognize the "real problem" that is causing such emotions. Once feelings such as depression, anger, muscle tension, nausea, or anxiety arise, the patient is instructed to use the mnemonic *"STOP and THINK"* as a means of inhibiting avoidance or impulsive problem-solving behavior. The THINK aspect of this phrase refers to the use of the various problem-solving steps. In addition, PST emphasizes that combining emotions and rational thinking (rather than relying solely on only one of these areas) leads to "wisdom," which represents effective, real-life problem solving. Note that accurately labeling a problem *as* a problem serves to inhibit the tendency to act impulsively or automatically in reaction to such situations. It also facilitates the tendency to approach or to confront problems rather than to avoid them.

Training in Rational Problem Solving

Problem Definition

This first rational problem-solving skill can be likened to "mapping" a guide for the remainder of the problem-solving process. The major focus of this task is to understand better the nature of the problem and to set clearly defined and reasonable goals. In other words, locating a specific destination on a map makes it easier to find the best route to get there. Training in problem definition focuses on the following tasks: gathering all available information about the problem, using clear language, separating facts from assumptions, setting realistic problem-solving goals, and identifying current factors that prevent one from reaching such goals.

Generating Alternatives

In generating alternative solutions to a problem, PST encourages broad-based, creative, and flexible thinking. In essence, patients are taught various brainstorming strategies (e.g., "The more, the better"; "Defer judgment of ideas until a comprehensive list is created"; "Think of a *variety* of ideas"). Using such guides helps to increase the likelihood that the most effective solution ideas will ultimately be identified or discovered.

Decision Making

Once a list of alternative options has been generated, the individual is taught systematically to evaluate the potential for each solution to meet the defined goal(s). Training in this skill helps the individual use the following criteria to conduct a cost–benefit analysis based on the utility of each alternative solution: the likelihood that the solution will meet the defined goal, and that the person responsible for solving the problem can actually carry out the solution plan optimally; personal and social consequences; and short- and long-term effects.

Solution Verification

This last rational problem-solving task involves monitoring and evaluating the consequences of the actual outcome after the solution plan is carried out. PST encourages the individual to practice the performance aspect of solution implementation as a means of enhancing the probability that it will be carried out in its optimal form. Once the plan is under way, the patient is encouraged to monitor the actual results. Using this information allows individuals to evaluate the results by comparing the actual outcome with their expectations or predictions about the outcome. Depending on the outcome, individuals are then either guided to troubleshoot where in the problem-solving process they need to extend additional effort, if the problem is not adequately resolved, or to engage in self-reinforcement, if the problem is solved.

Supervised Practice

After the majority of training has occurred, the remainder of PST should be devoted to practicing the newly acquired skills and applying them to a variety of stressful problems. Beyond actually solving stressful problems, continuous in-session practice serves three additional purposes: The patient can receive "professional" feedback from the therapist; increased facility with the overall PST model can decrease the amount of time and effort necessary to apply the various problem-solving tasks with each new problem; and practice fosters relapse prevention.

Clinical Illustration

In the following case, disguised to ensure confidentiality, PST was applied as the major clinical intervention for the treatment of depression.

Case Description

Bridget, a 57-year-old, retired probation officer and mother of three, previously had not sought counseling and reported a lack of any psychiatric history. In fact, Briget had always viewed herself as an extremely competent woman "who could be counted on to help others with their problems." She was self-referred due to extreme family stressors that focused primarily on her grown son Joe's cocaine addiction. At the time she sought counseling, she had symptoms of moderate to severe depression, with a profound sense of hopelessness.

Bridget and her husband Frank had been married for 38 years, a relationship that she described as fairly positive (e.g., "He's always right there with me"). She described their relationship with their other two children as close and supportive. During the initial session, Bridget described ongoing family struggles with Joe's addiction, which included his stealing behavior, frequent lies and excuses for his behavior, and, more recently, her former daughter-in-law seeking a court order to block Joe's unsupervised contact with his daughter due to the risk he posed. The son's reactions largely centered on seeing himself as a victim and had recently escalated in verbal aggression and property destruction (e.g., he recently had broken into the family home, stolen money, and called repeatedly with additional requests and insulting attacks toward family members when refused).

Initial Problem-Solving Assessment

Bridget was asked to complete the SPSI-R twice, in that there appeared to be discrepancies in how she rated her various problem-solving abilities. First, she was asked to complete the inventory with regard to how she *typically* solved problems. Next, she was asked to complete the measure with regard to how she viewed her problem solving related *specifically* to her family problems. As predicted, there was a marked difference, in that Bridget's opinion of her own problem-solving efforts had been shattered by the ongoing difficulties with her son, and she was beginning to question seriously her own self-image, abilities, and judgment. This resulted in striking vulnerabilities in her problem orientation. Other clinical and self-report measures confirmed the presence of significant symptoms of depression, hopelessness, and concomitant anxiety.

Adopting a Positive Problem Orientation

Bridget's sarcastic sense of humor and outward appearance as a strong and rather fearless woman masked a strong sense of vulnerability that surfaced when she began discussing her son's addiction and the resulting family distress. For example, she stated, "I could always be counted on to roll my sleeves up and manage family problems effectively—but, now, I am a complete failure!" She indicated that past worries regarding her other two children were always "normal, " describing, for example, only minor problems with how they performed in school, whether they stayed out too late, or their difficulties with peers. Her other son Jim worked as a police officer in a different town, and her daughter Kerry, a single mother, lived nearby and was often involved in the family difficulties with Joe.

Bridget's partnership with her husband was such that she made the rules at home and he supported her in these decisions. When someone needed help, or something went wrong, she sprang into action, finding the right information, making the necessary calls, and implementing what had to be done. She described their ongoing attempts to help her son rehabilitate in this way and additionally stated that her daughter often tried to help in much the same manner. However, Joe made frequent excuses for his lack of follow through, accused others of not understanding, and always came home to demand that the family bail him out. It was clear from her description that Bridget was doing all the work for her son, and consistent with her style of solving problems, believed that if she only worked harder, Joe would finally understand and "fall in line." When her efforts persistently failed to effect change and actually led to a worsening of the situation, Bridget questioned her own ability and her view of herself ("now useless"), others ("not helpful or understanding"), her son ("incapable of change"), and the future ("quite hopeless").

The visualization technique was first used to help Bridget adopt a positive problem orientation. Specifically, Bridget was asked to envision a future where "the current problems involving Joe were solved." Although this strategy generally results in a person's ability to describe a fantasy image of a future in which current problems are solved, Bridget actually experienced some initial difficulty and tearfully described seeing her son "laying in the morgue and having to identify the body." After being brought back to focus on a more positive image of the future (even if she currently thought it was unlikely), Bridget was able to describe a scene in which the entire family was at her home for a celebration and she had no worries of having money stolen or being lied to, and in which she was not compelled to control her son's interactions with others. Continuing to work with this strategy, Bridget was finally able to see herself as much less in need of controlling and managing everything, and was able to enjoy her family interactions. This represented a significant moment of insight for Bridget, in that she was able to see how her desire to "fix" things may have relayed a message to her son that she did not trust his ability or believe that he might effectively change his life. As a result, as the family became more and more involved in trying to solve things for him, his anger at their lack of confidence (as well as his own inability to see himself as even minimally instrumental) only served to increase his resentment and anger toward others. Armed with little else, Joe's addictive behavior was increasing. Bridget and Frank's well-meaning friends had suggested that they "cut him out of their life and refuse all contact." Although they had reached a point where they were willing to do this, it was doubtful that they would stay committed to such a plan. They viewed it as punishing themselves, because it would actually remove their son and granddaughter from their lives forever. Using cognitive change strategies to suggest greater flexibility in her orientation to the problem, Bridget's therapist was able to help her adopt the view that her past way of solving many other problems effectively was not working here, and that it would be better if she tried different alternatives that would place more responsibility on her son for change (e.g., Bridget was the one seeking counseling help, rather than her son, for his difficulties). Although this clearly involved changing her previous style of trying to "fix everything," the therapist emphasized many alternative ways for Bridget to communicate the need for Joe to take greater responsibility for his life, other than cutting him out of her life completely.

Defining the Problem

Bridget defined her "problem" as learning to allow her son to take more responsibility for his own rehabilitation and visitation with his daughter. She and her husband further defined the problem by stating some of the significant obstacles in the way, including the following:

- They had created a pattern in which Joe would always expect them to bail him out.
- He would be very angry with them and accuse them of not caring.

This always served to trigger their own sense of responsibility and, consequently, the need to provide money.

- Joe would try to engage his sister Kerry, if Bridget and Frank pulled back support.
- They were fearful that they would not be able to see their grandchild.

Generating Alternatives

Bridget, Frank, and Kerry generated as many alternatives as possible to improve the situation. Remembering that it was important to list as many alternatives as possible without judging, they were amazed to see the many possibilities other than giving up and cutting Joe out of their lives. These included (but were not limited to) the following:

- Provide a one-time investment of money for a rehabilitation program.
- Arrange visits between their granddaughter and their former daughter-in-law without Joe being present.
- Make attendance at family gatherings contingent on Joe's completion of drug rehabilitation.
- Turn off their telephone, so as not to receive difficult calls from Joe.
- Set up a family intervention meeting with a counselor.
- Attend family support groups to help commit to new contingencies they were putting into effect.
- Provide Joe with information to apply for Medicaid, as well as Medicaid-funded residential rehabilitation programs.
- Obtain a court order to prevent Joe's access to their home when high.
- Consult with local police to place a watch on their house when they were not at home.
- Participate in family therapy to help members change their patterns of taking all responsibility for Joe.
- Ask Joe's brother Jim to return for a family meeting and family counseling.

Decision Making and Carrying Out the Solution Plan

Whereas the listed alternatives do not include all of the family brainstorming activities, they do suggest many possible alternatives that the family had not previously considered. Better defining the problem was essential to their discovery of more effective solutions. For example, they had previously framed the problem as their inability to help Joe change. As a function of PST, they realized that the degree of responsibility they were taking, while allowing Joe to see himself as a victim and blame them for not helping enough, was worsening the situation. In many ways, it seemed as if Joe was trying to show them that they overestimated their own competencies by not responding to their attempts to help. This made all of the family members "failures."

After weighing the various alternatives and conducting a cost–benefit analysis, the family combined several alternatives to construct the following overall solution plan. They offered Joe initial assistance to help him complete the necessary applications for medical coverage and to attend a residential drug rehabilitation program for which only he would be responsible. The program involved participating in a group residence, where Joe would receive psychiatric care and therapy, drug counseling, and supervised job assistance. In addition, he and other residents were responsible for chores in the home. A family meeting was held with counselors from the program to indicate to Joe that family members were changing their past methods of taking responsibility. All family members—including Jim, Kerry, and Joe's former wife—attended, presenting a united front. Moreover, family members made arrangements with Joe's former wife to visit with their grandchild, independent of Joe's current restrictions. Joe had one failed attempt at the group residence and one arrest for disorderly conduct before he finally completed a successful 10-month stay at the residence. He is currently attending community college and working in a restaurant to secure his own apartment. He has recently begun unsupervised visits with his daughter for brief periods of time.

Monitoring and Verifying the Outcome

Although Joe has a long rehabilitative road ahead, Bridget and Frank now view his difficulties as "*his* life story" rather than their responsibility. Bridget is less hopeless and views the problems with her son in a more realistic way: The problem is neither immediately solvable by her nor hopeless. Instead, she views problems as an inevitable part of life and family, and is quick to point out that there are "no perfect solutions." When her first attempt to manage a situation effectively was not successful, she did not immediately jump to the extreme of seeing the situation as hopeless. As such, Bridget is less impulsive and self-critical in her decision making and one small step closer to the positive visualization she created earlier in therapy. Moreover, her initially high level of depression has decreased dramatically.

SUMMARY AND CONCLUSIONS

PST has been described as a positive clinical intervention that reduces and prevents stress and psychopathology by increasing positive problem-solving attitudes and skills, and promoting broad positive changes in coping performance and psychological well-being across a wide range of problematic situations. Empirical support for the theory and practice of PST comes from two areas of research: (1) studies supporting the relational/problem-solving model of stress and adjustment, and (2) investigations evaluating the efficacy of PST with a variety of different clinical and vulnerable populations. Despite the impressive body of research in these two areas, there are still a number of areas for future researchers to tackle regarding the efficacy and applicability of PST. Some of these are noted below.

PST for Positive Functioning

More research is needed on the role of PST in enhancing *optimal* or superior functioning that maximizes one's quality of life and place in society. Such research could focus on fostering exceptional performance, achievement, creativity, and invention in various areas of life and work, such as business and industry, medicine, public service, sports, and marriage and family.

Adolescents and Their Parents

Studies have identified a significant relationship between SPS deficits and serious psychological and behavioral problems in adolescents, including depression and suicidal ideation (Sadowski & Kelley, 1993; Sadowski et al., 1994), aggression and delinquency (Freedman, Rosenthal, Donahoe, Schlundt, & McFall, 1978; Jaffe & D'Zurilla, 2003; Lochman, Wayland, & White, 1993), substance abuse (tobacco, alcohol, marijuana) and high-risk automobile driving (Jaffe & D'Zurilla, 2003). As such, we recommend that more research on PST programs be developed to address these specific problem areas.

Individuals with Cardiovascular Disease

In recent years, PST has been successfully applied as a method for helping patients and their caregivers cope with serious medical conditions and their treatments. Whereas successful PST programs have been developed for cancer patients and their caregivers (e.g., Nezu et al., 2003), there are no studies on PST for cardiac patients. Like cancer, cardiovascular diseases and recovery from heart attacks and strokes require many difficult behavioral and lifestyle changes and adjustments, such as job adjustments, diet changes, taking daily medications, making time for exercise, and reducing stress in one's life. PST might be particularly useful and effective for helping cardiac patients cope more effectively with these difficult behavioral and lifestyle changes, thus improving their physical and psychological well-being (Nezu, Nezu, Cos, et al., 2006; Nezu, Nezu, & Jain, 2005).

Preventive Behavioral Health

A number of behavioral and lifestyle changes have also been recommended by medical professionals to *prevent* serious medical conditions, such as cancer and cardiovascular diseases. These changes include reducing and managing stress more effectively, changing eating habits, losing weight, stopping smoking, controlling alcohol intake, and increasing physical exercise. Hence, we recommend research on PST as a *preventive* intervention to help people overcome these obstacles to a healthy lifestyle.

Stress Reduction and Prevention in the Workplace

Except for senior citizens, most American adults spend at least half of their waking hours in the workplace. Hence, daily conflicts and problems at work are a major source of stress for most adults, resulting in adverse outcomes such as absenteeism, low productivity, occupational burnout, lost work days due to illness, high turnover rates, psychological disturbance, and health problems. PST can be an effective strategy for reducing and preventing stress and its negative effects in the workplace (D'Zurilla, 1990). However, there is a lack of research on the evaluation of PST workshops for managers, supervisors, and other employees. If they are proven to be effective, such workshops could have important psychological, health, and economic benefits for individual employees, business owners and executives, and society in general.

Mediators and Moderators of PST Outcomes

According to SPS theory, the major mediator of positive PST outcomes is SPS ability; that is, problem-solving training improves problem-solving ability and performance, which in turn produces more positive therapy outcomes. In support of this assumption, several outcome studies have found a significant relationship between improvements in SPS and positive changes in negative psychological conditions, including psychological stress (D'Zurilla & Maschka, 1988), depression (Nezu, 1987; Nezu

& Perri, 1989), and cancer-related distress (Nezu et al., 2003). However, more research is needed to identify *which* specific problem-solving dimensions are the most important mediators of PST outcomes for *which* particular patients with *which* particular adjustment problems. Whereas *mediators* are variables affected by PST that in turn influence or account for therapy outcomes, *moderators* are variables that interact with treatment to influence the magnitude of outcomes. Such variables to address might include age, gender, ethnicity, intelligence, educational level, and various personality traits. Research designed to identify moderator variables is important for determining which individuals might benefit most or least from PST.

New Methods for Implementing PST

The traditional mode of implementing PST in published outcome studies is face-to-face individual or group sessions lasting from 1 to 1½ hours. However, a few studies have successfully implemented innovative methods of service delivery, such as "telephone therapy" (e.g., Allen et al., 2002; Grant et al., 2002). Other possible alternative delivery methods include self-help manuals, bibliotherapy, and the Internet. To capitalize on advances in new communication technologies that might make PST more accessible, efficient, and cost-effective, more research is recommended on the efficacy of these alternative modes of intervention.

Concluding Comment

Since the publication of the original D'Zurilla and Goldfried (1971) conceptual paper, research on SPS and PST has increased at a rapid pace. In general, the results have provided significant support for the theory and practice of PST. Overall, research has indicated that effective problem-solving ability, assessed by several different measures, is related to positive psychological and behavioral functioning, whereas problem-solving deficits are associated with a variety of different forms of maladaptive functioning, including psychological distress, behavior deviations, and health problems. In addition, the evidence supports the perspective that PST is a useful and efficacious intervention for a variety of different clinical populations, including individuals with different kinds of psychological disorders, behavior disorders, and medical illnesses. Moreover, there is evidence that PST is also an effective preventive intervention with various vulnerable populations, such as individuals with high levels of life stress and those at risk for HIV. However, although the research to date has generally been supportive or promising, more work needs to be done to establish the true potential of SPS theory, research, and therapy.

REFERENCES

Allen, S. M., Shah, A. C., Nezu, A. M., Nezu, C. M., Ciambrone, D., Hogan, J., et al. (2002). A problem-solving approach to stress reduction among younger women with breast carcinoma: A randomized controlled trial. *Cancer, 94,* 3089–3100.

Aréan, P. A., Perri, M. G., Nezu, A. M., Schein, R. L., Christopher, F., & Joseph, T. X. (1993). Comparative effectiveness of social problem-solving therapy and reminiscence therapy as treatments for depression in older adults. *Journal of Consulting and Clinical Psychology, 61,* 1003–1010.

Barrett, J. E., Williams, J. W., Oxman, T. E., Frank, E., Katon, W., Sullivan, M., et al. (2001). Treatment of dysthymia and minor depression in primary care: A randomized trial in patients aged 18 to 59 years. *Journal of Family Practice, 50,* 405–412.

Barrett, J. E., Williams, J. W., Oxman, T. E., Katon, W., Frank, E., Hegel, M. T., et al. (1999). The Treatment Effectiveness Project: A comparison of the effectiveness of paroxetine, problem-solving therapy, and placebo in the treatment of minor depression and dysthymia in primary care patients: Background and research plan. *General Hospital Psychiatry, 21,* 260–273.

Beck, J. S. (1995). *Cognitive therapy: Basics and beyond.* New York: Guilford Press.

Bell, A. C., & D'Zurilla, T. J. (2009). Problem-solving therapy for depression: A meta-analysis. *Clinical Psychology Review, 29,* 348–353.

Bloom, B. L. (1985). *Stressful life event theory and research: Implications for primary prevention (DHHS Publication No. [AMD] 85-1385).* Rockville, MD: National Institute of Mental Health.

Burks, N., & Martin, B. (1985). Everyday problems and life change events: Ongoing vs. acute sources of stress. *Journal of Human Stress, 11,* 27–35.

Chang, E. C., Downey, C. A., & Salata, J. L. (2004). Social problem solving and positive psychological functioning: Looking at the positive side of problem solving. In E. C. Chang, T. J. D'Zurilla, & L. J. Sanna (Eds.), *Social problem solving: Theory, research, and training* (pp. 99–116). Washington, DC: American Psychological Association.

Chang, E. C., & D'Zurilla, T. J. (1996). Relations between problem orientation and optimism, pessimism, and trait affectivity: A construct validation study. *Behaviour Research and Therapy, 34,* 185–195.

Chang, E. C., D'Zurilla, T. J., & Sanna, L. J. (Eds.). (2004). *Social problem solving: Theory, research, and training.* Washington, DC: American Psychological Association.

Cuijpers, P., van Straten, A., & Warmerdam, L. (2007). Problem solving therapies for depression: A meta-analysis. *European Psychiatry, 22,* 9–15.

DeLongis, A., Coyne, J. C., Dakof, G., Folkman, S., & Lazarus, R. S. (1982). Relationship of daily hassles, uplifts, and major life events to health status. *Health Psychology, 1,* 119–136.

D'Zurilla, T. J. (1986). *Problem-solving therapy: A social competence approach to clinical intervention.* New York: Springer.

D'Zurilla, T. J. (1990). Problem-solving training for effective stress management and prevention. *Journal of Cognitive Psychotherapy: An International Quarterly, 4,* 327–355.

D'Zurilla, T. J., & Goldfried, M. R. (1971). Problem solving and behavior modification. *Journal of Abnormal Psychology, 78,* 107–126.

D'Zurilla, T. J., & Maschka, G. (1988, November). *Outcome of a problem-solving approach to stress management: I. Comparison with social support.* Paper presented to the Association for Advancement of Behavior Therapy, New York, NY.

D'Zurilla, T. J., & Nezu, A. (1980). A study of the generation-of-alternatives process in social problem solving. *Cognitive Therapy and Research, 4,* 67–72.

D'Zurilla, T. J., & Nezu, A. (1982). Social problem solving in adults. In P. C. Kendall (Ed.), *Advances in cognitive-behavioral research and therapy* (Vol. 1, pp. 202–274). New York: Academic Press.

D'Zurilla, T. J., & Nezu, A. M. (1990). Development and preliminary evaluation of the Social Problem-Solving Inventory (SPSI). *Psychological Assessment: A Journal of Consulting and Clinical Psychology, 2,* 156–163.

D'Zurilla, T. J., & Nezu, A. M. (1999). *Problem-solving therapy: A social competence approach to clinical intervention* (2nd ed.). New York: Springer.

D'Zurilla, T. J., & Nezu, A. M. (2007). *Problem-solving therapy: A positive approach to clinical intervention* (3rd ed.). New York: Springer.

D'Zurilla, T. J., Nezu, A. M., & Maydeu-Olivares, A. (2002). *Manual for the Social Problem-Solving Inventory—Revised.* North Tonawanda, NY: Multi-Health Systems.

D'Zurilla, T. J., Nezu, A. M., & Maydeu-Olivares, A. (2004). Social problem solving: Theory and assessment. In E. C. Chang, T. J. D'Zurilla, & L. J. Sanna (Eds.), *Social problem solving:Theory, research, and training* (pp. 11–27). Washington, DC: American Psychological Association.

Folkman, S., & Lazarus, R. S. (1988). Coping as a mediator of emotion. *Journal of Personality and Social Psychology, 54,* 466–475.

Freedman, B. I., Rosenthal, L., Donahoe, C. P., Schlundt, D. G., & McFall, R. M. (1978). A social-behavioral analysis of skill deficits in delinquent and non-delinquent adolescent boys. *Journal of Consulting and Clinical Psychology, 46,* 1448–1462.

Gagné, R. M. (1966). Human problem solving: Internal and external events. In B. Kleinmuntz (Ed.), *Problem solving: Research, method and theory* (pp. 128–148). New York: Wiley.

García-Vera, M. P., Labrador, F. J., & Sanz, J. (1997). Stress-management training for essential hypertension: A controlled study. *Applied Psychophysiology and Biofeedback, 22,* 261–283.

García-Vera, M. P., Sanz, J., & Labrador, F. J. (1998). Psychological changes accompanying and mediating stress-management training for essential hypertension. *Applied Psychophysiology and Biofeedback, 23,* 159–178.

Gellis, Z. D., & Kenaly, B. (2008). Problem-solving therapy for depression in adults: A systematic review. *Research on Social Work Practice, 18,* 117–131.

Gladwin, T. (1967). Social competence and clinical practice. *Psychiatry: Journal for the Study of Interpersonal Processes, 3,* 30–43.

Graf, A. (2003). A psychometric test of a German version of the SPSI-R. *Zeitschrift für Differentielle und Diagnostische Psychologie, 24*, 277–291.

Grant, J. S., Elliott, T. R., Weaver, M., Bartolucci, A. A., & Giger, J. N. (2002). Telephone intervention with family caregivers of stroke survivors after rehabilitation. *Stroke, 33*, 2060–2065.

Houts, P. S., Nezu, A. M., Nezu, C. M., & Bucher, J. A. (1996). A problem-solving model of family caregiving for cancer patients. *Patient Education and Counseling, 27*, 63–73.

Jaffe, W. B., & D'Zurilla, T. J. (2003). Adolescent problem solving, parent problem solving, and externalizing behavior in adolescents. *Behavior Therapy, 34*, 295–311.

Kant, G. L., D'Zurilla, T. J., & Maydeu-Olivares, A. (1997). Social problem solving as a mediator of stress-related depression and anxiety in middle-aged and elderly community residents. *Cognitive Therapy and Research, 21*, 73–96.

Kendall, P. C., & Hollon, S. D. (Eds.). (1979). *Cognitive-behavioral interventions: Theory, research, and procedures*. New York: Academic Press.

Lazarus, R. S. (1999). *Stress and emotion: A new synthesis*. New York: Springer.

Lazarus, R. S., & Folkman, S. (1984). *Stress, appraisal, and coping*. New York: Springer.

Lochman, J. E., Wayland, K. K., & White, K. J. (1993). Social goals: Relationship to adolescent adjustment and to social problem solving. *Journal of Abnormal Child Psychology, 21*, 135–151.

Londahl, E. A., Tverskoy, A., & D'Zurilla, T. J. (2005). The relations of internalizing symptoms to conflict and interpersonal problem solving in close relationships. *Cognitive Therapy and Research, 29*, 445–462.

Mahoney, M. J. (1974). *Cognition and behavior modification*. Cambridge, MA: Ballinger.

Malouff, J. M., Thorsteinsson, E. B., & Schutte, N. S. (2007). The efficacy of problem solving therapy in reducing mental and physical health problems: A meta-analysis. *Clinical Psychology Review, 27*, 46–57.

Maydeu-Olivares, A., & D'Zurilla, T. J. (1995). A factor analysis of the Social Problem-Solving Inventory using polychoric correlations. *European Journal of Psychological Assessment, 11*, 98–107.

Maydeu-Olivares, A., & D'Zurilla, T. J. (1996). A factor-analytic study of the Social Problem-Solving Inventory: An integration of theory and data. *Cognitive Therapy and Research, 20*, 115–133.

Maydeu-Olivares, A., Rodríguez-Fornells, A., Gómez-Benito, J., & D'Zurilla, T. J. (2000). Psychometric properties of the Spanish adaptation of the Social Problem-Solving Inventory-Revised (SPSI-R). *Personality and Individual Differences, 29*, 699–708.

Monroe, S. M., & Hadjiyannakis, K. (2002). The social environment and depression: Focusing on severe life stress. In I. H. Gotlib & C. L. Hammen (Eds.), *Handbook of depression* (pp. 314–340). New York: Guilford Press.

Nezu, A. M. (1986a). Cognitive appraisal of problem-solving effectiveness: Relation to depression and depressive symptoms. *Journal of Clinical Psychology*, *42*, 42–48.

Nezu, A. M. (1986b). Effects of stress from current problems: Comparisons to major life events. *Journal of Clinical Psychology*, *42*, 847–852.

Nezu, A. M. (1986c). Efficacy of a social problem-solving therapy approach for unipolar depression. *Journal of Consulting and Clinical Psychology*, *54*, 196–202.

Nezu, A. M. (1986d). Negative life stress and anxiety: Problem solving as a moderator variable. *Psychological Reports*, *58*, 279–283.

Nezu, A. M. (1987). A problem-solving formulation of depression: A literature review and proposal of a pluralistic model. *Clinical Psychology Review*, *7*, 121–144.

Nezu, A. M. (2004). Problem solving and behavior therapy revisited. *Behavior Therapy*, *35*, 1–33.

Nezu, A. M., & D'Zurilla, T. J. (1979). An experimental evaluation of the decision-making process in social problem solving. *Cognitive Therapy and Research*, *3*, 269–277.

Nezu, A. M., & D'Zurilla, T. J. (1981a). Effects of problem definition and formulation on decision making in the social problem-solving process. *Behavior Therapy*, *12*, 100–106.

Nezu, A. M., & D'Zurilla, T. J. (1981b). Effects of problem definition and formulation on the generation of alternatives in the social problem-solving process. *Cognitive Therapy and Research*, *6*, 265–271.

Nezu, A. M., & D'Zurilla, T. J. (1989). Social problem solving and negative affective conditions. In P. C. Kendall & D. Watson (Eds.), *Anxiety and depression: Distinctive and overlapping features* (pp. 285–315). New York: Academic Press.

Nezu, A. M., & Nezu, C. M. (in press). Problem-solving therapy. In S. Richards & M. G. Perri (Eds.), *Relapse prevention for depression*. Washington, DC: American Psychological Association.

Nezu, A. M., Nezu, C. M., & Cos, T. A. (2007). Case formulation for the behavioral and cognitive therapies: A problem-solving perspective. In T. D. Eells (Ed.), *Handbook of psychotherapy case formulation* (2nd ed., pp. 349–378). New York: Guilford Press.

Nezu, A. M., Nezu, C. M., Cos, T., Friedman, J., Wilkins, V. M., & Lee, M. (2006, November). *Social problem solving and depression among patients with cardiovascular disease*. Paper presented to the Association for Behavioral and Cognitive Therapies, Chicago, IL.

Nezu, A. M., Nezu, C. M., & D'Zurilla, T. J. (2007). *Solving life's problems: A 5-step guide to enhanced well-being*. New York: Springer.

Nezu, A. M., Nezu, C. M., Faddis, S., DelliCarpini, L. A., & Houts, P. S. (1995, November). *Social problem solving as a moderator of cancer-related stress*. Paper presented to the Association for Advancement of Behavior Therapy, Washington, DC.

Nezu, A. M., Nezu, C. M., Felgoise, S. H., McClure, K. S., & Houts, P. S. (2003). Project Genesis: Assessing the efficacy of problem-solving therapy for distressed adult cancer patients. *Journal of Consulting and Clinical Psychology,* *71,* 1036–1048.

Nezu, A. M., Nezu, C. M., Felgoise, S. H., & Zwick, M. L. (2003). Psychosocial oncology. In A. M. Nezu, C. M. Nezu, & P. A. Geller (Eds.), *Health psychology* (pp. 267–292). New York: Wiley.

Nezu, A. M., Nezu, C. M., Friedman, S. H., Faddis, S., & Houts, P. S. (1998). *Helping cancer patients cope: A problem-solving approach.* Washington, DC: American Psychological Association.

Nezu, A. M., Nezu, C. M., Houts, P. S., Friedman, S. H., & Faddis, S. (1999). Relevance of problem-solving therapy to psychosocial oncology. *Journal of Psychosocial Oncology, 16,* 5–26.

Nezu, A. M., Nezu, C. M., & Jain, D. (2005). *The emotional wellness way to cardiac health: How letting go of depression, anxiety, and anger can heal your heart.* Oakland, CA: New Harbinger.

Nezu, A. M., Nezu, C. M., & Lombardo, E. R. (2004). *Cognitive-behavioral case formulation and treatment design: A problem-solving approach.* New York: Springer.

Nezu, A. M., Nezu, C. M., & Perri, M. G. (1989). *Problem-solving therapy for depression: Therapy, research, and clinical guidelines.* New York: Wiley.

Nezu, A. M., Nezu, C. M., & Perri, M. G. (2006). Problem solving to promote treatment adherence. In W. T. O'Donohue & E. Livens (Eds.), *Promoting treatment adherence: A practical handbook for health care providers* (pp. 135–148). New York: Sage.

Nezu, A. M., Nezu, C. M., Saraydarian, L., Kalmar, K., & Ronan, G. F. (1986). Social problem solving as a moderator variable between negative life stress and depressive symptoms. *Cognitive Therapy and Research, 10,* 489–498.

Nezu, A. M., & Perri, M. G. (1989). Social problem solving therapy for unipolar depression: An initial dismantling investigation. *Journal of Consulting and Clinical Psychology, 57,* 408–413.

Nezu, A. M., Perri, M. G., & Nezu, C. M. (1987, August). *Validation of a problem a problem-solving/stress model of depression.* Paper presented to the American Psychological Association, New York, NY.

Nezu, A. M., Perri, M. G., Nezu, C. M., & Mahoney, D. J. (1987, November). *Social problem solving as a moderator of stressful events among clinically depressed individuals.* Paper presented to the Association for Advancement of Behavior Therapy, Boston, MA.

Nezu, A. M., & Ronan, G. F. (1985). Life stress, current problems, problem solving, and depressive symptomatology: An integrative model. *Journal of Consulting and Clinical Psychology, 53,* 693–697.

Nezu, A. M., & Ronan, G. F. (1988). Stressful life events, problem solving, and depressive symptoms among university students: A prospective analysis. *Journal of Counseling Psychology, 35,* 134–138.

Nezu, A. M., Wilkins, V. M., & Nezu, C. M. (2004). Social problem solving, stress, and negative affective conditions. In E. C. Chang, T. J. D'Zurilla, & L. J. Sanna

(Eds.), *Social problem solving: Theory, research, and training* (pp. 49–65). Washington, DC: American Psychological Association.

Nezu, C. M. (2003). Cognitive-behavioral treatment for sex offenders: Current status. *Japanese Journal of Behavior Therapy, 29,* 15–24.

Nezu, C. M., Fiore, A. A., & Nezu, A. M. (2006). Problem-solving treatment for intellectually disabled sex offenders. *International Journal of Behavioral Consultation and Therapy, 2,* 266–276.

Nezu, C. M., Nezu, A. M., & Aréan, P. A. (1991). Assertiveness and problem-solving training for mildly mentally retarded persons with dual diagnosis. *Research in Developmental Disabilities, 12,* 371–386.

Nezu, C. M., Palmatier, A., & Nezu, A. M. (2004). Social problem solving training for caregivers. In E. C. Chang, T. J. D'Zurilla, & L. J. Sanna (Eds.), *Social problem solving: Theory, research, and training* (pp. 223–238). Washington, DC: American Psychological Association.

Perri, M. G., Nezu, A. M., McKelvey, W. F., Schein, R. L., Renjilian, D. A., & Viegener, B. J. (2001). Relapse prevention training and problem solving therapy in the long-term management of obesity. *Journal of Consulting and Clinical Psychology, 69,* 722–726.

Perri, M. G., Nezu, A. M., & Viegener, B. J. (1992). *Improving the long-term management of obesity: Theory, research, and clinical guidelines.* New York: Wiley.

Sadowski, C., & Kelley, M. L. (1993). Social problem-solving in suicidal adolescents. *Journal of Consulting and Clinical Psychology, 61,* 121–127.

Sadowski, C., Moore, L. A., & Kelley, M. L. (1994). Psychometric properties of the Social Problem-Solving Inventory (SPSI) with normal and emotionally-disturbed adolescents. *Journal of Abnormal Child Psychology, 22,* 487–500.

Sahler, O. J. Z., Varni, J. W., Fairclough, D. L., Butler, R. W., Noll, R. B., Dolgin, M. J., et al. (2002). Problem-solving skills training for mothers of children with newly diagnosed cancer: A randomized trial. *Developmental and Behavioral Pediatrics, 23,* 77–86.

Sato, H., Takahashi, F., Matsuo, M., Sakai, M., Shimada, H., Chen, J., et al. (2006). Development of the Japanese version of the Social Problem-Solving Inventory—Revised and examination of its reliability and validity. *Japanese Journal of Behavior Therapy, 32,* 15–30.

Shaw, W. S., Feuerstein, M., Haufler, A. J., Berkowitz, S. M., & Lopez, M. S. (2001). Working with low back pain: Problem-solving orientation and function. *Pain, 93,* 129–137.

Siu, A. M. H., & Shek, D. T. L. (2005). The Chinese version of the Social Problem Solving Inventory: Some initial results on reliability and validity. *Journal of Clinical Psychology, 61,* 347–360.

van den Hout, J. H. C., Vlaeyen, J. W. S., Heuts, P. H. T., Stillen, W. J. T., & Willen, J. E. H. L. (2001). Functional disability in non-specific low back pain: The role of pain-related fear and problem-solving skills. *International Journal of Behavioural Medicine, 8,* 134–148.

van den Hout, J. H. C., Vlaeyen, J. W. S., Heuts, P. H. T., Zijlema, J. H. L., & Wijen, J. A. G. (2003). Secondary prevention of work-related disability in nonspecific low back pain: Does problem-solving therapy help? A randomized clinical trial. *Clinical Journal of Pain, 19*, 87–96.

Wakeling, H. C. (2007). The psychometric validation of the Social Problem-Solving Inventory—Revised with UK incarcerated sexual offenders. *Sex Abuse, 19*, 217–236.

Weinberger, M., Hiner, S. L., & Tierney, W. M. (1987). In support of hassles as a measure of stress in predicting health outcomes. *Journal of Behavioral Medicine, 10*, 19–31.

CHAPTER 4

Rational-Emotive
Behavior Therapy

Raymond A. DiGiuseppe

INTRODUCTION AND HISTORICAL BACKGROUND

Albert Ellis (1913–2007) considered himself the grandfather of cognitive-behavioral therapy (CBT) because of his early development of rational-emotive behavior therapy (REBT), one of the original forms of CBT. Ellis entered the profession in the 1940s and published his first article on rational therapy (1957a), and has had a major impact on psychotherapy in general, and on CBT in particular.

A survey of more than 2500 psychotherapists conducted by the *Psychotherapy Networker* (Cook, Bryyanova, & Coyne, 2009), reported that respondents rated Ellis as the sixth most influential psychotherapist. CBT was rated as the most popular theoretical approach to therapy. Although Carl Rogers remained the most influential psychotherapist, and Aaron Beck came in as number two, Ellis is recognized as a major icon in the field of psychotherapy.

When Ellis entered the profession in the late 1940s and began to publish on therapy in the 1950s, two major theoretical orientations dominated psychotherapy: psychoanalysis and client-centered therapy. Psychotherapy research was in a rudimentary stage. Most psychotherapy occurred in the therapy session. Therapists' relationships with their clients were defined by the passive, nondirective roles proscribed by the two major theoretical orientations to therapy. Ellis was instrumental in changing much of this. He was among the first psychotherapists to advocate psychotherapy research to evaluate the effectiveness of treatments. Ellis (1950) suggested that research-ers test the effectiveness of psychotherapy by the standards acceptable at that time. He also encouraged outcome research about specific therapy pop-ulations to help increase our knowledge (Ellis, 1956). Ellis's (1957b) first test of the effectiveness of what he then called rational therapy (RT) came between Eysenck's (1952) classic evaluation of the outcomes of psychoana-lytic treatments and Wolpe's (1961) pioneering report on the outcomes of behavior therapy.

Ellis was among the first psychotherapists to advocate actively chang-ing clients' present beliefs to induce emotional or behavioral change. Ellis was among the first to use between sessions assignments, including *in vivo* behavioral assignments. He provided workshops, lectures, books, and writ-ten assignments to identify, challenge, and replace irrational ideas and to reinforce the rational ideas that he covered in therapy. Ellis was amongst the first psychotherapy integrationists. Although his therapy had a strong cognitive focus, from the onset Ellis (1955) advocated many types of inter-ventions to help people change their disturbed emotions and behaviors. He encouraged the use of imagery, hypnosis, group sessions, family sessions, humor, psychoeducational readings, writing assignments, singing, behav-ioral rehearsal, action assignments, metaphors, parables, and cathartic expe-riences. The tasks of psychotherapy became any activity that could convince the client to change. Ellis and Harper's (1961) *A Guide to Rational Living* was one of the earliest self-help books. Ellis would follow with many more and helped the publishing revolution in self-help books promoting human change. Given these accomplishments, it seems that Ellis and REBT have had a profound influence on psychotherapy in general, and CBT in particular.

Before becoming a psychologist, Ellis, the true Renaissance man, sup-ported himself as an accountant while he pursued his interests. He read philosophy, wrote operas and other musical scores, authored several nov-els, and worked as a political activist. Many of Ellis's psychotherapy prin-ciples were actually recorded in his unpublished autobiographical novel (1933), which recounts his attempts to overcome his own shyness, anxi-ety, and shame about coming from a poor family (Warren, 2007). During these years, Ellis became interested in romantic and sexual relationships, and read voraciously on the topic. In 1941, he founded the nonprofit LAMP (Love and Marriage Problems) Institute to dispense advice on such topics, mostly to friends and relatives. On the advice of his lawyer to seek a profes-sional degree to provide some recognition of his expertise he enrolled in the doctoral program in clinical psychology at Columbia University at age 40 (McMahon & Viterito, 2007).

After graduating in the late 1940s, Ellis began psychoanalytic training and simultaneously practiced marital and sex therapy. He became discour-aged with the lack of effectiveness of psychoanalysis in the early 1950s. He discovered that clients in his relationship practice improved more than those he psychoanalyzed. Ellis recognized that after clients acquired insight, some still failed to improve. He concluded that insight into one's childhood experiences resulted in change for only a small percentage of individuals.

Ellis recognized that he behaved differently with clients in his marital and sex therapy practice. He actively taught these clients to change their attitudes. Ellis always had a long-standing interest in philosophy, including the works of great Asian and Greek thinkers. When freed from the constraining role that psychoanalysis placed on the therapist, Ellis freely provided advice to his clients based on these philosophical works. Ellis contemplated the Stoic philosophers' notion that people choose whether to become disturbed, or in the words of Epictetus (1996), "Men [*and women*] are not disturbed by things, but by the view which they take of them" (from the *Encheiridion*, p. 5). Ellis utilized philosophy as the foundation for his new therapy and always credited classical and modern philosophers as the source of his ideas. In 1955, he formulated his theory in a paper delivered at the American Psychological Association (Ellis, 1957a). Several years later, Ellis (1962/1994) published his first professional book, *Reason and Emotion in Psychotherapy.*

Ellis originally named his approach rational therapy because he focused on the role of cognitions. He later concluded that he had underemphasized the role of emotions, and he renamed it rational-emotive therapy. He changed the name again to rational-emotive behavior therapy (Ellis, 1999) at the urging of Corsini (1994), who noticed that Ellis always used behavioral interventions and had done so since the inception of his work. Corsini suggested that Ellis needed a name that better represented his actual practice and teachings.

Ellis founded the Institute for Advanced Study in Rational Psychotherapy in 1965 for professional training in rational-emotive therapy. It survives today as the Albert Ellis Institute. Affiliated centers offer REBT training for mental health professionals in Argentina, Australia, Canada, France, Germany, Israel, Italy, Japan, Mexico, the Netherlands, New Zealand, and Taiwan. The Institute or its affiliated centers have trained more than 13,000 therapists throughout the world.

Although REBT was one of the first forms of CBT, it differs from some forms of CBT in several distinctive ways. Ellis (2001, 2005a) often used the term *classic REBT* to refer to the distinctive feature of REBT, while using the terms *general REBT* to refer the use of these distinctive aspects plus the inclusion of other forms of CBT (Ellis, 2005b). Most REBT practitioners incorporate both the classic and distinctive features of REBT, while using the techniques of the wider field of cognitive and behavioral therapies (Ellis, 2001, 2005b). However, they usually try the classical or distinctive features first. In this chapter, I describe the classic REBT and its distinction features, strategies, and techniques. However, REBT is practiced as an integrative therapy that borrows all of the CBT techniques discussed in this book.

The REBT trademark emphasizes teaching people to learn their ABCs of emotional disturbance, identifying the Activating events, their Beliefs about those events, and the resulting emotional Consequences. REBT teaches that disturbed emotional and behavioral consequences result from irrational beliefs individuals hold rather than from activating events. The distinctive features of REBT (Dryden, 2008) are as follows: First, the A-B-C model focuses on underlying irrational beliefs and not on automatic thoughts. REBT would argue that automatic thoughts concern the probabilistic occurrence of negative reality. Whether overestimated or not, such thoughts are about the world and are part of the A. Second, rigidity is at the core of psychological disturbance, and flexibility is at the core of psychological health. Third, extreme beliefs are derived from rigid beliefs; nonextreme beliefs are derived from flexible beliefs. Fourth, the distinction between maladaptive and unhealthy negative emotions and adaptive or healthy beliefs are qualitative not quantitative. Fifth, self-esteem is a dangerous, elusive concept. Sixth, there is a distinction between ego and discomfort disturbance. Seventh, people get upset about their emotional experience; that is, emotional consequences can become activating events. Eighth, humans are biologically both rational and irrational.

Ellis's writings include his personal philosophy, a recommended philosophy of life, a theory of psychopathology, and a theory of psychotherapy. One might agree with some aspects of Ellis's writings, such as his theory of psychopathology, yet disagree with other aspects, such as his personal philosophy.

REBT rests on some philosophical assumptions. The first of these is commitment to the scientific method. Ellis believed that applying the scientific method to one's personal life results in less emotional disturbance and ineffectual behavior. People are better off if they recognize that all of their beliefs, schemas, perceptions, and cherished truths may be wrong. Testing one's assumptions, examining the validity and functionality of one's beliefs, and being willing to entertain alternative ideas promote mental health. Rigid adherence to a belief or schema of the world prevents one from revising one's thinking, and dooms one to behave as if the world is as one hopes it will be rather than the way it is. For Ellis, we are better off if we hold all beliefs *lightly*.

According to REBT (DiGiuseppe, 1986; Ellis, 1994), humans function best if they adopt the epistemology of the philosophy of science, specifically, the positions of Popper (1962) and Bartley (1987). Popper noted that all people develop hypotheses. Preconceived hypotheses distort the data that people collect and lead to confirmatory biases. As humans, we cannot stop ourselves from forming hypotheses, or from remembering data that fit them.

This renders objectivity in inductive reasoning an impossibility. The solution is to acknowledge our hypotheses and attempt to falsify them. Popper maintained that knowledge accumulates quickest when people deduce predictions from their hypotheses and attempt to disprove them. REBT recommends that we personally adopt the Popper model of falsifiablity for our emotional health and as professional therapists to help our clients. Bartley's epistemology of *comprehensive critical rationalism* adds that people should use not only empirical falsifiablity tests of their ideas but also any other argument they can muster to disprove their thinking. Following Bartley, Ellis believes that it is best to apply all means to challenge one's thinking as a theorist, a therapist, and an individual.

Ellis's philosophy contains elements of *constructivism*. Specifically, Ellis maintained that all humans create ideas of how the world is or ought to be. Ellis built his theory on Kelly's (1955) *The Psychology of Personal Constructs*. Accordingly, Ellis thought that people make up many of their beliefs. This explains why he abandoned searching for insights from the memories of clients' experiences or testing the veracity of automatic thoughts of past events. All these ideas could have been made up.

REBT proponents differ from postmodernist philosophers and contructivist cognitive therapists such as Mahoney (1974) and Neimeyer (1993) in two ways. First, these constructivist therapists believe that the sole criterion to assess beliefs is their utility or viability. Empirical reality is not a criterion. The extreme constructivists maintain that there is no knowable reality. REBT posits that empirical reality is an important criterion, and that one needs to assess the empirical veracity of one's beliefs, along with their utility and logical consistency. Second, constructivists believe that therapists should help clients examine the viability of their ideas. They should not provide alternative beliefs for clients, but should allow clients to develop alternatives on their own. As a philosophy of life, REBT posits that some rational alternative beliefs promote emotional adjustment. Learning though self-discovery is valued in REBT, but if the client fails to generate alternative beliefs, we offer alternatives and help them to assess the veracity and viability of these alternatives.

The values of the REBT philosophy of life that are posited to promote emotional adjustment and mental health appear in Table 4.1.

PHILOSOPHICAL AND THEORETICAL UNDERPINNINGS

REBT Theory of Psychopathology

REBT assumptions about psychopathology and psychotherapeutic change can be summarized in the six principles below. Cognitions or beliefs are the most proximate and identifiable cause of human disturbance. Irrational,

TABLE 4.1. REBT Values Thought to Promote Emotional Adjustment

Self-acceptance. Healthy people choose to accept themselves unconditionally rather than measure themselves, rate themselves.

Risk taking. Emotionally healthy people take risks and have a spirit of adventurousness in trying to do what they want, without being foolhardy.

Nonutopian. We are unlikely to get everything we want or to avoid all that we find painful. Healthy people do not strive for the unattainable or for unrealistic perfection.

High frustration tolerance. Healthy people recognize that they are likely to encounter only two sorts of problems: those they can and cannot do something about. Once this discrimination has been made, the goal is to modify those obnoxious conditions they can change, and accept those they cannot change.

Self-responsibility for disturbance. Healthy individuals accept a good deal of responsibility for their own thoughts, feelings, and behaviors.

Self-interest. Emotionally healthy people tend to put their interests at least a little above the interests of others. They sacrifice themselves to some degree for those for whom they care, but not completely.

Social interest. Most people choose to live in social groups. To do so comfortably and happily, they would be wise to act morally, protect the rights of others, and aid in the survival of the society in which they live.

Self-direction. Healthy people cooperate with others, but it is better that they assume primary responsibility for their own lives rather than demand or need considerable support or nurturance from others.

Tolerance. It is helpful to allow humans (the self and others) the right to be wrong. It is not necessary to damn the human for mistakes and failures.

Flexibility. Healthy individuals tend to be flexible thinkers. Rigid, bigoted, and invariant rules tend to minimize happiness.

Acceptance of uncertainty. We live in a world of probability and chance; absolute certainties probably do not exist. The healthy individual strives for order but does not demand certainty.

Commitment. Most people tend to be happier when vitally absorbed in something outside themselves. Strong creative interests and some important human involvement seem to provide structure for a happy daily existence.

---

illogical, and antiempirical beliefs lead to emotional disturbance. Rational beliefs lead to emotional adjustment and mental health. The most efficient strategy to change humans' emotional disturbance is to change their thinking. Humans have a biological predisposition to think irrationally and to become upset. Culture and family teach people the specific issues about which they will make themselves upset. Both nature and nurture influence how and whether people develop emotional disturbance. People remain upset because they rehearse their irrational beliefs and reindoctrinate themselves. Change is difficult, and people change only with repeated attempts to challenge their irrational thoughts and to rehearse new, rational thoughts. The sections below expand on these principles.

Adaptive and Maladaptive Emotions

REBT distinguishes between disturbed, dysfunctional emotions and normal motivating, albeit negative, emotions. Negative emotions are not evidence of psychopathology. If one experiences an activating event (A) and thinks irrationally (B), one will experience a disturbed emotion, such as anxiety, anger, or depression (C). If one then challenges this irrational belief, replacing it with a rational belief (a new B) a new emotional consequence (the new C) will emerge. If the unpleasant activating event is still present (and it usually is in our clients' lives), then it would be inappropriate to expect the person to feel good or even neutral after achieving cognitive change. What does one feel if the intervention is successful and one thinks rationally? The answer is a negative, nondisturbed, motivating emotion.

Most psychotherapies conceptualize therapeutic improvement as a quantitative shift in the emotion. Often therapists ask clients to rate their emotion on the SUDs (subjective units of discomfort) scale developed by Wolpe (1990), or on a self-report measure of a disturbed emotional state. Therapy is successful if the SUDs rating or the rating scale demonstrates less of the emotion or a lower score. According to this model, emotions differ along a continuum of their intensity of physiological arousal and phenomenological experience.

Ellis (1994; Ellis & DiGiuseppe, 1993) proposed that emotions have two continua, one for the disturbed emotion and another for nondisturbed emotion. When people think rational thoughts they actually experience a qualitatively different emotion that can differ in strength. The emotions generated by rational thoughts remain in the same family of emotions as the disturbed emotion. However, they differ in many aspects, such as phenomenological experience, social expression, problem-solving flexibility, and the behaviors they generate. Ellis posited that although irrational thinking leads to anxiety, depression, or anger, rational thinking will lead to concern, sadness, and annoyance, respectively. According to REBT (Walen, DiGiuseppe, & Dryden, 1992), clients can learn adaptive emotional scripts, and not just how to change the intensity of their feelings. As a result, therapists use words carefully to describe adaptive/functional emotions and to help clients choose which emotions they might feel in place of the disturbed emotion.

A good example of this principle might be Dr. Martin Luther King Jr.'s emotional response to racism. Dr. King had an *intense* but adaptive emotional reaction to racism. His intense emotion led to commitment, high frustration tolerance, problem solving, and goal-directed behavior. If he had encountered a psychotherapist who wished to help him experience a less intense emotion, would the world be a better place?

Recently Dryden (2008) suggested that perhaps there is some truth to both the traditional model of intense disturbed emotions and the REBT notion of two separate levels of emotional intensity. He noted that very intense emotions may cause cognitive constriction, reduce our ability to conceive of adaptive reactions, and leads to bodily harm. Perhaps a functional/adaptive emotion can only be so strong before the emotional arousal tips it into causing dysfunctional reactions. In Dryden's new model, intensity has a role in explaining disturbed emotions. However, disturbed emotions can vary substantially in intensity and still be defined as disturbed. Figure 4.1 displays the tradition model of emotions, Ellis's theory, and Dryden's proposed revision.

REBT theory posits that irrational beliefs lead to disturbed emotions, whereas rational beliefs lead to functional beliefs. Irrational beliefs lead to all disturbed emotions, including depression, anxiety, shame, and disturbed anger. Ellis's theory had not clearly defined how the combination of an activating event and an irrational belief could lead to such diverse disturbed emotions. David, Schnur, and Belloiu (2002) solved this problem. They suggested that the types of appraisals identified by Lazarus (1991) determine whether a person experiences an emotion in the depression/sadness, anxiety/concern, or anger/annoyance families, whereas the presence of irrational or rational beliefs determines whether the emotion is a disturbed or functional variant of that affective family.

Cognitive Mechanisms of Disturbance

Irrational beliefs were originally conceptualized as independent from the constructs of other cognitive theories because they were more evaluative in nature (Walen, DiGiuseppe, & Dryden, 1992). This distinction failed because some of Ellis's original irrational beliefs are factual errors. Irrational beliefs have the same characteristics as rigid, inaccurate schemas (DiGiuseppe, 1986, 1996; Ellis, 1994; Szentagotai et al., 2005). It may be more accurate to call them irrational schemas than to call them irrational

- Wolpe's SUDS/Traditional Model
    Functional   0-------------------100 Dysfunctional
- REBT Model
    Functional   0------------------100
    Dysfunctional 0------------------100
- Dryden's Revised REBT Model
    Functional   0------------------75 Actual Arousal
                   0------------------100 Phenomenological Experience
    Dysfunctional 0------------------75 Actual Arousal
                   0------------------100 Phenomenological Experience

FIGURE 4.1. Models of emotional arousal.

beliefs. REBT construes irrational beliefs as *tacit, unconscious,* broad-based schemas that operate on many levels. Rational/irrational schemas are sets of expectations about the way the world is and ought to be, and what is good or bad about what is and ought to be. Schemas help people organize their world by influencing (1) the information to which persons attend, (2) the perceptions that persons are likely to draw from sensory data, (3) the inferences or automatic thoughts that persons are likely to conclude from the data they perceive, (4) people's belief in their ability to complete tasks, (5) the evaluations people make of the actual or perceived world, and (6) the solutions that people are likely to conceive to solve problems.

Irrational beliefs/schemas influence other hypothetical cognitive constructs mentioned in other forms of CBT. Figure 4.2 demonstrates how irrational beliefs relate to other cognitive constructs and emotional disturbance. The model suggests that interventions aimed at the level of irrational beliefs/schemas will change other types of cognitions, as well as emotional disturbance; and that interventions aimed at other cognitive processes may, but do not necessarily, influence the irrational schema.

Originally, Ellis (1962/1994) identified 13 different irrational beliefs. According to current REBT theory, four types of irrational thinking lead to emotional disturbance: demandingness, awfulizing, frustration intolerance, and global condemnation of human worth. Maultsby (1975), one of Ellis's earliest students, defined three criteria for irrational beliefs. To be irrational, a belief is illogical, inconsistent with empirical reality, or inconsistent with accomplishing one's long-term goals. These are similar criteria to those that

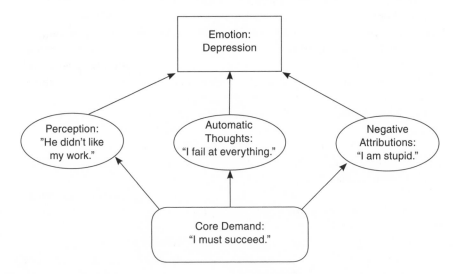

FIGURE 4.2. Irrational beliefs, other cognitions, and emotions.

Thomas Kuhn (1996), the historian of science, proposes scientists use to evaluate theories: logical consistency, empirical predictability, and heuristic or functional value. Ellis (1994) has revised his theory several times and now maintains that *demandingness,* or absolutistic, rigid adherence to an idea, is the core of disturbance and that the other types of irrational thinking are less important, and are psychologically deduced from or created from irrational demandingness. Below, I present each irrational belief and what makes it irrational.

Demandingness

REBT makes the distinction between preferences and demands. Preferences are neither rational nor irrational. They just are. Therapists do not attempt to change a person's "wants." REBT posits that no desire is a sign of pathology or normality. People's desires do not cause disturbance. However, when people insist that their preferences are reality, they become disturbed. However, how and why does demandingness lead to disturbance?

People construct schemas concerning the reality they encounter. Research has demonstrated that when people experience a discrepancy between their schema of the world and reality, they experience emotional arousal. We detect information that is inconsistent with our expectations. We call this the *reality–expectation discrepancy.* When people perceive this discrepancy, they attempt to resolve it. Piaget (1963) noted that people resolve this discrepancy by either assimilation or accommodation. A well-adjusted person becomes motivated by this emotional arousal and seeks out further information to revise his or her schema of the world. This is *accommodation. Assimilation* involves maintaining the schema in spite of the discordant information and changing the perception to keep the schema. The expectancy is maintained despite evidence that it is false. In science and in our personal lives, people do not change beliefs for every inconsistency that arises. However, when significant and substantial discrepancies exist, it may be best to change one's thoughts. REBT maintains that it is rigidity and a failure to change schemas, no matter what the evidence, that causes human disturbance. Thus, demandingness causes disturbance because people use assimilation to cope with the expectancy–reality discrepancy. This rigid attempt at assimilation results in the same expectation and the continued perception of a discrepancy between what people perceive and what they expect. This discrepancy continues to arouse emotions and a sense of frustration or threat.

For example, a man might tell himself, "My wife must always show me affection." Not only does he want his spouse to do as he desires, but he believes that because he wants it, his spouse must comply. He may be shocked when his wife behaves coolly toward him when he is hostile and inconsiderate, and he may continue to be hostile and inconsiderate despite all the feedback that his spouse provides. In addition, he may conclude, "Since she must behave affectionately toward me, I cannot stand it if she does not" or alternatively, "It is terrible and awful if my wife does not behave affectionately."

Ellis (1994) has identified English words such as *should, ought, must,* and *have to* as representing the demandingness. These words have several meanings in the *Oxford English Dictionary* (2008). One set of meanings concerns activities or things that are preferable, desirable, or beneficial. A second set of definitions identifies "shoulds" as the first premise in a conditional syllogism. If you want *X*, you should do *Y*. The third meaning refers to some reality (e.g., if you let go of the pen, it must drop down to the desk). In English, we use the same words to represent desirable events and reality. General semantics theory, which Ellis claimed as a basis for REBT, posits that humans become confused and dysfunctional when they use words imprecisely. This is most likely to occur when using a word with several meanings. Thus, people make preference into laws of physics.

Each year, professionals from around the world come to the Albert Ellis Institute for professional training. Over the last decade, I have asked colleagues from other countries whether their languages similarly use the same words for *should, ought, must,* and *have to* for preferences and realities. I have received affirmative responses from professionals speaking Arabic, Chinese, Croatian, Dutch, French, German, Hindi, Hungarian, Italian, Polish, Portuguese, Romanian, Russian, Serbian, Spanish, Thai, Ukrainian, Urdu, and Vietnamese. Humans all over the globe confuse preferences and reality, and use similar words such as *should, ought, must,* and *have to* in their languages to represent or confuse these two concepts.

Once people understand the irrationality of demandingness, we say that they "accept reality." The concept of acceptance has become popular in the therapy literature. A PsycINFO search for the word *acceptance* in the title of publications when psychotherapy appears in the abstract, produces some interesting results. Articles with the word *acceptance* appeared rarely before 1985. A large increase occurred in the 1990, and another jump occurred after 2000. Many of these publications have resulted from the recent popularity of Hayes's (2004) acceptance and commitment therapy (ACT). The word *acceptance* also appears often in articles about dialectical behavior therapy (DBT). Although some differences exist in Ellis' conceptualization of acceptance compared with the way ACT (Ciarrochi, Robb, & Godsell, 2005) and DBT (Robins & Chapman, 2004) conceptualize acceptance, these differences are small and reflect a clear influence of Ellis's ideas of acceptance in modern psychotherapy.

Awfulizing

Awfulizing is characterized by exaggerated negative evaluations and thoughts about oneself, others, or the world. It is represented in English by the words *terrible, awful,* or *catastrophic.* One might say, "It is awful if I do not have the approval of everyone around me." Rorer (1989) suggested that when people hold such a belief, they are unable to define just what *awful* or *terrible* is, or what catastrophe will occur. They are uncertain of the outcome and define it as extremely bad. Rorer believes awfulizing is definitional. People arbitrarily assign an extremely negative valence to an event and never test reality to see whether the occurrence of the event brings such dire consequences. The empirical argument against awfulizing thinking is best summarized by Mark Twain, who said, "I have survived many a catastrophe that never occurred." Rational thinking would allow one to acknowledge that some things are bad but stress that they are survivable.

Challenging awfulizing beliefs can lead to an alliance rupture, because the client may erroneously conclude from therapist comments that the therapist does not understand or empathize. Clients who have experienced trauma are particularly sensitive to feeling invalidated when therapists challenge such ideas. It is best to target these thoughts when the stimulus evaluation is extreme, not a belief concerning a real trauma.

Frustration Intolerance

Ellis (2005a, 2005b) originally called this type of irrational belief *low frustration tolerance,* or LFT. Such beliefs imply that an individual cannot stand something he or she finds frustrating, or that the individual does not have the endurance to survive in its presence. For example, someone who has many e-mails in his or her inbox might say, "I cannot stand having to respond to all these people. It is too hard to have all this work to do." These beliefs are illogical because, short of dying, one has actually tolerated whatever one claims one cannot stand. The term *frustration intolerance* appears more appropriate than Ellis's term LFT. The Australian psychologist Marie Joyce pointed out that the term LFT can invalidate clients' difficulties. In working with parents of neurologically disabled children, Joyce found that the parents had difficulty following behavior management plans. They often complained that the strategies were too hard. They could not stand being so consistent with their children when they misbehaved. When Joyce challenged the parents' LFT, they felt misunderstood. Joyce admitted that these parents had more difficulty raising their children than did most other parents. In fact, they had been tolerating more frustration than most parents had. The problem was not that the parents had LFT, but that they did not have sufficient frustration tolerance to accomplish a most difficult goal.

They needed to have greater frustration tolerance than the average parent to get their children to behave better. Joyce suggests that REBT change the name of this type of irrationality to *frustration intolerance* (FI). It represents the unwillingness to sustain or tolerate the degree of frustration necessary to achieve one's goals. This prevents therapists from invalidating the difficulties of people who are intolerant of the frustration needed to accomplish their goals but have experienced more frustration than most people.

Global Condemnation of Human Worth

Global negative evaluations of human worth can result in depression or guilt, if one applies the evaluations to oneself, or in anger and contempt, if one applies the evaluation to another. These beliefs in human worthlessness cannot be true; a person cannot be rated as either good or bad, because people are so complex that it is not possible to be completely good or bad (Ellis, 1994, 2005c). Instead, ratings should be restricted to people's behaviors. It is more logical and certainly healthier simply to state, "I performed poorly on my teaching," instead of saying, in addition, "Therefore, I am a bad person." Ellis's position is a philosophical one. He proposes that people take seriously the Preamble to the U.S. Constitution or the Judeo–Christian religious tradition, both of which state that all persons are created equal, the former by government and the latter by God. REBT tries to teach people to rate their deeds and not themselves. As the proverb goes, "Hate the sin, but love the sinner." Self-evaluations are replaced with what Ellis calls unconditional self-acceptance (USA).

REBT very much opposes programs that attempt to build a person's self-esteem. Self-esteem is a combination of two different cognitive processes. The first is self-efficacy, which is belief in one's own ability to perform a task. An examination of the items on self-esteem scales reveals that many items reflect this type of statement. The second cognitive process is self-evaluation. This involves conclusions about one's worth as a person. Laypeople and psychotherapists often get these two concepts confused and evaluate their worth, or lack of it, based on perceived self-efficacy or lack of it.

Self-esteem interventions either teach people that they are special or good people because they are efficacious, or directly teach people unwarranted self-efficacy. REBT points out two difficulties with such interventions. First, they teach people that they have self-worth because of self-efficacy. This may work for the moment, but what if their skills falter or they are surpassed by their peers? The mental health of people who receive such interventions may be on a roller coaster; they feel good when they perform well, and worthless when they perform badly. Second, self-esteem interventions often teach self-efficacy beyond people's skills. They are likely to collapse emotionally when they can no longer receive feedback that they are effective. Third, self-esteem programs fail to provide coping strategies for poor performance. Because most people fail some of the time on the way to success, or fail more often than they succeed, people need to cope with doing poorly. Thus, REBT works at self-acceptance.

Primary versus Secondary Disturbance

REBT posits that irrational beliefs can yield two types of disturbances. Primary emotional–behavioral disturbance arises from irrational beliefs about concrete activating events. Secondary emotional disturbance is the result of irrational beliefs about one's primary emotional–behavioral disturbance; that is, the emotional consequence of a primary ABC becomes an activating event for a new ABC. Because people reflect on their own cognitions, emotions, and behaviors, irrational beliefs about their own thoughts, feelings, and actions often lead to secondary emotional disturbance. People can get depressed about being depressed, anxious about their anxiety, and angry with themselves for getting angry. Secondary emotional disturbance maintains or escalates the disturbed state. Considerable research supports the importance of this secondary emotional disturbance in the area of anxiety disorders, especially panic disorder.

When a client presents with secondary disturbance, the theory posits that the therapists should intervene at the level of the secondary disturbance first, and that interventions aimed at the primary disturbance usually fail. When people think about how they upset themselves or the strategies they can use to overcome their primary disturbance, they elicit their catastrophic thinking or FI about that emotion and escalate it into secondary disturbance. REBT suggests that therapists treat the secondary disturbance first, and when finished, then treat the primary disturbance (Dryden, DiGiuseppe, & Neenan, 2003; Ellis & Dryden, 1997; Walen, DiGiuseppe, & Dryden, 1992).

Several other therapists have come to similar conclusions and recommend that clients learn to tolerate their emotional disturbance as a means of preventing further escalation of their problems (Hayes, Strosahl, & Wilson, 1999; Jacobson, 1992). Barlow (1991) has stated that all emotional disorders may be secondary disturbance. He believes that people often produce secondary disturbance after they experience nondisturbed emotions because of FI over experiencing the nondisturbed emotions.

The Therapeutic Model

Practical versus Emotional Solutions

REBT makes a distinction between practical and emotional solutions (Ellis, 1994; Walen et al., 1992). A *practical solution* involves a problem-solving or skills development approach that helps the client change the activating event. An *emotional solution* attempts to change the client's emotional reaction to the activating event. Practical solutions try to change the A's; emotional solutions try to change the C's. REBT recommends that therapists seek an emotional solution first, for reasons that were apparent in the preceding section. Often there are not practical solutions, and clients must "bite the bullet" and learn to cope with harsh realities. Clients are more likely to learn problem-solving and behavioral skills after they have calmed down.

Some therapists misinterpret the REBT strategy of working on the emotional solution first to mean that REBT only attends to the emotional solution. They think that helping clients achieve the practical solution is selling out the Stoic philosophical roots of REBT. However, a goal of REBT is to help clients lead happier lives. People can accomplish this best if they can tolerate and handle hassles. It is not consistent with the theory that people should tolerate frustration when it is unnecessary. Helping clients change their A's is an acceptable goal of therapy. However, REBT recommends that this intervention be done after an emotional solution, in case no practical solution exists, and because clients are better able to pursue practical solutions when they remove their emotional disturbance.

Philosophical/Elegant versus Inelegant Solutions

According to REBT, therapists best achieve emotional solutions by changing clients' core irrational beliefs instead of changing their perceptions or automatic thoughts. Ellis refers to interventions aimed at irrational beliefs as *the elegant solution*. Ellis considers the philosophical/elegant solution preferable, because it provides a coping strategy that clients can use in a wide variety of possibly negative activating events. Philosophical solutions are thought to promote more generalizable change across a wider array of situations.

REBT recommends that therapists avoid interventions focused on changing perception through reattribution or reframing, or correcting negative automatic thoughts. Ellis calls such interventions *inelegant*. They are considered inelegant because they do not require a major philosophical change, and they provide a coping strategy for a particular activating event, but not for a wide range of situations. Also, the reattribution, reframing, and changing of the automatic thought may be inconsistent with reality; that is, clients' perceptions and inferences about reality may be accurate.

Six Insights into the Change Process

Rational-emotive behavioral theory identifies six basic insights into the human change process. Cognitions or beliefs are the most proximate and identifiable cause of human disturbance. Irrational, illogical, and antiempirical beliefs lead to emotional disturbance. Rational beliefs lead to emotional adjustment and mental health. The best way to change our emotional disturbance is to change our thinking. Although nature and nurture influence how and whether people develop emotional disturbance, the reason people stay upset is because they rehearse their irrational beliefs and reindoctrinate themselves with what they were taught. Change is difficult, and people change only with repeated efforts to challenge their dysfunctional thoughts and rehearse new, rational, adaptive modes of thinking. One could add that according to REBT, beliefs are influences by many factors, including verbal discussion and challenge to their logic, empirical correctness, and functionality. People can learn new rational beliefs through psychoeducational teaching, reading, Socratic discussion, and modeling of the thoughts of others. People can rehearse new, rational beliefs by reciting verbal self-statements, rehearsing imaginal scenes of the activating event and pairing the new belief with an adaptive or a new behavior. Acting against irrational beliefs not only helps to strengthen the new behavior but also undermines the irrational belief and supports the new, rational belief.

In the process of REBT, therapist tasks include the following:

1. Establish a therapeutic alliance with the client, including an agreement on the goals of therapy.
2. Identify the client's activating events and dysfunctional emotions.
3. Identify the client's maladaptive cognitions (the demands and the derivatives).
4. Actively and persuasively challenge the client's maladaptive/irrational cognitions.
5. Help the client formulate alternative adaptive/rational beliefs to replace maladaptive/irrational beliefs.
6. Provide the client practice by actively challenging his or her maladaptive cognitions and rehearsing the new alternative adaptive/rational beliefs through readings, rehearsal, and imagery.
7. Collaborate with the client to design homework that helps him or her identify, evaluate, and/or challenge and replace maladaptive cognitions and behave in ways inconsistent with the disturbance.

More details of the therapeutic process are discussed below.

EMPIRICAL EVIDENCE

Several areas of research are relevant to support rational-emotive behavior theory. The first hypothesis is that irrational beliefs correlate with or predict psychopathology. Several scales have been constructed to assess irrational beliefs and many attempts have been made to relate these to measures of psychopathology. Overwhelmingly, hundreds of studies of this type have been consistent with Ellis's theory (see David, Freeman, & DiGiuseppe, 2009). Irrational beliefs have been associated with concepts of emotional disturbance, such as depression (Macavei, 2005), which is also measured by self-report and physiological measures of inflammation process among apparently healthy individuals (Papageorgiou et al., 2006). The majority of research in this area assesses irrational beliefs by self-report questionnaire. However, these scales often do not include the same subscales. This makes for difficulty in making comparisons across studies and promotes confusion over what the theory espouses. Although the theory has identified irrational beliefs as tacit cognitions that are often outside of awareness, most researchers continue to rely on self-report assessment strategies, which may not be best for accessing tacit cognitions. Other strategies that are better designed to access tacit thoughts, such as the Articulated Thoughts in Simulated Situations procedure, have also found a clear relationship between irrational beliefs and disturbance (Eckhard & Jamison, 2002).

An important REBT hypothesis states that functional and dysfunctional emotions can be discriminated in research, rational beliefs lead to functional beliefs, and irrational beliefs lead to dysfunctional emotions. Several studies exploring this hypothesis have demonstrated that endorsement of rational beliefs triggers what Ellis termed *adaptive/functional emotions*, and that irrational beliefs trigger disturbed emotions (David et al., 2002; David, Schnur, & Birk, 2004; David, Montgomery, Macavei, & Bovbjerg, 2005).

REBT hypothesizes that demandingness is the core of human disturbance. This centrality has led to several hypotheses. The first is that demandingness is the cause of other irrational beliefs, such as FI, self-denigration, and awfulizing. Few studies have attempted to test this hypothesis. If this were true, we might expect that demandingness would emerge first on exploratory factor analyses of irrational belief scales. One would also then expect that other irrational beliefs would mediate the effect of demandingness on measures of disturbance. Finally, one might expect structural equation modeling to find that in the best-fitting model, demandingness would lead to all other irrational beliefs, and that these other beliefs would have an effect on disturbance. No research has tested Ellis's hypothesis on the centrality of demandingness in these ways. Thus, we do not know whether demandingness is the most central irrational belief.

If this is true, irrational beliefs should account for more variance in disturbance than other cognitive variables or effect disturbance through automatic thoughts and other construct developed by other forms of CBT. Although irrational beliefs have a direct effect on disturbance, they may also have an effect by causing or activating these other cognitive constructs. Very little research has appeared in this area. However, some research has identified irrational beliefs as playing such a role in constructs of cognitive content and on a measure of cognitive process. Szentagotai and Freeman (2007) found that the effects of irrational beliefs on distress are partially mediated by automatic thoughts. Thus, irrational beliefs lead to the automatic thoughts that lead to emotional distress. The process of thought suppression has been shown to affect emotional disturbance. Szentagotai (2006) showed with mediational analysis that the impact of irrational beliefs on distress is completely mediated by thought suppression. Irrational beliefs did not mediate the effects of thought suppression. Once irrational beliefs are triggered, thought suppression may intervene as a way of controlling unwanted/intrusive thoughts and emotions, thus mediating the impact of irrational beliefs on distress. It is easy to imagine that a high level of irrational beliefs (e.g., expressed as "I cannot stand ...," " "This is awful,") may lead to thought suppression. These results, along with other research findings in the literature, support the REBT hypothesis that the primary appraisal mechanism in distress is based on irrational beliefs, which might mediate the impact of a stressful event on distress (Montgomery, David, DiLorenzo, & Schnur, 2007).

Most important is research supporting the efficacy and effectiveness of REBT. In one of the first comparative reviews of the effectiveness of psychotherapy, Smith and Glass (1977) concluded that rational-emotive therapy (as it was called then) was the second most effective psychotherapy, after systematic desensitization. Since that review, 16 other reviews of REBT outcome literature have appeared, including reviews by DiGiuseppe, Miller, and Trexler (1977), Engels, Garnefski, and Diekstra (1993), González et al. (2004), Gossette and O'Brien, (1992, 1993), Haaga and Davison (1989), Hajzler and Bernard (1990), Jorm (1989), Lyons and Woods (1991), Mahoney (1991), McGovern and Silverman (1984), Oei, Hansen, and Miller (1993), Polder (1986), Tripp, Vernon, and McMahon (2007), Silverman, McCarthy, and McGovern (1992), and Zettle and Hayes (1980). Most of these have been narrative reviews; four have been meta-analyses (i.e., Engels et al., 1993; Lyons & Woods, 1991; Polder, 1986; Tripp et al. (2007). Most have included studies of adults and children. Others have focused only on adults (Gossette & O'Brien, 1992; Zettle & Hayes, 1980), and three have focused only on research with children and adolescents (González et al., 2004; Gossette & O'Brien, 1993; Hajzler & Bernard, 1990; Tripp et al. (2007). Most reviewers included both articles published in peer-reviewed journals and unpublished dissertations. Others have included a majority of unpublished dissertations in their review (Gossette & O'Brien, 1992, 1993).

More than 280 studies appear these 16 reviews. However, the reviewers rarely included the same studies. Only 13 studies were mentioned in five reviews, three studies were included in six reviews, and 124 studies were mentioned in just one review. Reviewers had very low agreement on which studies they included when they covered the same period, type of study, or type of population. Most of the reviews ignored, excluded, or failed to uncover a sizable number of studies from the period they selected. The most inclusive reviews were the two by Silverman and colleagues (McGovern & Silverman, 1984; Silverman et al., 1992).

Because of the uneven coverage in these reviews, Terjesen, Esposito, Ford, and DiGiuseppe (2008) have attempted a more exhaustive search of the REBT outcome literature. So far, we have uncovered more than 430 studies. We have begun a meta-analytic review and have coded the studies on various characteristics and calculated effect sizes. The final data analysis is not yet complete. The list of studies is available on the Web (Terjesen et al., 2008).

The number of studies supporting the efficacy and effectiveness of REBT is substantial. However, many problems exist with this group of studies. Many were done as dissertations by authors who produced one study. As a result, very few studies were by researchers with sustained progressive research programs that expand our knowledge of REBT. Many of the studies are old and were done before the field developed the present methodological standards for efficacy studies. Many of the studies have substantial methodological flaws. Many selected the participants by scores above a specified cutoff rate and meeting criteria for diagnostic disorders. Despite these flaws, this large number of studies represents strong support for the effectiveness of REBT across a large number of samples with many diverse problems, including anxiety, depression, difficulty with public speaking, substance abuse, anger, conduct problems, and stuttering.

The best test of a psychotherapy is not comparison to placebo or to no-treatment control conditions but to the most efficacious treatments of the specific disorder. David, Lupu, Cosman, and Szentagotai (2009) conducted a randomized clinical trial to compare the efficacy of REBT and two well-established treatments for depression: cognitive therapy and pharmacotherapy with a selective serotonin reuptake inhibitor (SSRI; fluoxetine) in the treatment of patients diagnosed with major depressive disorder. Patients were randomly assigned to 14 weeks of REBT, 14 weeks of cognitive therapy (CT), or 14 weeks of pharmacotherapy. Results indicated that there were no differences among treatment conditions at posttest. A larger effect of REBT (significant) and CT (nonsignificant) over pharmacotherapy at 6-month follow-up was noted on the Hamilton Depression Rating Scale but not the Beck Depression Inventory. This well-controlled methodologically sophisticated study clearly demonstrates that REBT is as efficacious as the better research interventions for depression. Similar comparisons of REBT with established treatments for anxiety have shown REBT to be equal or superior to standard behavioral treatments of anxiety (Terjesen et al., 2008). Overall, considerable research supports the basic tenets of REBT and its effectiveness.

CLINICAL PRACTICE

The 13 Steps of REBT

Dryden et al. (2003) identified 13 steps that normally occur in a REBT psychotherapy session. They developed these steps by working closely with Ellis and reviewing their own and Ellis's advice to trainees in supervision. Therapists new to REBT could follow these steps to avoid mistakes and ensure that they practiced the crucial aspects of the model. Some trainees keep a checklist to remind them of the steps and to guide them through a session. Figure 4.3 presents the 13 steps in a session note format that can be used to record the specific information revealed at each step.

Step 1 is to ask clients what problems they want to discuss in the session. Sometimes clients present problems that are unrelated to topics discussed in previous sessions, but mostly they present examples of the primary referral problem. Knowing what the client wishes to discuss in the session helps to establish agreement on the goals of the session and maintain the therapeutic alliance. Step 2 is to agree formally on the goal of the session. Clients may present entirely new issues, unrelated to those discussed in previous sessions. Therapists may prefer to continue with ongoing topics before switching to a new topic. As a result, there may not be agreement on what to cover in the session and before continuing. If these events occur, the therapist discusses the pros and cons of pursuing each topic until agreement is reached. In addition, clients often express the goal of the session as changing the A, while therapists see it as changing the C. Because REBT recommends working on emotional problems first, agreement on the goals aspect of the therapeutic alliance may break down. A consensus on what problem to tackle is crucial for the session to continue.

Steps 3, 4, and 5 involve assessing the C, assessing the A, and assessing for secondary emotional disturbance, respectively. At Step 6, the therapist teaches the client the B–C connection. Clients often present vague examples of the A. We try to get them to present a specific example of an A. This helps in generating the exact C and B they need to change. We do this by asking them to pick the most upsetting, recent, or prototypical example of an event they can recall.

In Step 7, we assess the client's irrational beliefs. Remember that irrational beliefs are tacit, unconscious, schematic cognitions. They are not experienced in the stream of consciousness, although they can become available to our consciousness. Most therapists ask clients, "What were you thinking

REBT SESSION NOTE AND GUIDE

Client: _____ Session #: _____ Date: _____

Persons Present: _____

Step 1:   Ask the client about the problem.

Step 2:   Define and agree on the goals of therapy.

Step 3:   Assess the emotional and behavioral consequences.

Step 4:   Assess the A.

Step 5:   Assess the existence of any secondary emotional problems.

Step 6:   Teach the B–C connection.

Step 7:   Assess the irrational beliefs.

Step 8:   Connect the irrational beliefs to the disturbed emotions, and connect the rational beliefs to the nondisturbed emotion.

Step 9:   Dispute irrational beliefs: Circle all that you have done: logical, empirical, heuristic, design new rational alternative beliefs, didactic, Socratic, metaphorical, humorous.

Step 10: Prepare your client to deepen his or her conviction in the rational belief.

Step 11: Encourage your client to put new learning into practice with homework.

Step 12: Check homework assignments.

Step 13: Facilitate the working-through process.

FIGURE 4.3. The 13 steps of rational-emotive behavior therapy in session note format.

when you got upset?" Such questions elicit automatic thoughts but not irrational beliefs. DiGiuseppe (1991a) suggests that there are two primary strategies to assess irrational beliefs. The first is inference chaining. Automatic thoughts are inferences that people draw from the perceptions they make and are prepared to make based on the core schema or irrational beliefs they hold. Following the logic of the inferences, one can uncover the core irrational belief. Inference chaining involves a series of follow-up questions to the automatic thoughts. Clients are asked to hypothesize that their automatic thought is true. If it is true, what would happen next, or what would it mean to them? Clients usually respond with other automatic thoughts. The therapist continues with the same type of questions until an irrational belief, a "must," an awfulizing statement, an "I can't stand it," or a global evaluation is uncovered. Inference chains keep clients emotionally aroused, because with each question the therapist gets closer to the real, emotionally triggering event. This strategy also uses a high degree of self-discovery as clients generate the response to each question. Despite the increase in emotional arousal as the therapy proceeds down the inference chain, clients feel relieved to get their core beliefs out in the open. The Eureka! experience at the end of the chain often produces a bonding experience between the therapist and client.

The second primary strategy is based on the awareness that not all clients are capable of putting their tacit schematic irrational beliefs into language, because such thoughts are stored in episodic not verbal memory. DiGiuseppe (1991a) suggests that all therapists develop hypotheses about their clients' irrational beliefs. Rather than let clients struggle to try to become aware of their core irrational beliefs, therapists can offer hypotheses to clients. To do this effectively, therapists should (1) be sure to use suppositional language, (2) ask the client for feedback on the correctness of the hypotheses, (3) be prepared to be wrong, and (4) revise the hypotheses based on the responses of the client. Dryden (2008) has developed another approach. He listens to the client's automatic thoughts, then constructs a rational and an irrational thought that follow from the automatic thought. He presents these to the client and asks him or her to identify which is closest to what he or she is thinking. The client usually identifies the irrational belief. Then they discuss how the client can put that belief into his or her own words.

In Steps 8, the therapist links the irrational beliefs with the client's emotional disturbance and begins disputing the irrational beliefs (Step 9). Disputing irrational beliefs is the most difficult task in REBT. Ellis has always used the term *disputing*. Some therapists object to the term and view it as harsh or adversarial. The point is that therapist and client work at evaluating the truth or falsity of the beliefs. To accomplish this process requires a good therapeutic alliance, with explicit agreement on the goals and tasks of therapy. DiGiuseppe (1991b) has detailed the disputing process after dissecting many hours of Ellis's therapy videotapes. One can dispute an irrational belief by challenging its logic, by testing its empirical accuracy, and by evaluating the functionality of the consequences that follow from holding it. In addition, the therapist needs to propose an alternative rational idea. These rational alternatives are based on the philosophy of REBT. After proposing a rational alternative belief with which the client agrees, the therapist challenges it with the same arguments to assess whether it fares any better.

In addition to adjusting the type of argument, DiGiuseppe (1991b) suggests that a therapist can vary the rhetorical style of his or her disputing. One can use didactic (direct teaching) strategies, Socratic strategies, metaphors, or humor. Kopec, Beal, and DiGiuseppe (1994) have created a grid, with each cell representing a type of argument and a type of rhetorical style. They recommend that therapists generate the disputing statements for each cell in the grid before each therapy session. Their data suggest that this activity increases trainees' self-efficacy in disputing. To learn better disputing techniques, the reader can try this activity for several weeks with several clients. Another important component of disputing is the use of imagery. Therapist and client can construct scenes of the client approaching the activating event and rehearsing the new rational coping statement, experiencing adaptive emotions, and behaving appropriately.

Step 10 in the model involves deepening the client's conviction in his or her rational beliefs. Clients often report that they know the irrational belief is incorrect, but they believe it. The therapist tries to accomplish the client's conviction to not just knowledge of the rational alternative belief. This is accomplished through continued disputing, and by defining how the client would behave differently if he or she actually held the new rational belief (Step 11), and agreeing to actual homework between sessions to achieve the goals (Step 12).

Homework may include having the client complete REBT homework sheets that guide him or her through disputing an irrational belief, the rehearsing of imagery, or engaging in a behavioral activity. In behavior homework, it is important that clients actually confront the A and not practice avoiding it. For example, I recently supervised a therapist treating a client with panic disorder. This client had developed secondary fears of traveling the New York City subway, where he had experienced panic attacks. While riding the subway, the client was flooded with thoughts that he would have a panic attack, look silly, and people would laugh at him, which would be awful. The therapist had the client ride the subway while rehearsing the thoughts that the panic attacks were under control and that he would not look silly. These exercises did not have the desired effect. I suggested that the client actually confront his fears and look silly on the subway. The client agreed that the next time he rode the subway, he would feign a panic attack and, as he said, "look like a sicko." This assignment had him face his fears, and it worked. Ellis usually recommended flooding-type homework assignments and believed that graduated exposure assignments inadvertently taught clients that the emotion associated with exposure was *too* painful to bear.

Step 13, the final step, is to review other examples of activating events about which the client has been upset to promote generalization. The client is encouraged to go through the same steps with other situations to generalize his or her reactions.

Case Illustration

Ray Richie, a 34-year-old European American man, sought therapy for prolonged attachment to an ex-girlfriend and fear of dating. Ray had developed Tourette's syndrome as a youngster. His tics were extremely serious. He recalled peers teasing him throughout junior and senior high school. He was isolated, spit upon, and ridiculed. After years of medications, therapy, and even some hospitalizations, his tics abated when he was in his 20s. He developed obsessive–compulsive disorder (OCD) in his 20s. He had received behavioral treatment for this, which was very successful. Ray repeated some short phrases three or four times when he spoke, mostly when he was nervous or stressed. By all accounts, his tics and obsessions were at a manage-able level, and Ray believed that he could live with them.

Ray had secured a civil service job with the help of his parents, to whom he had remained very close. He had a handful of close friends. At work, he felt accepted, and he was sociable and outgoing. He attended a weekly OCD self-help group. During high school and his early 20s, Ray had not dated. He reported that he believed no woman would ever want him. He had survived his adolescents and being tormented by his peers with an enduring sense of self-loathing and worthlessness. At the age of 25, Ray met a woman named Nancy, with whom he had had his only romantic relation-ship. Although he had loved Nancy, he reported that she had been quite cruel to him. She made him sleep on the floor, ridiculed his tics, and mocked him for his civil service, blue-collar job. Ray reported numerous incidences where Nancy treated him badly. Ray was unable to kiss Nancy, because he had an extreme fear of saliva, which he reported having had since peers had spit at him in high school. He reported that he stayed with Nancy because of his belief that no other woman would have him. Eventually Ray left Nancy when she became physically abusive toward him. He returned to live with his parents and, of course, told them about the abusive relationship with Nancy. After about a year, Ray moved out on his own. When he sought therapy, he had not dated any other women. He reported that at work, social, and community events, he could talk to married women, because he knew he would not date them. He avoided all single women or place where singles would meet. Ray's primary goal was to meet women, date, and, he hoped, marry and have a family.

Ray spent considerable time in therapy discussing his relationship with Nancy and avoiding the topic of meeting women. In an early session, we had identified the A as meeting new women, and the C as fear. Asked what ideas were triggered by the thought of meeting women, Ray said that they would reject him. While using the inference chain technique, I had asked Ray what would happen if all women rejected him. He responded, "Go back to Nancy." Ray secretly desired to rekindle his relationship with Nancy. Despite the abusive way she had treated him, he still loved her and thought that seeing other women would be like cheating on her. I encour-aged him to talk about what it would be like to see her, and what feelings he experienced when entertaining those fantasies.

A flood of emotions emerged. First, Ray felt shame. What would I think of him for still loving Nancy after all the horror stories he had revealed about her? In addition, what did it reveal about him that he could still love someone who had mocked and beaten him? Second, he felt fear. Since leav-ing Nancy, he had recounted the stories of the relationship to his parents. They, of course, thought the worst of her. We immediately went about look-ing at the beliefs he had for each of these emotional issues. I had a choice to make. I could have told Ray that, of course, I accepted him even as he loved Nancy. That would have been the inelegant solution. Therefore, I asked him to imagine the worst. What if even his therapist thought badly of him for continuing to love some who abused him? He had had several good therapists in the past who had helped him with other issues. He was happy with his life except for this one issue, and he would be OK even if he never mastered this issue. I helped him accept himself even the people around him, even me, thought he was foolish.

Next we worked on his shame for still loving Nancy. Ray thought about her regularly. He revealed that he had maintained weekly phone contact with her. He would never see her because he thought that would make him crazy. It appeared that Ray's shame over loving Nancy had prevented him from moving on. Here was a classic example of the secondary emotional problem. Whenever Ray thought of Nancy, he triggered thoughts about how sick and worthless he was for loving such an abusive person. This interfered with his evaluation of Nancy and their relationship. The shame about the love seemed to make the love continue. So I encouraged Ray to experience his love for Nancy. He reported that although she abused him, he had many good memories of their relations. I helped him accept the fact that he did love her, and that this feeling was real. It was neither good nor bad. It just was. Moreover, if it meant that he had a crazy relationship or a constant unrequited love, so be it. He would accept that and make the best of his life.

Next, Ray revealed that we wished to see Nancy. Now that he accepted loving her, why not act on it? Therefore, we planned his stepping from weekly phone friend to face-to-face romance. Ray was unable to call Nancy to plan a visit. He feared that his parents would reject him. Ray's parents were a major factor in his life. Throughout his ordeal with Tourette's syndrome, they had been exemplary parents. They did everything to love and support Ray when the world had taunted and mocked him. Ray was sure that they would disapprove of his reunion with Nancy. He thought that because they knew all the bad things in his relationship with Nancy, they would turn their back on him because of this self-defeating love.

Here, again, was that choice. From all the information Ray had revealed to me about his parents, which I had no reason to doubt, they were supportive, loving people. I could easily muster sufficient evidence to show that he could count on their continued love and support. However, I chose the elegant solution instead. I asked him to imagine his worst nightmare coming true. Could he imagine his parents rejecting him because he chose to love Nancy, whom they had learned to detest? This aroused strong negative feelings in Ray, and he questioned whether he could become independent of his parents. As we explored his belief that he needed them to lean on, other information was revealed. Ray avoided other things because he feared his parents' disapproval. These ranged from speaking about his choice of politi-cal candidates to sharing some food preferences. What if they knew and disapproved? We also discussed the issue that they had gotten older. They, unfortunately, were mortal and would not live forever. Whether they disap-proved of him now or died later, he would still have to accept living his life without them. Ray finally accepted two new rational philosophies. First, he would be his own person and live life his way, even if significant others, such as his parents and his therapist, disapproved. It was worse to pretend to be someone else, and it was not so awful to be rejected. He had endured a lot of that in his life. He turned his survival of childhood taunting into evidence that he was a strong survivor, not a weakling. Second, Ray recognized that he had to make his own way in the world, and face his parents' eventual death. He accepted that life might involve some risk, and that fear was part of life. To avoid it was to stagnate.

Ray decided he had had enough of the cognitive interventions. Ray decided to act. He met with Nancy. After seeing her several times, he told his parents. Two things happened. Ray's parents said that it was his life and he had to do what made him happy. I was right. They would accept him no matter what. Nevertheless, he felt freer. He loved and appreciated them but did not feel captured by their love. Once Ray concluded that he could live his life even if they disapproved of his actions, he pursued Nancy more ardently. We then switched our attention to two issues. First, was he allowed to love her, even if he found these feeling unacceptable? Second, did he need to have Nancy to have a loving life? He quickly learned to accept his feelings for her. When one needs someone and must have him or her, there is no choice. Once Ray freely accepted his feelings for Nancy and examined whether he needed her, he decided he did not want her. He saw her as demanding, criti-cal, arbitrary, and impossible to please. He decided he did not want her even if he loved her. Within a month of seeing her, Ray's love for her dissipated. I had become, like Irving Yalom (1989), love's executioner.

Ray took a month or so off from therapy. He returned with a renewed effort to work on his fear of women's rejection. Once again, the choice pre-sented itself. Do I teach him better social skills to become a better pursuer of women, or do I help him accept that the path to love is littered with rejections? Again, I chose the latter and worked at helping Ray accumulate rejections. The goal was to reach at least 100 hundred in a year. Following this work, we did discuss the social skills he needed to meet women. After several months, Ray dated a physician. After several dates, he decided that he did not like her. Nevertheless, he was proud that someone with so much more education than he would date him. He started to meet other women. He was on his way. One other thing changed. Since Ray no longer needed his parents' approval, he wanted to give up the security of a civil service job to start his own business. He was sure they would disapprove, but he was going to do it anyway. Of course, they were not happy with his choice, but they supported him. He contacts me once a month. He still has not met the right woman. However, he is having fun accumulating the required 100 rejections.

SUMMARY AND CONCLUSIONS

The death of Albert Ellis deeply affected those who worked to develop REBT and the hundreds of practitioners who knew him well. The question for any theory after the death of its founder is what the theory will become without its most forceful proponent. REBT seems alive and thriving. There has been renewed interested in testing the tenets of the theory and the efficacy of the therapy developed during Ellis's several-year illness leading up to his death. Training in REBT continues to grow the worldwide.

The specific challenges that face REBT are still large. Ellis was primarily a clinician. He often made theoretical statements without the considering the specificity that would be needed to test his notions. The primary research that remains is investigations to tests Ellis's hypothesis that demandingness is the core irrational belief. He proposed that all other irrational beliefs derive from a person's demandingness. Part of this hypothesis is that the cognitive constructs identified in other cognitive models of psychopathology and psychotherapy are psychologically derived from demandingness. According to Ellis's model, demanding ideas then generate other irrational beliefs, such as FI, global evaluations of self- or others' worth, and awfulizing. In addition, demands generate negative automatic thoughts; global, stable, and internal attributions of failure; poor problem solving; and negative self-talk. Let us take an example of a person who recently failed to secure a job after an interview. If the person had the irrational belief that he had to have the job, the failure to attain it would have generated the following: (1) automatic thoughts, such as "I never get what I need," "I will always be a failure," "I cannot do anything right," and "If I cannot get this job, I will be unable to get any job"; (2) ideas that reflect global, stable, and internal attribution for the failure; (3) other irrational beliefs, such as "It's terrible that I did not get this job. This proves that I am a worthless person" or "I cannot stand not having a job"; (4) seeing the situation as hopeless and failing to engage in problem solving to get another job.

As I mentioned earlier, research strategies to test this hypothesis have not been forthcoming. Such a test would require a multivariate study that measures of all these constructs in a large clinical sample. REBT supporters need more studies like this before they can claim Ellis's theory to be sound.

More outcome research is needed to support the efficacy of REBT. Although a large number of studies do support the therapy, the majority were done before modern methodological standards for outcomes studies existed. Such studies need to include clients with diagnosed disorders and be compared to well-established interventions. The real test of REBT involves continued therapy gains, failure to relapse, or the development of happiness and increased well-being after the goals of therapy have been accomplished. Ellis always acknowledged that other forms of CBT work. He even admitted that other, non-CBT forms of psychotherapy work, albeit inefficiently. However, he held that the deep philosophical change of accepting reality and working hard toward achieving one's preferences is the key to adjustment. Testing this idea requires a longitudinal design. People who receive REBT will benefit more in the end. Follow-up designs demonstrating improved outcomes are the true test of Ellis's philosophical model.

Over the years, REBT had been synonymous with Ellis's personality. Some people found his style and directiveness abrasive. Since Ellis's 1959 debate with Carl Rogers on the nature of the therapeutic relationship, people have erroneously concluded that Ellis and REBT place little value on the therapeutic relationship. Recall that Rogers (1957) hypothesized that unconditional acceptance of the client by the therapist is a necessary and sufficient condition of psychotherapeutic change. Ellis (1959) disagreed. He reported that unconditional acceptance was not necessary, and that humans improve under a wide range of conditions. True to his nature, he was against any overgeneralized rule or conclusion. However, he did believe that unconditional acceptance was highly desirable, and that it greatly helped the client trust, like, and respect the therapist, which would greatly enhance the chances of all other therapeutic interventions working.

Ellis had great respect for his clients, and research has demonstrated that REBT as practiced by Ellis and others at his institute, resulted in a strong therapeutic relationship (DiGiuseppe & Leaf, 1993). Recently books and training manuals on REBT have begun to espouse formally the importance of the therapeutic alliance in REBT (Dryden et al., 2003; Ellis & Dryden, 1992). In fact, given the active and directive nature of this form of therapy, failure to attend to the components of the therapeutic relationship would lead to dropout or therapy failure. More research on this aspect of REBT is needed.

Despite these limitations, REBT remains a philosophical form of psychotherapy with deep roots in classic, modern, and Asian philosophy. Ellis spent thousands of hours with suffering clients to derive it. The theory and practice of this form of therapy is general enough to serve as a platform to treat clients presenting with a wide range of disorders and problems. However, the practice of this model is flexible enough to allow the incorporation of other techniques when they have value to help the clients. The philosophical basis, breadth of application, and flexibility of the technique has been and remains the hallmark of REBT.

REFERENCES

Barlow, D. H. (1991). Disorders of emotion. *Psychological Inquiry, 2*(1), 58–71.

Bartley, W. W. (1987). In defense of self-applied critical rationalism. In G. Radnitzky & W. W. Bartley (Eds.), *Evolutionary epistemology, theory of rationality and sociology of knowledge* (pp. 279–312). LaSalle, IL: Open Court.

Ciarrochi, J., Robb, H., & Godsell, C. (2005). Letting a little nonverbal air into the room: Insights from acceptance and commitment therapy: Part 1: Philosophical and theoretical underpinning. *Journal of Rational-Emotive and Cognitive Behavior Therapy, 23*(2), 79–106.

Cook, J. M., Bryyanova, T., & Coyne, J. (2009). Influential figures, authors, and books: An Internet survey of over 2000 psychotherapists. *Psychotherapy: Theory, Research, Practice, Training, 46*(1), 42–51.

Corsini, R. J. (Ed.). (1994). *Encyclopedia of psychology* (2nd ed.). New York: Wiley.

David, D., DiLorenzo, T., & Montgomery, G. H. (in press). Relations between irrational beliefs and response expectancies in predicting anticipatory psychological distress in exam-related situations. A brief research report. *Journal of Rational-Emotive and Cognitive Behavior Therapy.*

David, D., Freeman, A., & DiGiuseppe, R. (2009). Rational and Irrational Beliefs: Implications for psychotherapy. In D. David, S. Lynn, & A. Ellis (Eds.), *Rational and irrational beliefs in human functioning and disturbances*. London: Oxford University Press.

David, D., Lupu, V., Cosman, D., & Szentagotai, A. (2008). Rebt versus cognitive therapy versus medication in the treatment of major depressive disorder: A randomized clinical trial Post-treatment outcomes and six-months follow-up. *Journal of Clinical Psychology.*

David, D., Montgomery, G. H., Macavei, B., & Bovbjerg, D. H. (2005). An empirical investigation of Albert Ellis's binary model of distress. *Journal of Clinical Psychology, 61*(4), 499–516.

David, D., Schnur, J., & Belloiu, A. (2002). Another search for the "hot" cognitions: Appraisal, irrational beliefs, attributions, and their relation to emotions. *Journal of Rational-Emotive and Cognitive-Behavior Therapy, 20,* 94–131.

David, D., Schnur, J., & Birk, J. (2004). Functional and dysfunctional feelings in Ellis' cognitive theory of emotion: An empirical analysis. *Cognition and Emotion, 18*(6), 869–880.

DiGiuseppe, R. (1986). The implications of the philosophy of science for rational emotive theory and therapy. *Psychotherapy, 23*(4), 634–639.

DiGiuseppe, R. (1991a). A rational emotive model of assessment. In M. E. Bernard (Ed.), *Doing rational emotive therapy effectively* (pp. 151–172). New York: Plenum Press.

DiGiuseppe, R. (1991b). Comprehensive disputing in rational emotive therapy. In M. E. Bernard (Ed.), *Doing rational emotive therapy effectively* (pp. 173–195). New York: Plenum Press.

DiGiuseppe, R. (1996). The nature of irrational beliefs: Progress in rational-emotive behavior therapy. *Journal of Rational-Emotive and Cognitive-Behavior Therapy, 14*(1), 5–28.

DiGiuseppe, R., & Leaf, R. (993). The therapeutic relationship in rational-emotive therapy: Some preliminary data. *Journal of Rational-Emotive and Cognitive-Behavior Therapy,* 11(4), 223–233.

DiGiuseppe, R., Miller, N. J., & Trexler, L. D. (1977). A review of rational emotive psychotherapy outcome studies. *The Counseling Psychologist,* 7, 64–72.

Dryden, W. (2008). *Rational emotive behaviour therapy: Distinctive features.* Hove, UK: Routledge.

Dryden, W., DiGiuseppe, R., & Neenan, M. (2003). *A primer on rational-emotive behavioral therapy* (2nd ed.). Champaign, IL: Research Press.

Eckhard, C., & Jamison, T. R. (2002). Articulated thoughts of male dating violence perpetrators during anger arousal. *Cognitive Therapy and Research,* 26(3), 289–308.

Ellis, A. (1933). *Youth against the world: A novel.* Unpublished manuscript. New York: The Albert Ellis Institute.

Ellis, A. (1950). Requisites for research in psychotherapy. *Journal of Clinical Psychology,* 6, 152–156.

Ellis, A. (1955). New approaches to psychotherapy techniques. *Journal of Clinical Psychology,* 11, 207–260.

Ellis, A. (1956). The effectiveness of psychotherapy with individuals who have severe homosexual problems. *Journal of Consulting Psychology,* 20(3), 191–195.

Ellis, A. (1957a). Rational psychotherapy and individual psychology. *Journal of Individual Psychology,* 13, 38–44.

Ellis, A. (1957b). Outcome of employing three techniques of psychotherapy. *Journal of Clinical Psychology,* 13, 344–350.

Ellis, A. (1959). Requisite conditions for basic personality change. *Journal of Consulting Psychology,* 23(6), 538–540.

Ellis, A. (1994). *Reason and emotion in psychotherapy: A comprehensive method of treating human disturbance: Revised and updated.* New York: Birch Lane Press. (Original work published 1962)

Ellis, A. (1999). Why rational-emotive therapy to rational emotive behavior therapy? *Psychotherapy: Theory, Research, Practice and Training,* 36(2), 154–159.

Ellis, A. (2001). The rise of cognitive behavior therapy. In W. T. O'Donohue, D. A. Henderson, S. C. Hayes, J. E. Fisher, L. J. Hayes, & L. J. (Eds.), *A history of the behavioral therapies: Founders' personal histories* (pp. 183–194). Reno, NV: Context Press.

Ellis, A. (2005a). Why I (really) became a therapist. *Journal of Clinical Psychology,* 61(8), 945–948.

Ellis, A. (2005b). Discussion of Christine A. Padesky and Aaron T. Beck, "Science and philosophy: Comparison of cognitive therapy and rational emotive behavior therapy." *Journal of Cognitive Psychotherapy: An International Quarterly,* 19(2), 181–185.

Ellis, A. (2005c). *The myth of self-esteem: How rational emotive behavior therapy can change your life forever.* Amherst, NY: Prometheus Books.

Ellis, A., & DiGiuseppe, R. (1993). Appropriate and inappropriate emotions in rational emotive therapy: A response to Craemer and Fong. *Cognitive Therapy and Research,* 17(5), 471–477.

Ellis, A., & Dryden, W. (1992). *The practice of rational emotive therapy* (2nd ed.). New York: Springer.

Ellis, A., & Harper, R. (1961). *A guide to rational living*. Seacacus, NJ: Lyle Stuart.

Engels, G. I., Garnefski, N., & Diekstra, R. F. W. (1993). Efficacy of rational emotive therapy: A quantitative analysis. *Journal of Consulting and Clinical Psychology, 61*, 1083–1090.

Epictetus. (1996). *The Enchiridion*. Raleigh, NC: Alex Catalogue. Also available as an e-book from *classics.mit.edu/epictetus/epicanth1b.txt*.

Eysenck, H. J. (1952). The effects of psychotherapy: An evaluation. *Journal of Consulting Psychology, 16*(5), 319–324.

González, J., Nelson, J. R., Gutkin, T. B., Saunders, A., Galloway, A., & Shwery, C. S. (2004). Rational emotive therapy with children and adolescents: A meta-analysis. *Journal of Emotional and Behavioral Disorders, 12*(4), 222–235.

Gossette, R. L., & O'Brien, R. M. (1992). The efficacy of rational emotive therapy in adults: Clinical fact or psychometric artifact. *Journal of Behavior Therapy and Experimental Psychiatry, 23*, 9–24.

Gossette, R. L., & O'Brien, R. M. (1993). Efficacy of rational emotive therapy with children: A critical re-appraisal. *Journal of Behavior Therapy and Experimental Psychiatry, 24*, 15–25.

Haaga, D. A., & Davison, G. C. (1989). Outcome studies of rational emotive therapy. In M. E. Bernard & R. DiGiuseppe (Eds.), *Inside rational emotive therapy: A critical appraisal of the theory and therapy of Albert Ellis* (pp. 155–197). San Diego: Academic Press.

Hajzler, D. J., & Bernard, M. E. (1990). A review of rational emotive education outcome studies. *School Psychology Quarterly, 6*, 27–49.

Hayes, S. C. (2004). Acceptance and commitment therapy, relational frame theory, and the third wave of behavioral and cognitive therapies. *Behavior Therapy, 35*(4), 639–665.

Hayes, S. C., Strosahl, K. D., & Wilson, K. G. (1999). *Acceptance and commitment therapy: An experiential approach to behavior change*. New York: Guilford Press.

Jacobson, N. (1992). Behavioral couples therapy: A new beginning. *Behavior Therapy, 23*, 491–506.

Jorm, A. F. (1989). Modifiability of trait anxiety and neuroticism: A meta-analysis of the literature. *Australian and New Zealand Journal of Psychiatry, 23*, 21–29.

Kelly, G. (1955). *The psychology of personal constructs* (Vol. 1). New York: Norton.

Kopec, A. M., Beal, D., & DiGiuseppe, R. (1994). Training in rational emotive therapy: Disputation strategies. *Journal of Rational-Emotive and Cognitive-Behavior Therapy, 12*(2), 47–60.

Kuhn, T. (1996). *The structure of scientific revolutions* (3rd ed.). Chicago: University of Chicago Press.

Lazarus, R. S. (1991). *Emotion and adaptation*. London: Oxford University Press.

Lyons, L. C., & Woods, P. J. (1991). The efficacy of rational emotive therapy: A quantitative review of the outcome research. *Clinical Psychology Review, 11*, 357–369.

Macavei, B. (2005). The role of irrational beliefs in the rational emotive behavior theory of depression. *Journal of Cognitive and Behavioral Psychotherapies,* 5(1), 73–81.

Mahoney, M. (1974). *Cognition and behavior and behavior modification.* Cambridge, MA: Ballinger.

Maultsby, M. C. (1975). *Help yourself to happiness through rational self-counseling.* Oxford, UK: Herman.

McGovern, T. E., & Silverman, M. S. (1984). A review of outcome studies of rational emotive therapy from 1977 to 1982. *Journal of Rational-Emotive Therapy,* 2(1), 7–18.

McMahon, J., & Viterito, J. (2007). LAMP unto our feet: The light of Albert Ellis shines in the work of John Gottman. In E. Velten (Ed.), *Under the influence: Reflections of Albert Ellis in the work of others.* Tucson, AZ: Sharp Press.

Montgomery, G. H., David, D., DiLorenzo, T. A., & Schnur, J. B., (2007). Response expectancies and irrational beliefs predict exam-related distress. *Journal of Rational-Emotive and Cognitive Behavior Therapy,* 25(1), 17–34.

Neimeyer, R. (1993). Constructivistic psychotherapies: Some concepts and strategies. *Journal of Cognitive Psychotherapies,* 7(2), 159–171.

Oei, T. P. S., Hansen, J., & Miller, S. (1993). The empirical status of irrational beliefs in rational-emotive therapy. *Australian Psychologist, 28,* 195–200.

Oxford English Dictionary (2nd ed.). (2008). Oxford, UK: Oxford University Press.

Papageorgiou, C., Panagiotakos, D. B., Pitsavos, C., Tsetsekou, E., Kontoangelos, K., Stefanadis, C., et al. (2006). Association between plasma inflammatory markers and irrational beliefs: The ATTICA epidemiological study. *Progress in Neuro-Psychopharmacology and Biological Psychiatry,* 30(8), 1496–1503.

Piaget, J. (1963). *The origins of intelligence in children.* New York: Norton.

Polder, S. K. (1986). A meta-analysis of cognitive behavior therapy. *Dissertation Abstracts International, B47,* 1736.

Popper, K. (1962). *Conjecture and refutation.* New York: Harper.

Robins, C. J., & Chapman, A. L. (1994). Dialectical behavior therapy: Current status, recent developments, and future directions. *Journal of Personality Disorders,* 18(1), 73–89.

Rogers, C. R. (1957). The necessary and sufficient conditions of therapeutic personality change. *Journal of Consulting Psychology,* 21(2), 95–103.

Rorer, L. (1989). Rational-emotive theory: II. Explication and evaluation. *Cognitive Therapy and Research, 13,* 531–548.

Silverman, M. S., McCarthy, M., & McGovern, T. (1992). A review of outcome studies of rational emotive therapy from 1982–1989. *Journal of Rational-Emotive and Cognitive-Behavior Therapy, 10,* 11–175.

Smith, M. L., & Glass, G. V. (1977). Meta-analysis of psychotherapy outcome studies. *American Psychologist, 32,* 752–760.

Szentagotai, A. (2006). Irrational beliefs, thought suppression and distress—A mediation analysis. *Journal of Cognitive and Behavioral Psychotherapies,* 6(2), 119–127.

Szentagotai, A., & Freeman, A. (2007). An analysis of the relationship between irrational beliefs and automatic thought in predicting distress. *Journal of Cognitive and Behavioral Psychotherapies,* 7(1), 1–9.

Szentagotai, A., Schnur, J., DiGiuseppe, R., Macavei, B., Kallay, E., & David, D. (2005). The organization and the nature of irrational beliefs: Schemas or appraisal? *Journal of Cognitive and Behavioral Psychotherapies, 5*(2), 139–158.

Terjesen, M., Esposito, M., Ford, P., & DiGiuseppe, R. (2008). A meta-analytic review of REBT outcome studies. Manuscript in preparation. A list of the studies used in this review can be found at *www.albertellisinstitute.org/rebtoutcome_studies_bibliography.*

The top 10 most influential therapists. (2007, March/April). *Psychotherapy Networker,* pp. 24–68.

Tripp, S., Vernon, A., & McMahon, J. (2007). Effectiveness of rational-emotive education: A quantitative meta-analytical study. *Journal of Cognitive and Behavioral Psychotherapies, 7*(1), 81–93.

Walen, S., DiGiuseppe, R., & Dryden, W. (1992). *A practitioners' guide to rational-emotive therapy* (2nd ed.). New York: Oxford University Press.

Warren, R. (2007). Modern cognitive-behavioral treatment of anxiety disorders began in 1933. In E. Velten (Ed.), *Under the influence: Reflections of Albert Ellis in the work of others.* Tucson, AZ: Sharp Press.

Wolpe, J. (1961). The prognosis in unpsychoanalysed recovery from neurosis. *American Journal of Psychiatry, 118,* 35–39.

Wolpe, J. (1990). *The practice of behavior therapy.* Needham Heights, MA: Allyn & Bacon.

Yalom, I. (1986). *Love's executioner and other tales of psychotherapy.* New York: Basic Books.

Zettle, R., & Hayes, S. (1980). Conceptual and empirical status of rational emotive therapy. *Progress in Behavior Modification, 9,* 125–166.

CHAPTER 5

Acceptance and Commitment Therapy

Thomas J. Waltz
Steven C. Hayes

[We are like] dwarfs perched on the shoulders of giants.... We
see more and further than our predecessors, not because we have
keener vision or greater height, but because we are lifted up and
borne aloft on their gigantic stature.

—JOHN OF SALISBURY (1159)

INTRODUCTION AND HISTORICAL BACKGROUND

Acceptance and Commitment Therapy (ACT—said as a single word) is a
treatment based on a philosophical tradition that distinguishes this therapy from most other cognitive-behavioral therapies (CBT). All therapeutic
approaches have implicit and explicit assumptions regarding what counts
as an explanation for clinical phenomena. These assumptions guide clinical
practice and the methods of science used to develop and test the treatments
employed in clinical practice. Before describing the more immediate influences on the development of ACT, it is useful to place the approach in its
appropriate historical context.

Brief Review of the Role of Theory in CBT

Early behavior therapy tested the generalizability of learning theories based
on basic animal research (Franks, 1964). The learning theories of this era
attempted to develop a scientifically based collection of principles adequate
for the analysis of all behavior (Leahey, 2004). A variety of learning theo-

ries were developing their own sets of principles and concepts, and there was constant debate between the different approaches. Thus, early behavior therapy was not a single approach but a confederation of applied learning theories. Part of what drew them together was the commitment to scientific evaluation of therapeutic interventions and resistance against empirically weak clinical traditions (Eysenck, 1952). Over time, this commitment weakened an interest in the role of theory, particularly as the pressure to account for more complex phenomena increased. Leaders in behavior therapy began to advocate the abandonment of theory as a guide to clinical practice in favor of using empirically supported techniques independent of their origin, underlying rationale, or theoretical clarity, so long as they produced meaningful behavior change (e.g., Lazarus, 1967).

Today the CBT tradition is primarily united by a devotion "to the relief of human suffering using methods that have been shown to work" (Association for Behavioral and Cognitive Therapies [ABCT], 2007). It has been proposed that the most central identifying feature of CBT is "the high value we place on demonstrating effectiveness of our methods in randomized controlled trials and other controlled studies" (Persons, 2003, p. 225).

While the shift in emphasis was understandable, in the long run it was probably not progressive. The history of science suggests that empiricism alone is not enough for science to progress. The progress of science is dependent on the synergy between theory and empirical observations. Given the decreased emphasis on the role of theory in CBT over the last 50 years, we view this volume as a step in the right direction.

The Importance of Theory and Philosophy for Therapeutic Practice

Philosophy of science refers to the acknowledgment and systematization of those assumptions adopted for analytic purposes. Theory refers to the construction and systematization of concepts that describe events and their interrelationships. Defined this way, theory and philosophy influence therapist behavior either implicitly or explicitly. They influence all aspects of the therapeutic process: how psychological health and distress are characterized, how these are assessed, what course of treatment and what treatment techniques are called for, whether techniques studied for one population are likely to be useful with another, why one abandons the use of one technique to try another, and how to measure outcomes. The ultimate purpose of theory and philosophy is to guide the behavior of the therapist through new territory. Without the guidance of theory, the therapist is in the position of having to apply techniques without guiding principles. Personal experience and intuition have a role in clinical practice, but research has shown that these are not reliable guides for the individual therapist (Dawes, 2000).

Our view is that "the goal of science is the construction of increasingly organized systems of verbal rules that allow analytic goals to be accomplished with precision, scope, and depth, and based on verifiable experience" (Hayes, 2004, p. 36); that is, science codevelops with theories, and these theories have particular characteristics.

"Precision means that a limited number of concepts are relevant to a given phenomenon given a specific analytic goal" (Biglan, 1993, p. 252). Precise theories can effectively guide therapists to assess and address specific problems.

"Scope means that a wide range of phenomena can be analyzed with a limited number of concepts" (Biglan, 1993, p. 252). Theories with scope can effectively guide therapists to apply the theory to new problems or domains, without the need to invoke a separate theory for every new problem encountered. Therapists who can apply a theory with scope and fidelity separate themselves from practitioners who are mere technicians and thus limited in their ability to improvise or be guided by the conceptual relevance of disparate techniques.

Depth means that the various analytic concepts within the theory comport with scientific knowledge developed at other levels of analysis. What is well established at the level of psychology should not contradict what is well known at the level of neurobiology, for example.

Verifiable experience refers to replicable systematic observations. Verifiable theories can specify the means by which therapists can assess (1) the relevance of the theory to particular clients or problem domains, (2) changes in variables the theory posits as important to clinically relevant outcomes, and (3) outcomes deemed important to the theory.

That leaves the key issue of goals, and here the different approaches within psychology differ. Predicting and influencing behavior are at the center of therapeutic practice and these are the primary analytic goals of *functional contextualism*, the philosophy of science underlying ACT (Biglan & Hayes, 1996; Hayes, 1993). In practical terms, they are shared by CBT in general, but some wings of CBT adopt scientific assumptions that test the adequacy of knowledge by the ability of models to correspond with events. This approach puts relatively more importance on prediction: Influence is presumed to flow from adequate knowledge rather than being an essential measure of it. As an applied matter, prediction without influence is of marginal use for reliably improving the human condition. Effective practice relies on both, and a scientific theory that leads to both is of unparalleled value.

Historical Roots

The grand learning theories that influenced the development of CBT had two distinct approaches to science. These different approaches are important, because ACT and some other approaches (Functional-Analytic Psychotherapy; Behavioral Activation; Dialectical Behavior Therapy, to a degree) are based on an approach that is not fully adopted by the rest of CBT. The assumptions of these approaches are sufficiently different that it is impossible to understand ACT without understanding how the assumptions of this approach differ from the rest of CBT. The separation begins with a division in the approach to science called *positivism*, which generally holds that science is limited to objectively quantifiable observable events.

PHILOSOPHICAL AND THEORETICAL UNDERPINNINGS

The Foundations for the Greater CBT Tradition

Positivism was originally an effort to describe the world in mathematical terms. Observations by the senses were quantitatively described (e.g., using standardized measurement), and metaphysical explanations were specifically avoided. Logical positivism developed to take positivism beyond merely describing the world in mathematical terms. From this perspective, the foundations of science remain in objectively quantifiable observations; however, they can also be accompanied by theoretical explanatory terms. Formal rules of logic were used to regulate the relationship between observations and theoretical terms. As this was carried into psychology, theoretical terms were based on operational definitions (Bridgman, 1927) that supposedly described the essential features of sense data (observations), with the goal of allowing scientists to reliably replicate one another's observations. When adequate description was provided, it was hoped that this would allow the truth of theoretical terms to be established through consensus or agreement. Consensus was assumed to mitigate the problems of individual history and context that are implied by a psychological approach to epistemology. In other words, logical criteria for determining truth were prioritized over pragmatism.

Logical positivism and operationism became the tools for most of the behavioral science that forms the foundation for most of present-day CBT. The echo of its influence can be seen in the tradition of calling for "operational" definitions rather than simply "definitions." This practice allowed for any term to be used in science provided that it could be "operationalized." As motivational constructs were "operationalized," these formerly unobservable constructs were equated with descriptions of the operations that were purported to investigate them (e.g., the hunger drive increases as the duration of food deprivation increases). Later, this strategy was employed to include the scientific investigation of theoretical terms related to cognition.

Within psychology, this general strategy is reflected in the stimulus–

mediator–response (S-M-R) approach. *Mediators* are operationalized intervening variables that account for how a stimulus or the external environment causes some response to occur. Researchers typically avoid dualism by conceptualizing their mediators (e.g., drives, cognitions) as ultimately physiological processes (e.g., brain activity), but they are not directly measured at this level. Rather, physiological measures are used to provide an apparent naturalistic basis for inferred events. For example, referring to different levels of neural activation employed in particular "cognitive" tasks allows the researcher to use reaction time data as a measure of inferred cognition. This is a comfortable inference when cognitive processes are considered synonymous with brain processes. The reductionism that is explicit in this approach is not usually disturbing, because S-M-R analyses are most commonly based on the idea that the job of scientific understanding is to model how parts, relations, and forces combine to create complexity. Mediating variables are supposedly simpler elements that cause behavior. Thus, for example, schemas are ultimately brain processes that cause behavior. Successful outcomes are thought to depend on changes in these mediating variables.

The Foundation for ACT

The physicist, mathematician, and philosopher of science Ernst Mach (1838–1916) took positivism in a different direction. "For Mach, complete description is all one can ask of science; any attempt at explanation that goes beyond the bounds of description is to be eschewed as metaphysical" (Smith, 1986, p. 35). Most of the scientific postulates with which Mach disagreed were those logically deduced to fill in gaps in either time or space between sensory experiences of the scientist. For example, scientists could readily observe that light traveled from a source (e.g., candle) to an object (e.g., a painting on a wall). The scientist could not observe how the light got from the candle to the painting. Since all things are known to get from one point to another by some means, it was logically deduced that the light of the candle must travel through some medium to reach the painting (e.g., luminiferous ether). Mach saw this want for explanations involving hypothetical materials that causally push or pull entities toward some effect as a pseudoproblem caused by the arbitrary requirement that there be no gaps in space or time when accounting for cause–effect correlations.

Mach's radical positivism was not interested in these types of causes, nor did it assume that public agreement over sensory observation could ensure truth (i.e., he was familiar with sensory illusions). Instead, he advocated using description to identify recurring patterns in observable phenomena. The pattern of events/observations that reliably covaried with a given phenomenon were called *functional relations*, and it was considered the task of the scientist to describe these functional relations as economically as possible (Moore, 2003). For Mach, functional relations served an adaptive purpose: They were useful in that they allowed the scientist to adaptively predict and influence nature. He considered the quest for objective Truth as a metaphysical crime that seduces the scientist to seek explanations beyond the data that form the foundation of knowledge (Leahey, 2004). From this perspective, the usefulness of the functional descriptions among observed events was all the truth science needed.

Skinner's approach to the study of behavior differed from the logical positivism of many of his behavioristic contemporaries. He applied Mach's radical positivism to the study of behavior. In *The Operational Analysis of Psychological Terms*, Skinner (1945) clarified his approach as an alternative form of operationism involving the efficient characterization of the features of the world as they functionally affect behavior, without appeal to mentalistic constructs or mediational events (Hineline, 1984). Like Mach, Skinner emphasized the identification of functional relationships instead of causes. Skinner's explanations were historical and contextual rather than cause–effect. Unlike those of the logical positivist tradition, who viewed thoughts and feelings as mediators in a S-M-R causal chain, radical behaviorists view thinking and feeling as activities influenced by antecedent and consequential functional relations (antecedent–behavior–consequence, A-B-C). They are better conceptualized as behaviors to be accounted for ("behaviors" not in the sense of muscle movement but in the sense of actions of the organism) than as causes of other actions of the organism.

Basic research for the A-B-C approach involves predicting and influencing environment–behavior functional relations under tightly controlled conditions (often, but not necessarily, with nonhumans). As reliable relations are identified, they are tested in increasingly less restrictive situations. When behavior analysts speak of basic research supporting an analysis of complex human behavior, they specifically mean that the functional relations being invoked to explain complex behavior involve the same theoretical terms refined by the identification of functional relations in tightly controlled studies. In contrast to the causal mediators of the S-M-R tradition, functional relations need to be demonstrated to be useful for both the prediction and influence of behavior patterns. The theoretical terms used to characterize these functional relations undergo careful refinement to maximize their precision, scope, and depth of integration with the overall theoretical approach.

The concepts and principles that provide the analytic foundation of this approach gradually emerged over 75 years of basic and applied research. As additional research suggests further useful behavior–environment functional relations (often by observing order at different time scales) these are incorporated into the approach. Skinner's Behavior Analysis is an integrated science and the terms used to describe the various functional relations complement one another as part of an ever-maturing theory.

ACT is based on a contemporary behavior analytic understanding of the behavior–environment functional relations involved in language. At its most intricate level, this analysis rests on Relational Frame Theory (RFT; Blackledge, 2003; Hayes, Barnes-Holmes, & Roche, 2001) and the functional analysis of rule-governed behavior (Catania, Matthews, & Shimoff, 1982; Hayes, Brownstein, Zettle, Rosenfarb, & Korn, 1986; Shimoff, Catania, & Matthews, 1981; Zettle & Hayes, 1982). The focus on cognition and emotion was not, however, mentalistic or mediational, because these were viewed as actions, and the relationship of these actions to overt behavior were argued to be contextually regulated rather than directly causal (Hayes & Brownstein, 1986). This approach was supported empirically both by a functional analysis of the social context for psychological distress and behavior change (Rosenfarb & Hayes, 1984), and basic behavioral principles and the molar behavioral dynamics derived from basic behavior analytic research (Drossel, Waltz, & Hayes, 2007; Hayes et al., 2007).

The philosophical and theoretical underpinnings of the form of modern behavior analysis that underlies the ACT treatment model has been described in many places (Hayes, 1986, 1993, 1997; Hayes & Brownstein, 1986; Hayes, Hayes, & Reese, 1988). The term *functional contextualism*, used to clarify the philosophy of modern behavior analysis, was borrowed from Stephen Pepper's (1942) analysis of worldviews (Hayes et al., 1988). This was done in part to sidestep the misunderstanding that accompanies the term *radical behaviorism*. Many non-behavior analysts interpret *radical* to imply an extreme form of Watsonian behaviorism rather than an extension of Mach's radical functionalism to the study of behavior. Furthermore, the approach is also radical in that it extends the functional analysis to the behavior of the scientist and scientific knowing itself, which overturns most of Watson's philosophical views (Skinner, 1945). It also brought much greater clarity to the importance of the specification of analytic goals (Hayes, 1993), as well as providing a rationale for the flexible use of different terms for different purposes in different contexts (Hayes, 1984), both of which are key to ACT.

Direct Influences on the Development of ACT

Although ACT emerged more from the desire to find a new way forward in the application of behavioral thinking to language and cognition, it would not have made sense to do so if the existing approaches to cognition in the behavioral and cognitive therapies had been fully successful when measured against functional contextual goals. We were seriously interested in cognitive therapy (A. T. Beck, Rush, Shaw, & Emery, 1979) but were frustrated by its theoretical approach. We conducted both conceptual and empirical analyses of cognitive therapy (CT; Hayes, Korn, Zettle, Rosenfarb, & Cooper, 1982; Zettle & Hayes, 1987), focusing particularly on one treatment component of CT, cognitive distancing. It was of interest because it seemed to overlap with some aspects of more Eastern traditions and resonated with functional–behavioral thinking. "The process of regarding thoughts objectively is labeled *distancing*" (A. T. Beck, 1976, p. 243). Any technique that facilitates a client's ability to hold thoughts as hypotheses (distantly) rather than as representing literal truths is hypothesized to be useful in CT. A sample of these techniques includes reattribution, alternative conceptualizations, imagining an identical situation happened to a friend, core belief challenging metaphors, and imagining realistic levels of distress at distant time intervals (A. T. Beck et al., 1979; J. S. Beck, 1995). The focus of distancing in CT is to gain greater objectivity when evaluating thoughts.

Cognitive distancing was subjected to a conceptual functional analysis (Hayes, 1987), which suggested that the model was unnecessarily restrictive. Cognitive distancing as a technique in CT is to be applied to each dysfunctional thought as it occurs (e.g., "Can you hold that thought as a hypothesis rather than as a fact?"). The behavior analysis of language suggests that there is nothing special about each particular dysfunctional thought, and that thoughts alone cannot directly cause psychological distress or ineffective behavior. In the ACT model, and in behavior analysis more generally, thoughts and feelings are treated not as causes but as behaviors under contextual influence. This means that to change the impact of thoughts and feelings, one needs to change their context. From a functional–contextual perspective, distancing techniques establish a less literal context that can weaken the behavior regulatory impact of language.

This fit with what behavior analysts were learning at the time about the negative impact of verbal rules. Rules are often repertoire-narrowing influences that reduce the sensitivity of behavior to programmed contingencies (for a book length review, see Hayes, 1989). The core idea was to construct ways to reduce excessive regulation by verbal rules, and to increase the impact of long-term contingencies. We did that by amplifying distancing, and by confronting unworkable rules that we thought artificially sustained the behavior regulatory impact of private experiences by encouraging experiential avoidance.

To test this model, a treatment (now called ACT—then called *Comprehensive Distancing*) was developed and compared to CT in a small, randomized trial (Zettle & Hayes, 1986). ACT led to better outcomes and decreased the believability but not the frequency of depressogenic thoughts relative to CT. A second study in group form (Zettle & Rains, 1989) found marginally significant differences on the Beck Depression Inventory (BDI). However, while the CT group's decreases in depression were accompanied by decreases in the frequency of dysfunctional attitudes, the ACT group's improvements were not accompanied by decreases in dysfunctional attitudes. We compared ACT to CBT for pain (Hayes et al., 1982) and found better outcomes. That study was put aside, however, and only published 17 years later (Hayes, Bissett, et al., 1999).

It was not published because, having shown that our approach was useful, we stopped doing outcome research and turned toward the principles needed for a broader understanding of these methods. We spent over a dozen years on model development, measures, and research on the functional analysis of language as we tried to understand what a verbal rule was and how to bring that knowledge into the clinical arena. Over time this led to RFT and, finally, to the description of ACT in its modern form (Hayes, Strosahl, & Wilson, 1999).

That development approach is not common in empirical clinical psychology, but it is characteristic of behavior analysis, in which there is a continuous and mutual interplay between basic principles and application. We have discussed this more recently under the label *contextual behavioral science*, which is an explication and modernization of the behavior analytic development strategy (Hayes, Levin, Plumb, Boulanger, & Pistorello, in press; Vilardaga, Hayes, Levin, & Muto, 2009).

Influences on the Developer of ACT

The Early Days

The structure of this volume requires a description of various influences on the developer of the methods covered by chapters. Although there were many hands in the development of ACT, and the first book-length treatment was authored with the help of Kirk Strosahl and Kelly Wilson, the original work can be traced to Steven C. Hayes. To avoid awkward sentences, this section on influences is phrased in the third person, despite the fact that the initial developer is a coauthor of this chapter.

Steven C. Hayes grew up in southern California, attending high school and college there in the 1960s, and being influenced by the heyday of the hippie counterculture. He came to psychology with an interest in its impact on human development and well-being, as described in Maslow's self-actualization approach. He found in B. F. Skinner's (1948) utopian novel *Walden Two* a way of combining that interest with science. Like many in the counterculture, he developed an interest in Eastern philosophy and lived for several months in an Eastern religious commune in Grass Valley, California.

As a student at Loyola Marymount University in Los Angeles in 1966, he was exposed to behavior therapy and gravitated toward it. His first undergraduate paper was on the possibility of applying exposure methods to emotions, not just situations. He completed an honor's thesis comparing response prevention, shaping, and observation in the reduction of avoidance behavior in rats. Getting into graduate school proved to be unexpectedly difficult due to a poor letter from a faculty member who objected to his hippie appearance, but after 2 years of failure he was accepted into the doctoral program in clinical psychology at West Virginia University (WVU).

WVU's psychology department was (and remains to this day) one of the strongholds of behavior analysis. The faculty with whom Hayes worked, who were behavior analysts or cognitive-behavioral therapists included John Cone, Rob Hawkins, Andy Lattal, Nathan Cavior, John Krapfl, and Hayne Reese. Hayes published both human and animal work as a graduate student.

Academic Genealogy: Behavior Analytic from Beginning to End

Other than Skinner, Hayes's biggest influences were his undergraduate advisor, Irving Kessler; his major advisor at WVU, John D. Cone; his internship advisor at Brown University, David Barlow; his early colleagues at University of North Carolina–Greensboro (UNC-G), Rosemery O. Nelson and Aaron J. Brownstein; a sabbatical year with A. Charles Catania; and his colleague Dermot Barnes-Holmes. All of these people can be linked to functional-behavioral thinking. Kessler was an early behavior therapist, completing a dissertation on eye blink conditioning at the University of Southern California in 1966. John D. Cone founded the journal *Behavioral Assessment* and studied under the psychometrician Allen Edwards, who studied under A. R. Gilliland, who completed his degree at the University of Chicago while it was still heavily influenced by the functionalist and contextualistic thinking of such faculty members as James Rowland Angell, J. R. Kantor, and John Dewey. Gilliland was also a well-known psychometrician but had published some of the earlier well-developed work on the law of effect in the 1930s. Hayes completed his clinical internship under David Barlow, who studied under Harold Leitenberg, who studied under basic behavior analyst James Dinsmoor, who studied under William Nathan ("Nate") Schoenfeld. Schoenfeld, along with Fred S. Keller (a roommate, fellow graduate student, and close friend of B. F. Skinner at Harvard), coauthored the first major textbook in behavior analysis in 1950. Rosemery Nelson was trained in behavior therapy at State University of New York–Stony Brook in the late 1960s; Aaron Brownstein in basic behavior analysis in the late 1950s at Missouri; and A. Charles Catania in behavior analysis at Harvard with Skinner and Richard Herrnstein. Barnes-Holmes was trained by Michael Keenan, whose lineage traces through Julian Leslie and Jock Millenson to Fred Keller and Nate Schoenfeld.

Significant Achievements to Date

Hayes has received numerous research awards, including the Don F. Hake Award for Exemplary Contributions to Basic Behavioral Research and Its Applications from Division 25 (Behavior Analysis) of the American Psychological Association; the Impact of Science on Application Award for basic contributions to applied psychology from the Society for the Advancement of Behavior Analysis, and the Lifetime Achievement Award from ABCT.

He has served as president for Division 25 (Experimental Analysis of Behavior), the Association for Applied and Preventive Psychology, the Association for the Advancement of Behavior Therapy, and the Association for Contextual Behavioral Science.

An author of over 400 scholarly papers and 32 books, he was named in 1992 by the Institute for Scientific Information as the 30th highest-impact psychologist in the world from 1986 to 1990, and in 2007 as the ninth most productive clinical psychologist in the United States during 2000–2004.

Theory of Psychopathology

At the core of many psychological syndromes is the personal attempt to alter the intensity, form, frequency, or duration of unwanted private events (e.g., thoughts and feelings) even when doing so causes behavioral problems. This struggle has been conceptualized as a functional class of behavior called *experiential avoidance* (Hayes, Wilson, Gifford, Follette, & Strosahl, 1996). Experiential avoidance tends to persist for two reasons. First, immediate attempts at distracting oneself from or changing historically produced private events often result in their immediate reduction, which negatively reinforces the process. Unfortunately, these efforts tend to increase the importance, salience, and behavior regulatory impact of these private events and the avoidance-based rules related to them. Thus, this immediate relief is often only temporary (for a review, see Wegner, 1994).

The second reason experiential avoidance tends to persist has to do with language and culture. Cultures (especially Western culture) often support linguistic contexts that can facilitate a continued struggle with trying to avoid undesirable thoughts and feelings. The flow of literal verbal events increases with every technological advance. Feeling good is upheld as the goal of living by commercial culture. Reason giving is continuously demanded, and private events, such as thoughts and feelings (e.g., "I did it because it seemed like a good idea at the time," or "I stayed in bed because I was too depressed to get up") are often accepted as sufficient causal explanations.

The result of these contextual features is *cognitive fusion*, which is the domination of behavioral regulation by verbal events due to contexts that support their being taken literally. Therapeutic techniques that promote more flexibly with respect to verbal behavior are described as promoting *defusion*, which involves the ability to flexibly notice, observe, and suspend the compulsion to take immediate action with respect to private verbal events.

Cognitive fusion leads to other overextensions of language, including loss of contact with the present moment and the tendency to take stories about the self literally. This can interfere with the ability to behave in accord with one's values. From this perspective psychological health is a form of psychological flexibility: "changing behavior when change is needed and persisting when persistence is needed—so as to accomplish desired ends" (Hayes, Strosahl, Bunting, Twohig, & Wilson, 2004, p. 24).

To understand the rationale for the ACT treatment conceptualization it helps if we review some of the research on which this conceptualization is based. Much of the ACT model emerged from the basic research on rule-governed behavior (for a book-length review, see Hayes, 1989). This research included studies (e.g., Hayes, Brownstein, Haas, & Greenway, 1986; Hayes, Brownstein, Zettle, et al., 1986) in which human subjects pressed keys on a computer keyboard to earn points. The requirements to earn the points changed without notice during the course of the experiment. In one condition, subjects needed to respond quickly to earn points; in the other, points could only be earned by responding slowly. The researchers found that if subjects were given a rule, they tended to follow that rule even after they stopped earning points when the task's requirements changed (without notice). Subjects who were given more flexible instructions (i.e., "Sometimes you will have to respond quickly to earn points and sometimes you will have to respond slowly") were more likely to change their behavior when the point requirements changed.

This research was seen to have direct implications for conceptualizing how verbal behavior can contribute to clinical presentations. In the basic research, the rule (e.g., press fast) was initially credible in that it efficiently characterized what the subject had to do to earn the most points. When conditions changed, the subject behaved as if the conditions described by the rule were still in effect. The more fused individuals are to the literal content of verbal behavior, the less likely they are to be able to respond to the changing demands of their situation. A reoccurring theme that emerges in the ACT treatment conceptualization involves the need to undermine fusion and promote functional flexibility.

Treatment Conceptualization

ACT was developed to address verbal barriers to pursuing meaningful life directions. Thus, ACT targets psychological distress related to experiential avoidance and fusion. The behavior analytic theory behind ACT holds that to change the behaviors involved in fusion and experiential avoidance, it is the task of the therapist to change the context for those behaviors—and for verbal behavior more generally. The previous section outlined the cultural context that supports these patterns of verbal behavior, and any techniques employed in ACT are used for the purpose of undermining the contextual variables that support fusion and experiential avoidance.

Theory has a central role in guiding the therapist through all aspects of clinical activity. One difficulty is that ACT is based on basic behavioral principles, molar behavioral dynamics, the functional analysis of rule-governed and social behavior, and RFT. This means that to take advantage of the full breadth of the theory underlying ACT, a newcomer to the tradition would have to become familiar with over 75 years of basic and applied behavioral research to facilitate the functional/flexible understanding of the theoretical terms that were progressively refined to their present day use. This gives ACT work its intellectual depth, but it is also a burden.

ACT has adopted a pragmatic but risky dissemination strategy to overcome these problems: the development of a theory of intervention using accessible "middle-level" terms, including *acceptance, defusion, present moment focus, self as perspective, values,* and *committed action.* Metaphorically the ACT model of treatment is a kind of operating system that stands atop the programming language of basic behavioral principles and RFT. It is pragmatic in that it focuses on providing therapists with rather abstract rules (i.e., the six core processes and their goal of psychological flexibility) to facilitate functionally flexible behavior while providing therapy. This strategy seems to produce effective ACT therapists (Lappalainen et al., 2007; Strosahl, Hayes, & Bergan, 1998), but it is important also to note the risk of these middle-level terms being taken to be equivalent to the functional processes that underlie them.

The four core processes of acceptance, defusion, self as perspective, and contact with the present moment are conceptualized as mindfulness and acceptance processes; those of self as perspective, contact with the present moment, values, and committed action are conceptualized as commitment and behavior change processes (Hayes, Strosahl, Bunting, et al., 2004).

These are considered "middle-level" processes in that they seem to provide functionally flexible rules for both guiding therapist behavior and evaluating patterns of clinically relevant client behavior. These six processes are intended to facilitate the broad and functionally flexible application of techniques (scope), while mitigating the risk of excessive (or misplaced) precision that can accompany more concrete rules for practice (e.g., observe problem X, implement technique Z). The six processes overlap and interrelate, but the distinct emphasis of each seems to be useful.

Acceptance

Acceptance-oriented techniques aim to undermine the ubiquity of social support for behaving as if private events cause behavior, and that these must be controlled before other meaningful life outcomes can be pursued. The therapist actively creates a context in which the client is given the opportunity to experience private events without engaging in any behavior directed at controlling the private events. The deliberate disengagement from the struggle to control private events, described as *willingness*, helps to highlight that acceptance involves an active process with a purpose. While the struggle to control private events typically narrows an individual's repertoire to focusing exclusively on that struggle, willingness (through repeatedly choosing to disengage with the struggle to control) broadens the range of response alternatives so that other outcomes can be pursued.

Willingness is to be distinguished from resignation and stoicism. *Resignation* involves inactive submission. This may seem to capture the key aspect of discontinuing the struggle with private events, but it fails to take the next important step—taking action in the presence of undesirable private events. *Stoicism* may appear to capture the importance of taking action independent of private events, but it places an unnecessary premium on striving to be free from undesirable private events altogether. Acceptance requires an agnostic stance toward private events: They are neither scorned nor held in high esteem; they just are.

Defusion

Whereas acceptance-oriented techniques undermine the social convention that private events cause action, defusion techniques more specifically target undermining the social and other contextual supports for treating thoughts as causes for behavior. One of the core goals of ACT is to disarm the power of language when it presents as a barrier to functional flexibility. "Defusion involves a change in the normal use of language and cognition such that the ongoing process of thinking is more evident and the normal functions of the products of thinking are broadened" (Luoma & Hayes, 2003, p. 71). Recall the earlier discussion of how literal rule following can function to restrict an individual's sensitivity to changing environmental conditions. Defusion exercises aim to broaden the context of language more generally through providing opportunities to interact with language in a variety of nonliteral ways. These unconventional opportunities undermine the exclusivity of the social community's support for the literality of language (i.e., undermine fusion). This broader nonliteral context affords greater functional flexibility with respect to language and can facilitate greater sensitivity to changing environmental conditions.

Strosahl, Hayes, Wilson, and Gifford (2004) noted that fusion can be undermined by focusing on four different levels of literality. The first level involves highlighting the basic properties of language and focuses on undermining the literality of individual words. The second level focuses on undermining the literality that accompanies the practice of reason giving. The third level focuses on undermining the literality of evaluations that accompany reason giving. The fourth and final level focuses more broadly on the process of thinking and the ability to dispassionately observe the ongoing verbal process. Because the literality of language is so pervasive in these levels, it is useful to spend some time addressing each of the four levels with every client. One of the more entrenched domains involving the literality of language concerns conceptualization of the self.

Self as Perspective

Fusion with conceptualizations of the self can interfere with functional flexibility. Taken literally, "I am _____" can narrow the range of possible actions a person can take. Thus, the aspiring executive cannot also be a good parent or spouse, or the trauma survivor cannot also live a vital life, or the statement "I cannot handle another loss" necessitates engaging in experiential avoidance. There is an inherent danger in the inflexibility that accompanies the conceptualization of the self as being literally anchored to the content of that description. Even positive self-conceptualizations can restrict the flexibility of responding in detrimental ways (Hayes, 1995). For example, the self-conceptualized saintly person may be unable to provide unfavorable feedback to others, even though that feedback may actually benefit the saint and/or the recipient of the feedback.

An alternative conceptualization involves viewing the self as a matter of perspective, not in the sense of an opinion or point of view, but in the sense of viewing events from I–here–now. To cultivate this conceptualization a variety of exercises are used to highlight how the self as a locus or point of perspective remains consistent, although particular roles, thoughts, emotions, behaviors, and experiences have changed over time (child–adult, student–teacher, lover–estranged, etc.). The perspective broadens the conceptualization of the self beyond the literal aspects of any particular label (Hayes, 1984). The self is the context where life events unfold and is contrasted with the self as being considered synonymous with any particular label or experience. Thus, another common name for this aspect of the model is "self-as-context." Basic research in RFT is increasingly showing that this aspect of the self is based on the fluency of the relational frames I–you; here–there; and now–then (e.g., McHugh, Barnes-Holmes, & Barnes-Holmes, 2004; Weil, Hayes, & Capurro, 2008).

Contact with the Present Moment

One of the beneficial roles of language is that it facilitates our ability to describe and evaluate the past and plan for the future. With this comes the liability that our current behavior may be disproportionately influenced by past- and future-oriented rules, and less influenced by the present context. ACT employs a variety of techniques that function to reorient the individual to the present context. Many of the exercises employed in the service of this goal function to unmask how language can bring the past and future into the present. When the literal aspects of language interfere with attending to the present context, defusion techniques are used to facilitate increased control by the present situation.

The present moment can be misunderstood as an unending succession of moments. The philosophy underlying ACT emphasizes that context and ongoing patterns matter more than isolated moments. Language tends to narrow the focus of attention to particular thoughts, evaluations, or descriptions to the exclusion of other potentially important aspects of the environment. Thus, in some situations, particular verbal barriers become the dominant context for behavior. Exercises that facilitate contact with the present moment can broaden the context for behavior beyond the content of any verbal barrier. Thus, the ability to defuse from language processes can promote functional flexibility by opening the door for additional contextual variables to influence behavior. However, it is important to remember that flexibility in and of itself is not a virtue. Flexibility needs to be useful for obtaining some preferred type of outcome, and this is why ACT has focused on the identification and clarification of values.

Values Identification and Clarification

Up to this point, the core processes of ACT have primarily focused on undermining the literality of language. Values identification and clarification in ACT involve the exploration of abstract outcomes that can be used to guide behavior once the literality of barriers has been undermined. Values are like broad and abstract rules that are difficult to interpret literally and thus afford greater functional flexibility than particular concrete goals. These abstract values are not something that can be possessed or achieved *once and for all*. Rather, they are adverbs and gerunds that have a temporal extension. For example, "being a loving partner" is not something that you can do just once. It involves an ongoing pattern of a wide variety of behaviors—any of which instantiate their related value. Furthermore, no specific commitment to a single member of that pattern is required (e.g., going on a date every weekend). Clients are encouraged to be quite inclusive regarding the types of activities that they consider as part of a particular pattern of valued living (e.g., excelling at one's place of employment can be framed as facilitating financial stability that brings a desirable sense of security to a marriage). It is useful to encourage the itemization of multiple concrete goals related to a value. However, these goals should always be framed as being subordinate to abstract values to maintain functional flexibility.

The literality of language still places values and goals at risk for becoming rigidly followed rules rather than flexible guidelines. In addition, there is always the risk that a client may identify and work toward values that "sound good" to the therapist or other people who are important to the client. It is important to guide the client always to use *workability* as a criterion when evaluating commitment to any particular value-related activity (e.g., Does doing all of the cooking and cleaning in the household impact your partner in loving ways, or does it result in the partner feeling like a guest in his or her own home?). What is important is the actual impact that patterns of valued living have on the client, and not whether particular activities *should* produce a particular impact.

Values are most often addressed in therapy after the mindfulness- and acceptance-based processes have already been addressed to some degree. Some therapists choose to address values earlier in therapy, because doing so can increase a sense of purpose for engaging in mindfulness- and acceptance-based work. If this latter path is taken, then values often provide much of the language content that is addressed through the mindfulness- and acceptance-based processes.

Committed Action

The overall goal of ACT is to help individuals engage in value-congruent behavior and persist in that engagement even when undesirable private events make that journey difficult. Thus, whereas committed action may appear to be one of the end points of therapy, it often is just the beginning. Committing to a course of action brings with it all the liabilities of language that we discussed earlier. Committed action involves an active willingness to experience undesirable private events. It also presupposes all of the mindfulness–defusion skills needed to act in functionally flexible ways. For this to occur, action is either something an individual does or does not execute. "Trying" without action is one way language can provide the illusion that action is actually occurring when it is not.

Reason giving can also be a barrier to taking action. As we discussed earlier, the wider verbal community supports treating reasons as causes for behavior, and this history influences current behavior. Likewise, reasons can also be grounds for not engaging in behavior. Action provides the opportunity to contact aspects of the current situation that are relevant to valued outcomes. ACT focuses on teaching clients to choose to take action *with* reasons instead of *for* reasons. If action is taken *for* reasons, then action apparently needs to change if those reasons are compromised. In contrast, if action is taken *with* reasons, then action can persist, independent of those reasons. It is equally important that a particular course of action can be discontinued if necessary, without the implication that the related value "must not matter." Difficulties in this area often emerge when it becomes obvious that a client has been engaging in mindfulness and acceptance work in the hope of *feeling* better instead of *living* better.

The role of the therapist in committed action is very important. People are more likely to follow through with committed action if that commitment is made publicly (Hayes et al., 1985; Hayes & Wolf, 1984; Rosenfarb & Hayes, 1984; Zettle & Hayes, 1983). The therapist is an important audience that holds the client accountable for value-congruent patterns of action. That the client reports back to the therapist regarding whether he or she has been engaging in committed action is typically sufficient if it increases the likelihood of value-congruent behavior. The therapist should not adopt a "one up" or law enforcement position. Some clients find any social accountability for their actions uncomfortable, and reporting to the therapist may place a strain on the therapeutic relationship. It is important for the therapist to emphasize that commitment is about engaging in a process and not about being able to achieve particular goals or outcomes. Fusion with the need to produce a particular outcome for the therapist can be a barrier to functional flexibility, just like any other narrowly prescribed role. All barriers to engaging in committed action should be addressed by using the five other processes covered earlier in therapy.

The concept of workability provides an inroad for discussing problems with commitment. If a particular path of action is not as congruent with a value as anticipated, or if it unexpectedly conflicts with a different value, then that particular path is abandoned and another is taken. Values identification and clarification, and committed action involve an iterative process whereby putative values lead to committed action. Particular courses of committed action are more or less congruent with their related values. If the relationship between the action and the value proves unworkable for reasons other than private barriers to engagement, then that course of action can be abandoned for workability reasons rather than some other rationale. Thus, workability can be used to emphasize flexibility, without abandoning the need to actually take value-congruent action.

Workability can be a difficult metric early in therapy, when behavior may be more sensitive to more immediate goals related to values. ACT aims to help clients build patterns of committed action. It often helps to begin with the smallest goals and a commitment to the process of applying the mindfulness and acceptance processes to the barriers that emerge when the first attempts at taking action occur. Clients are expected to "commit and slip," and to take responsibility for that process rather than being victimized by it. This aspect of therapy has a lot in common with behavior therapy in general, in that therapists encourage clients to notice any incremental progress in this journey. The goal is to build larger and larger patterns of value-related committed action, using the acceptance and mindfulness processes to accommodate the barriers that inevitably emerge along the way.

The six processes in ACT are complementary, and this becomes especially clear with committed action. Committed action provides the opportunity to practice skills relevant to all of the other processes. This involves a lifelong practice of orienting to these six processes whenever the individual notices that private events (i.e., thoughts, emotions, and evaluations related to these) serve as barriers to engaging in value-congruent action.

Ongoing Challenges to the ACT Treatment Conceptualization

It is important to remember that ACT specifically addresses verbal barriers to engaging in effective action. Clients often have skills deficits and require skills training to engage effectively in value-congruent committed action. ACT is a model of how to do behavior therapy, and literally nothing that is known about behavioral methods should be put aside. It is a dreadful mistake for a therapist to continually assume that a client's only possible barriers to taking effective action are fusion- or experiential avoidance-based. It is also possible that the individual has never had the skills to behave effectively in certain situations. Perhaps the best way to assess this is to have the client engage in role play or other *in vivo* exercises with the therapist. The broader theory underlying ACT can be an effective guide for assessing and remediating these more practical skills deficits, although a review of this broader approach (Behavior Analysis) is beyond the scope of this chapter. Those who choose to understand more comprehensively the basic behavioral principles, behavioral dynamics, and the functional analyses of more complex social and verbal behavior underlying ACT will find this theory's ability to guide the treatment of skills deficits very rewarding.

EMPIRICAL EVIDENCE

Outcome Studies

Since ACT targets processes that transcend typical DSM categories, it has been applied to a wide variety of forms of psychological distress. Research only began in earnest after the publication of the first ACT book less than a decade ago (Hayes, Strosahl, et al., 1999), and since then over two dozen controlled investigations have appeared and several more are currently under review. ACT is part of the empirically supported treatment (EST) movement and appears at least to meet criteria for a *Probably Efficacious Treatment* (see Chambless & Hollon [1998] on the defining features of EST) for anxiety disorders, chronic pain, depression, habit disorders, psychotic symptoms, and substance use. Studies that are currently under review, if accepted, would establish ACT as a *Well-Established Treatment* in the area of anxiety disorders, chronic pain, depression, psychotic symptoms, and substance use. Table 5.1 specifies the studies that support ACT receiving EST status in these areas. Individual researchers can question the methodological features of these studies (e.g., Öst, 2008), and EST status can be formally established only by properly constituted committees, so Table 5.1 reflects our judgments. It should be noted, however, that the purpose of the methodological recommendations of Chambless and Hollon (1998) are to ensure that experimental results can be interpreted as being due to treatment-specific effects (as opposed to general treatment effects). The great majority of the studies in Table 5.1 include process measures, allowing for discussion of the relevance of these to the various presenting problems that define the populations receiving treatment. In this sense, many of these studies are able to speak more directly to the central concerns that the methodological recommendations of Chambless and Hollon were intended to address.

Evidence for the effectiveness of ACT is growing in several other behavioral health areas, such as anorexia (Heffner, Sperry, & Eifert, 2002), cancer (Branstetter, Wilson, Hildegrandt, & Mutch, 2004; Paez, Luciano, & Gutiérrez, 2007), epilepsy (Lundgren, Dahl, Melin, & Kies, 2006; Vowles & McCracken, 2008), and type 2 diabetes management (Gregg, Callaghan, Hayes, & Glenn-Lawson, 2007). ACT has also been used to address areas of social importance, such as stigma and prejudice, where the barriers to action may also involve private events (see Hayes, Bissett, et al. [2004] for therapist stigma toward clients; Luoma et al. [2007] for self-stigma in substance abuse; Masuda et al. [2007] for stigma toward the mentally ill). ACT has also proven useful in reducing the struggle with undesirable private events in high-stress populations in areas such as the workplace (Bond & Bunce, 2000) and with parents of autistic children (Blackledge & Hayes, 2006).

Process Studies

Although it is important to demonstrate the effectiveness (discussed previously) and efficacy (see Lappalainen et al., 2007; Strosahl, Hayes, & Bergan, 1998) of ACT, the model of science on which ACT is based requires more than blind empiricism and technique-based studies for support. The approach specifically holds that as the cultural support for treating private events as causal is undermined in the therapeutic relationship, the ability of these private events to function as barriers to value-congruent action

TABLE 5.1. Suggested Empirical Status of ACT by Disorder

Domain—status by Chambless & Hollon (1998) criteria	Support	Outcome
Anxiety disorders— well-established treatment	*ACT compared to other treatments:* Forman, Herbert, Moitra, Yeomans, & Geller (2007)	Effectiveness randomized controlled trial (RCT): ACT equivalent to cognitive therapy (CT)
	Lappalainen et al. (2007)	Effectiveness RCT: ACT superior to traditional CBT in anxiety and mood disorders.
	Paez et al. (2007)	Small RCT: ACT equivalent to CT at posttreatment and superior to CT at 1-year follow-up in women diagnosed with breast cancer.
	Campbell-Sills, Barlow, Brown, & Hofmann (2006)	Component RCT with patients with anxiety and mood disorders. Better response to anxiety-provoking material with ACT intervention than with control-based intervention.
	Levitt et al. (2004)	Component RCT with patients with panic disorder. Better response to exposure with ACT intervention than with control-based intervention.
	Zettle (2003)	RCT: No significant difference between ACT and systematic desensitization on math anxiety, better outcomes with high experiential avoiders.
	Roemer, Orsillo, & Salters-Pedneault (2008)	Small RCT for GAD: Large, about 70% ACT and all ACT-consistent. Large effect sizes.
	ACT pre–post no active comparison: Dalrymple & Herbert (2007)	Open trial for social phobia: Large effect sizes.
	Ossman, Wilson, Storaasli, & McNeill (2006)	Large effect sizes
	ACT time-series design: Twohig, Hayes, & Masuda (2006a)	Multiple baseline for OCD: Large improvement.
	Zaldivar Basurto & Hernández López (2001)	Improvement
	Huerta, Gomez, Molina, & Luciano (1998)	Improvement
	Hayes (1987)	Improvement

(*continued*)

TABLE 5.1. (continued)

Chronic pain—well-established treatment	*ACT compared to other treatments:* McCracken, MacKichan, & Eccleston (2007)	ACT for severe patients showed better outcomes than standard care for normal patients.
	Vowles, McNeik, et al. (2007)	RCT with low back pain: Comparing acceptance, pain control, and practice. Better outcomes for ACT-based intervention.
	Dahl, Wilson, & Nilsson (2004)	Small RCT: ACT superior to medical treatment as usual (TAU) alone.
	Wicksell, Ahlqvist, Bring, Melin, & Olsson (2008)	Small RCT: Comparing ACT to TAU with whiplash patients; good outcomes.
	Pre–post no active comparison: Vowles & McCracken (2008)	Large effectiveness trial: Large effect sizes and strong process–outcome relation.
	Vowles, McCracken, & Eccleston (2007)	Large effectiveness trial with large effect sizes.
	Wicksell, Melin, & Olsson (2007)	Large effect sizes
	McCracken, Vowles, & Eccleston (2005)	Large effect sizes
	Time-series design: Luciano, Visdomine, Gutiérrez, & Montesinos (2001)	Improvement
Depression—well-established treatment	*ACT compared to other treatments:* Forman, Herbert, Moitra, Yeomans, & Geller (2007)	Effectiveness RCT: ACT equivalent to CT.
	Lappalainen et al. (2007)	Effectiveness RCT: ACT superior to traditional CBT in anxiety and mood disorders.
	Paez et al. (2007)	Small RCT: ACT equivalent to CT at posttreatment and superior to CT at 1-year follow-up in women diagnosed with breast cancer.
	Zettle & Raines (1989)	Small RCT: ACT did not significantly differ from CT at posttreatment; ACT superior to CT at 8-week follow-up.
	Zettle & Hayes (1986)	Small RCT: ACT significantly better than CT at posttreatment and 8-week follow-up.
	Petersen & Zettle (2008)	Small RCT: Comparing ACT to TAU with inpatients with comorbid depression/alcohol use disorders. Lower depression in ACT and quicker time to release.

(continued)

TABLE 5.1. (continued)

	Time-series designs:	
	Blackledge & Hayes (2006)	Improvement
	Lopez Ortega & Arco Tirado (2002)	Improvement after failure to respond to CT.
	Luciano & Cabello (2001)	Improvement
Habit disorders— probably efficacious	*Pre–post no active comparison:* Woods, Wetterneck, & Flessner (2006)	Large effect sizes
	Time-series designs: Flessner, Busch, Heidemann, & Woods (2008)	Improvement
	Twohig, Hayes, & Masuda (2006a)	Improvement
	Twohig, Hayes, & Masuda (2006b)	Improvement
	Twohig & Woods (2004)	Improvement
	Hayes (1987)	Improvement
Psychotic symptoms— well-established treatment	*ACT compared to other treatments:* Gaudiano & Herbert (2006)	Small RCT: ACT superior to enhanced TAU (medium effect size).
	Bach & Hayes (2002)	RCT: ACT superior to TAU (medium effect size).
	Time-series design: García Montes & Perez Alvarez (2001)	Improvement
Substance use— well-established treatment	*ACT compared to other treatments:* Gifford et al. (2004)	Large RCT: ACT equal to nicotine replacement therapy (NRT) at posttreatment and ACT superior to NRT at 1-year follow-up.
	Hayes, Wilson, et al. (2004)	RCT: ACT equal to intensive 12-step facilitation (ITSF) and superior to methadone maintenance (MM) at posttreatment. ACT increasingly superior to MM and ITSF at 6-month follow-up.
	Gifford et al. (in press)	Large RCT: ACT + FAP + Zyban equal to Zyban at posttreatment and superior at follow-up.
	Smout et al. (2008)	RCT: ACT equal to CBT for methamphetamine abuse.
	Pr-post no active comparison: Brown et al. (2008)	Open trial with distress-intolerant smokers; improvement.
	Time-series designs: Twohig, Shoenberger, & Hayes (2007)	Improvement
	Batten & Hayes (2005)	Improvement in substance abuse and posttrauamtic stress disorder symptoms.
	Luciano & Gomez (2001)	Improvement

decreases. Thus, the treatment model is agnostic regarding the importance of changing the form or frequency of these undesirable private events so long as they lose their function (e.g., literality).

Various studies have looked at the relationships between ACT processes and a variety of related measures and outcomes. A common measure used in ACT research is the Acceptance and Action Questionnaire (AAQ; Hayes, Strosahl, Wilson, et al., 2004). Item construction for this instrument was guided by the conceptualization that many psychological problems are the result of struggles related to experiential avoidance. Thus, items include things like "I am able to take action on a problem even if I am uncertain what is the right thing to do" and "When I feel depressed or anxious, I am unable to take care of my responsibilities." Such items are used to access the degree to which private events function as barriers to action. Generally, high levels of experiential avoidance, as measured by the AAQ, correlate with higher levels of psychological distress and lower quality of life (Hayes, Strosahl, Wilson, et al., 2004). Other research has included domain-specific AAQ-derived measures for smoking (Avoidance and Inflexibility Scale [AIS]; Gifford, 2002; Gifford et al., 2004), chronic pain (Chronic Pain Acceptance Questionnaire [CPAQ]; McCracken, Vowles, & Eccleston, 2004), diabetes management (Acceptance and Action Diabetes Questionnaire [AADQ]; Gregg et al., 2007), and auditory hallucinations (Voices Acceptance and Action Scale [VAAS]; Shawyer et al., 2007), among others.

Other ACT-related process measures have looked at the literality of language by asking questions about the believability of thoughts. Prepublication versions of the Automatic Thoughts Questionnaire (ATQ, Hollon & Kendall, 1980) included client ratings of the frequency and believability of a variety of thoughts. Although the ATQ, as published, has focused on the frequency of thoughts, ACT researchers have continued to use the Believability scale (ATQ-B), because the underlying theory suggests that changes in believability should be more important than changes in the frequency of thoughts. The ATQ-B was included in the first Comprehensive Distancing Study (Zettle & Hayes, 1986). Subsequent studies (e.g., Gaudiano & Herbert, 2006) have constructed specific assessment items that inquire about the believability of various psychological barriers, including the Stigmatizing Attitudes—Believability Scale (SAB; Hayes, Bissett, et al., 2004).

Although a comprehensive review of studies supportive of the underlying ACT model is beyond the scope of this chapter, Hayes, Luoma, Bond, Masuda, and Lillis (2006) provide a recent review of this literature. In lieu of review, a sampling of relevant studies is presented in Table 5.2.

Limitations to the Theory

ACT addresses private events that function as barriers to value-congruent action. Not every instance of psychological distress is the result of such

TABLE 5.2. Process of Change Evidence

Study	Population	Result
Studies where ACT-related processes provided statistical mediation		
Zettle & Hayes (1986)	Depression	ACT and CT differed in Automatic Thoughts Questionnaire—Believability scale (ATQ-B) and a reason-giving measure. ATQ-B mediated outcomes (as reanalyzed in Hayes et al., 2006).
Zettle & Rains (1989)	Depression	ACT and CT differed in ATQ-B. ATQ-B mediated outcomes (as reanalyzed in Hayes et al., 2006).
Bond & Bunce (2000)	Workers	Acceptance and Action Questionnaire (AAQ) mediated General Health Questionnaire (GHQ) changes.
Gifford et al. (2004)	Chronic smokers	Avoidance and Inflexibility Scale (AIS) mediated abstinence.
Hayes, Bissett, et al. (2004)	Therapists	Stigmatizing Attitudes—Believability scale (SAB) mediated therapist burnout and stigmatizing attitudes in the ACT group but not in the multicultural training or biological education groups.
Gaudiano & Herbert (2006)	Psychotics	"Believability" mediated frequency of hallucinations and their associated distress.
Gregg et al. (2007)	Type 2 diabetics	Acceptance and Action Diabetes Questionnaire (AADQ) and self-management behaviors mediated blood glucose outcomes.
Forman et al. (2007)	Anxiety and depression	Using an exploratory mediational analysis, the AAQ and three of the four subscales of the Kentucky Inventory of Mindfulness Skills (KIMS) mediated outcomes for ACT.
Lundgren et al. (2006); Lundgren, Dahl, & Hayes (2008)	Seizure disorder	Epilepsy-specific AAQ mediated seizure duration, and a values measure mediated a quality-of-life measure; both measures mediated a well-being outcome measure. AIS mediated abstinence; measure of the therapeutic relationship also mediated abstinence. Further analysis suggested that acceptance had an indirect effect on the therapeutic relationship measure.

(continued)

TABLE 5.2. (*continued*)

Study	Population	Result
Vowles, McCracken, & Eccleston (2008)	Chronic pain	Chronic Pain Acceptance Questionnaire (CPAQ) mediated the effect of catastrophizing on patient functioning.
Lillis, Hayes, Bunting, & Masuda (2009)	Overweight and obese	Weight loss mediated weight-related AAQ.
Gifford et al. (in press)	Smoking	Smoking-related psychological inflexibility mediated smoking outcomes.

Studies where ACT-related processes were correlated with outcomes

Bach & Hayes (2002)	Psychotics	No rehospitalization of psychotics who both admitted symptoms and rated them low on believability.
McCracken et al. (2005)	Chronic pain	CPAQ correlated with improvements in depression, pain-related anxiety, physical disability, psychosocial disability, and improvements in a behavioral measure.
Woods et al. (2006)	Trichotillomania	AAQ scores correlated with changes in hair pulling.

Experimental/analogue studies (examples from over 30 studies)

Feldner, Zvolensky, Eifert, & Spira (2003)	College students	Those scoring high on the AAQ reported greater anxiety when presented CO_2-enriched air than did those scoring low on the AAQ.
Gutierrez, Luciano, Rodriguez, & Fink (2004)	College students	Subjects in the high pain context increased pre–post pain tolerance with ACT training but decreased pain tolerance with cognitive control training; believability of the pain decreased for the ACT group.
Levitt, Brown, Orsillo, & Barlow (2004)	Panic disorder	Greater use of acceptance strategies was related to greater willingness to receive a second CO_2 challenge (panic-inducing).
McCracken et al. (2004); McCracken & Eccleston (2005, 2006)	Chronic pain	Greater acceptance was correlated with better physical and psychological functioning, improved work status, and lower medication use.
McCracken & Vowles (2008)	Chronic pain	Acceptance of pain and values-based action correlated with greater emotional, physical, and social functioning.

(*continued*)

TABLE 5.2. (*continued*)

Study	Population	Result
Masuda & Esteve (2007)	College students	Acceptance training produced greater distress tolerance for cold pressor task than suppression and pain education conditions.
Forman, Hoffman, et al. (2007)	College students	Acceptance training resulted in less subjective distress and less difficulty resisting food cravings for subjects who scored high on a scale related to factors influencing food-related impulsivity. Control-based strategies worked well for those who scored low on food-related impulsivity.

barriers. Zettle (2003) provides a good example of this problem. In this study, college students with math anxiety were treated with either ACT or systematic desensitization for 6 weeks. Overall, ACT and desensitization were equally effective in reducing math anxiety (and desensitization was more effective for trait anxiety) except for those subjects who scored high on experiential avoidance, where ACT was superior. This study highlights that when experiential avoidance is not the primary barrier to effective action, other approaches should be used to address the problem.

However, therapists have long noted that clients often "resist" treatment. When this resistance is the result of verbal barriers to engaging in the change process, ACT can provide a useful place to begin therapy, and there is evidence (Levitt, Brown, Orsillo, & Barlow, 2004) that it empowers existing methods. Thus, ACT is a model and not just a technique. This strategy allows therapist and client to be able to address barriers to engaging in empirically supported therapeutic activities of any kind, so long as these other therapeutic activities and ACT do not obviously contradict one another.

CLINICAL PRACTICE

There are now dozens of treatment protocols, self-help books and workbooks, and therapist training guides for the application of ACT to a variety of presenting problems. Readers with interest in the application of ACT to particular types of presenting problems should search for relevant resources. A compilation of ACT-relevant guides and resources can be found at *www.contextualpsychology.org*.

Case Example

Cindy, a 28-year-old, single, white female, has attractive features and, at 240 pounds, qualifies as being obese. She is employed as a midlevel manager at a local bank. Cindy is seeking therapy because she has lost her lust for life. She has felt depressed ever since several of her lifelong friends moved out of state a few years ago. She used to be a social person, but now she spends most of her time alone and is finding social interactions more difficult. She attributes her weight gain to being an "emotional eater," and excessive afterwork eating distracts Cindy from her loneliness.

Cindy scored a 32 on the AAQ-II. Scores of 48 and below are associated with poor acceptance and greater psychological distress. Her score on a conventional depression instrument suggested moderate depression. Cindy's scores on the ATQ-B indicated a high frequency of negative thoughts and that such thoughts were experienced as highly believable. Her moderate score on the Five-Factor Mindfulness Questionnaire (FFMQ; Baer, Smith, Hopkins, Krietemeyer, & Toney, 2006) suggests that language processes often interfere with her ability to engage fully in the present moment.

The early sessions of ACT with Cindy focused on problem identification. Cindy was encouraged to describe the various ways she has tried to manage her depression and loneliness. In this phase of therapy, the therapist adopted a curious, nonjudgmental stance and inquired about how these strategies have worked. Several examples of fusion were observed. Cindy believes that she has to present with a positive attitude or others will not like her. Similarly, she holds the view that negative thoughts are unproductive and must be eliminated for her to get better. She also holds several self-critical evaluations, such as no one would want to be friends with someone so overweight, and no one would like the "real" Cindy. She also described several patterns of experiential avoidance. In the evenings, Cindy watches television and eats to avoid feeling lonely. She also reports avoiding interpersonal interactions, because when she is interacting with others, she is constantly evaluating herself negatively.

In these early sessions, the therapist encouraged Cindy to describe her fusion and experiential avoidance-based strategies. She was also encouraged to evaluate how well they have worked. The therapist was careful to appeal to Cindy's experiences with their workability rather than the therapist's own preconceptions of workability or logic. On many occasions, however, the therapist asked Cindy to distinguish between the short-term and long-term usefulness of the strategies. Many strategies (e.g., eating in front of the television) provided her with temporary respite from loneliness but were viewed more as a distraction than as a long-term solution. Cindy also found that avoiding interpersonal interactions was a useful way to avoid many of her negative self-evaluations, but she noted that this also makes the problem worse, because she cannot make new friends without interacting with others.

This first phase of therapy is called creative hopelessness. The goal of creative hopelessness for Cindy was to introduce workability as an evaluative guide for behavior. In this phase, she started to develop a healthy skepticism toward her unworkable emotional and evaluative control strategies. Most people continue to struggle with their control strategies as therapy progresses toward introducing acceptance and defusion strategies. The following is an example:

T: Our minds have been programmed by our loved ones, teachers, television, and more with all kinds of stuff. And the mind just spits it back out. Try this, Twinkle, twinkle, little...

C: Star?

T: Good. Now was it really important to you that you remember that?

C: No, I probably haven't thought of that since my niece was little.

T: Does it mean something special to you that *star* seems to leap right out after I say twinkle, twinkle?

C: No, it's just kind of automatic.

T: That's right. Our minds automatically spit out all kinds of stuff. Sometimes it is useful, like while trying to remember the things we need while grocery shopping. Other times it is stuff like *star*. However, often the stuff that automatically comes out is harder to sit with than *star*. When you thought *star*, did you want to make that thought go away?

C: No, I was kind of surprised by how automatic it was—but that's normal, right?

T: It's one of the things the mind does, but it doesn't always seem normal. Let's just try something. I'd like you to say whatever pops into your mind after I say something. [*Client nods head.*] Red.

C: Blue.

T: Five.

C: Seven.

T: Television.

C: Waste of time.

T: Dad.

C: Works too much.

T: Work.

C: Fake.

T: Friends.

C: Too busy.

T: Loneliness.

C: Weak.

T: So what just happened in this exercise?

C: I don't like how it ended. I shouldn't think that way. I know that it is not productive.

T: So what changed as we shifted from colors and numbers to places, people, and emotions?

C: Well, at first it seemed like a silly game, then it got serious. I felt like I was criticizing my dad, friends, and myself.

T: How easy was it to notice how automatically the mind works when I said colors and numbers?

C: Easy, but those didn't seem important.

T: And how easy was it to notice how automatically the mind works with places, people, and emotions?

C: I didn't really notice. I wanted them to go away. Then I started blaming myself for getting bothered by this.

T: So here's the tough part to notice. Was your reaction to what your mind said—like you're weak—something you planned or automatic?

C: Automatic. If I had a plan, it would be to stop the negative thoughts from happening at all.

T: And how well has that plan worked so far?

C: Obviously not very well—it keeps happening.

T: So do you remember what it is like just to notice the automatic colors and numbers?

C: Yes.

T: Are you able to *just* notice the negative stuff when it comes up?

C: I might for just a second, but then more negative stuff comes up.

T: Almost automatically, right—but you could just notice that too.

C: Maybe, but I usually try to make it go away.

T: And how well does that work (*sarcastic tone*)?

C: I usually start criticizing myself more and more.

T: So would you be willing to take a step back and notice all this automatic stuff?

C: I could try, but I usually just react.

T: That's right—and for much of what the mind does the automatic stuff works just fine. But for this more emotional and evaluative stuff, it can be useful to distinguish between what's called clean and dirty discomfort.

C: I don't know. Isn't it all bad?

T: Well, try this. What does loneliness feel like for you?

C: Horrible.

T: OK, but that's already an evaluation of that feeling. What does loneliness *feel* like?

C: Well, its like wanting something you can't have (pause) … and that wanting exhausts you, and you just want to curl up, hide, and wait for things to change or be different. But I—

T: Wait on the *but* part. You were just able to describe what loneliness is like for you, before getting swept up by all the evaluations and *buts* that follow. We call that feeling of loneliness clean pain. It's clean in the sense that it directly comes from your experience of missing your friends and not having developed any new relationships. It isn't a logical conclusion or the right or wrong way to be. In the moment, you're not working to make loneliness happen. It just is.

C: OK, but how do I make it go away?

T: You could criticize yourself for being negative or unproductive (*sarcastic tone*).

C: Yeah, that's what I usually do, and I end up feeling worse.

T: We call that feeling worse dirty pain, because it is the additional distress we experience on top of the clean pain when we try to make the clean pain go away.

C: I've noticed that before. Then I start criticizing myself, for criticizing myself and it all gets so frustrating. So how do I make all of this stop?

T: Well, making it stop sounds like using brute force to gain control over your thinking and feelings. How has that strategy worked so far?

C: Not so well.

T: So I'm going to ask you to experiment over the next week and try something that is counterintuitive. I'd like you to try to stick with feeling the clean pain, and notice when you have switched into control mode and you have added dirty pain to the situation.

C: OK, but that won't be easy.

T: It won't be easy at all. And the point of the homework is not for you to get it right or that clean pain is somehow good, while dirty pain is bad. For now, it is important to work on noticing the difference between the two. This noticing will provide the foundation for what we will work on later.

Subsequent sessions would build on noticing the difference between clean and dirty discomfort. If Cindy reported difficulty noticing the difference while out of session, then subsequent sessions would focus on training mindfulness skills. If she reported doing well with noticing, then subsequent sessions would focus on defusion and acceptance skills.

Cindy actually did well with the noticing homework, so therapy progressed through acceptance and defusion techniques. A common exercise intended to foster acceptance was used with Cindy (i.e., physicalizing). The therapist asked her to describe unconventional elements of loneliness (size, color, speed, smell, etc.). The intended function of having her describe the nonaffective aspects of loneliness was to broaden her noticing skills while that emotion was salient. This can loosen the restrictive effect of language while the emotion is present. The theory underlying ACT notes that such private events can be barriers because of how they narrow the individual's repertoire. It is important to make sure that the client is not using the irrelevant aspects of the emotion as a form of distraction. The goal is to have an increased range of action in the presence of emotion. This theory contrasts with S-M-R assumptions, which suggest that the rationality of the emotions or emotion-related thoughts should be addressed. This also contrasts with the assumptions of Experiential Therapy, where the goal of therapy is to promote adaptive and integrative self-organizations (Greenberg, Lietaer, & Watson, 1998). In both of these accounts, one aspect of language is used to try to limit, reframe, or otherwise directly tame problematic private events and to use language in specific ways. ACT aims to loosen the grip of language more generally.

When the therapist was debriefing Cindy after the physicalizing exercise, she asked whether the trick was to try to think of the physical dimensions of loneliness instead of the emotion. It is very common for clients to try to use exercises to control undesirable thoughts and emotions. Like most clients, Cindy required multiple examples of acceptance and defusion exercises before she started to understand this stance as being distinct from the thought–emotion control agenda.

One area where Cindy got particularly stuck was developing a self as perspective. She had severely negative evaluations about her weight that interfered with her ability to engage with others socially. In social situations she assumed that others were judging her harshly for being overweight and barely engaged with them. When invited to events, she would say she would attend, but she did not. Cindy always assumed that people only extended invitations to her because they were being polite.

Cindy also benefited from several exercises that illustrated the self-as-perspective orientation as an alternative to being fused with her judgments about herself. When Cindy first started exploring self as perspective, she made the common mistake of thinking that this perspective was her "true self." This orientation can be problematic, because it implicitly evaluates all other experiences of the self either as wrong or otherwise faulty, thus supporting the literality of language and any struggle to control those experiences. The self as perspective is presented as a potentially useful stance to take when private events function as barriers to engaging in value-relevant activities. It is also not a place to escape to and stay in lieu of engaging in value-relevant action. As with every exercise used in

ACT, the function of the experience is more important than experiencing per se.

The latter phases of therapy addressed values and commitment. Cindy enjoyed the values clarification process and needed little assistance in reframing her values statements so they involved descriptions of processes instead of discrete goals. For example, Cindy indicated that she valued development of caring relationships filled with humor and mutual respect. She also identified several goals related to that value: attending events to which she is invited, and extending an invitation to someone she would like to know better at least once every 2 weeks. She also specified that it was important to work out three times a week. This last goal relates to her relationship goal in four ways: Cindy prefers to take classes at the gym, so working out creates an opportunity to meet people; she has more energy when she is in better shape, and she wants to bring more energy (in contrast with depression) to her friendships; she used to enjoy going dancing and hiking, but her current weight makes participating in these activities more difficult; and increased fitness may bring an increased sense of self-respect to the relationships she is trying to develop.

Once values clarification and commitment have begun, it is common to have to revisit all of the earlier processes addressed in therapy. Up to this stage in therapy, the amount of behavior change required from everyday living has been relatively small. We now rejoin the dialogue between the therapist and Cindy:

T: So how was your first week of committed action homework?

C: Well, the day after we met was great. I went to the gym and took a really hard kickboxing class. Then I walked on the stair machine for 30 minutes.

T: Wow, that was a big first day for someone who has not been working out.

C: No kidding! I felt so sore the next morning I could barely move. I wasn't able to go to the gym for the rest of the week.

T: How did you do on the rest of your goals?

C: Well, nobody invited me out, and I didn't reach out to anyone either. But instead of watching television I set up a profile on a social networking website. I figured that even if I'm not getting out I could try to connect with old friends. I did network with a friend from high school, Marne, and we typed back and forth on each other's pages a couple of times. It was fun.

T: What a great idea.... Now is networking on the Web something you want place as higher priority than your other goals that involve interacting with people in person?

C: Well ... I think I should still work on meeting with people in person.

T: So is that *should* about looking good when you come to our meetings, or is it about something else?

C: I know you're going to ask me about how I did, but I really want to have direct interactions with friends too.

T: OK, I just want you to know that it's perfectly all right to revise your goals and values as you try things out. This is a learning process, and many folks are surprised by what they learn as they explore their goals and values. Switching things up is only a problem if that seems to be what you do every week. At some point it is important to commit to sticking to one thing for a few weeks, just to give it a chance. Speaking about giving things a chance, how about your workout?

C: I did great that first day, but I was really too sore to go again. My legs were so tired, it hurt to walk for four days!

T: Well, was that hurting something that comes with starting a new exercise routine or do you think you injured yourself?

C: I'm better now, so I guess it was just from overdoing it.

T: Have you ever tried to get back into shape after not working out for a long time?

C: No, I was always much more active when I took classes at the gym before. But back then I only went when I felt like it—so it wasn't like I had a real routine or anything. This was my first time working out in 3 years.

T: You should probably talk to your instructor or a personal trainer for some advice on how to safely get into an exercise routine. If you are doing a safe beginners' routine, then you can use the acceptance and commitment techniques we have covered with the normal aches and pains. I just don't want us to use those if they lead you to the point of getting injured. A professional should be able to help you with understanding which types of aches and pains are safe, and which signal injury.

C: My gym comes with two 30-minute trainer consultations a month. I could use those to make sure I'm doing things safely.

T: So when will you call to schedule an appointment with the trainer?

C: On my lunch break tomorrow.

T: And what other goals will you be working on this week?

C: Meeting with people in person.

T: Any plans or prospects?

C: Well, there's a group of people from work that go out for a beer every Thursday. They used to invite me to come along, but after I didn't show up several times they just stopped asking. I could invite myself to come along this week.

T: So, what are the potential barriers that might get in the way of that goal?

The rest of the session focused on the verbal and emotional barriers that have historically interfered with social interactions. Acceptance, defusion, and self as perspective were revisited in relation to taking action on this particular goal. Additional action options were explored that would allow for optional action if the group was not meeting this week.

It took several weeks before Cindy reliably arranged for social outings with others. She did not make a new "best friend," but she enjoyed interacting with others, and they seemed to enjoy interacting with her. Cindy's good sense of humor was an asset in forging new social relationships. She continued to struggle with fusion in the form of self-critical thoughts, but she was getting better at accepting these. They no longer served to keep her isolated from others; she could have those negative thoughts and still have meaningful interactions with others.

There are several important things to notice about this latter phase of therapy for Cindy. Although Cindy initially failed to follow through with one of her goals (i.e., asking others to go out), she did initiate social activity over the Internet. The therapist could have addressed this as a potential way for Cindy to avoid her original goal, since Internet social networking does not involve direct interpersonal interaction. This path was not taken, because it was an opportunity to encourage value-related flexibility. However, if a pattern of choosing activities that did not involve interpersonal interaction had developed over the next few sessions, then potential avoidance functions of these activities would have been explored.

Cindy's case also illustrates that some problems can be due to skills deficits. The deficit addressed in the sample involved her not having the experience to know the difference between normal workout aches and pains, and pain due to injury. It was also clear that Cindy was unable to select realistic workout goals for herself. Thus, she was advised to seek consultation with a personal trainer.

Other skills deficits were addressed with Cindy as well. She had difficulty initiating conversations with others. This was partially due to her unyielding barrage of negative self-evaluations. However, she was also awkward when practicing conversation initiation *in vivo* with the therapist. Cindy usually had a relaxed, smooth conversational style, but while practicing *in vivo*, her voice became strained and she stumbled over her words. The therapist used behavioral modeling and response-contingent feedback to improve her delivery.

As a functional contextual (i.e., behavior analytic) therapy, skills-based interventions can easily be worked into ACT. It is common for ACT therapists to work with their clients on two fronts. This was illustrated with Cindy when acceptance, defusion, and self-as-perspective skills were used to disarm the negative self-evaluations that had previously served as barriers to her initiating conversations. Then, behavioral skills training was included to improve the quality of her interactions.

SUMMARY AND CONCLUSIONS

Although many of the techniques used in ACT may serve as useful tools for clinicians interested in the approach, a clinician is not doing ACT until he or she is applying the theoretical model to the case. ACT therapists have borrowed from and modified techniques from a wide variety of approaches. However, this should not be confused with the type of technical eclecticism advocated by Lazarus (1967).

ACT is a model of how to do behavioral and cognitive therapy. It is based on a theoretical tradition that distinguishes it from most other contemporary cognitive-behavioral therapies, and that distinguishes the treatment development strategy from a traditional manualized package for syndromes approach. This philosophical tradition has more than 75 years of basic and applied research supporting the utility of its analytic concepts.

Although this chapter has focused on reviewing middle-level theoretical processes that emphasize scope and function (specifically for guiding therapist behavior) over precision and depth, the foundations of the approach are the use of inductive functional methods to develop high-precision/high-scope principles of behavior. The concepts underlying ACT are functional, and to be used at their best they need to be used flexibly. This can be done to some degree without understanding basic behavioral principles; that was the purpose of adopting middle-level concepts. The theory also suggests specific ways to assess the relevance of presenting problems to experiential avoidance or cognitive fusion, and there are measures in use (see process studies section) that allow therapists to monitor the change processes that mediate positive client outcomes. But these concepts and methods can only go so far in a given case. Study of the basic concepts and principles of behavior analysis, molar behavioral dynamics, and RFT allow therapists to apply this treatment approach better to novel presenting problems. A broader conceptual foundation also helps to ensure that the focus of treatment is functional, not topographical.

In terms of treatment development, ACT has several unusual or even unique features compared to other cognitive and behavioral methods. ACT developers have been willing to wait until basic principles were developed, greater philosophical clarity was reached, or evidence of effectiveness was obtained, because the goal of ACT is not just another labeled therapy that can reside in lists of empirically supported treatments, but the development of a better model of behavioral and cognitive therapy, linked to a progressive research program in applied and basic psychology. The inductive, bottom-up approach of contextual behavioral science is inherently slow, but it can be speed up with broader and increased participation by clinicians, basic scientists, students, and researchers. This in fact is what seems to be happening. Twenty years ago, there were a few dozen people interested in ACT and its basic research program. Now there are several thousand. Where that interest will take the field is anyone's guess, but it will be interesting to find out.

REFERENCES

ABCT. (2007). *About the Association for Behavioral and Cognitive Therapies: What is ABCT*. Retrieved December 8, 2007, from *www.aabt.org/about*.

Bach, P., & Hayes, S. C. (2002). The use of acceptance and commitment therapy to prevent the rehospitalization of psychotic patients: A randomized controlled trial. *Journal of Consulting and Clinical Psychology, 70*(5), 1129–1139.

Baer, R. A., Smith, G. T., Hopkins, J., Krietemeyer, J., & Toney, L. (2006). Using self-report assessment methods to explore facets of mindfulness. *Assessment, 13*(1), 27–45.

Batten, S. V., & Hayes, S. C. (2005). Acceptance and commitment therapy in the treatment of comorbid substance abuse and post-traumatic stress disorder: A case study. *Clinical Case Studies, 4*(3), 246–262.

Beck, A. T. (1976). *Cognitive therapy and the emotional disorders*. New York: International Universities Press.

Beck, A. T., Rush, A. J., Shaw, B. F., & Emery, G. (1979). *Cognitive therapy of depression*. New York: Guilford Press.

Beck, J. S. (1995). *Cognitive therapy: Basics and beyond*. New York: Guilford Press.

Biglan, A. (1993). A functional contextualist framework for community interventions. In S. C. Hayes, L. J. Hayes, H. W. Reese, & T. R. Sarbin (Eds.), *Varieties of scientific contextualism* (pp. 251–276). Reno, NV: Context Press.

Biglan, A., & Hayes, S. C. (1996). Should the behavioral sciences become more pragmatic?: The case for functional contextualism on human behavior. *Applied and Preventive Psychology: Current Scientific Perspectives, 5*, 47–57.

Blackledge, J. T. (2003). An introduction to relational frame theory: Basics and applications. *The Behavior Analyst Today, 3*(4), 421–433.

Blackledge, J. T., & Hayes, S. C. (2006). Using acceptance and commitment training in the support of parents of children diagnosed with autism. *Child and Family Behavior Therapy, 28*(1), 1–18.

Bond, F. W., & Bunce, D. (2000). Mediators of change in emotion-focused and problem-focused worksite stress management interventions. *Journal of Occupational Health Psychology, 5*(1), 159–163.

Branstetter, A. D., Wilson, K. G., Hildegrandt, M. J., & Mutch, D. (2004, November). *Improving psychological adjustment among cancer patients: ACT and CBT*. Paper presented at the 38th meeting of the Association for Advancement of Behavior Therapy, New Orleans, LA.

Bridgman, P. W. (1927). *The logic of modern physics*. New York: Macmillan.

Brown, R. A., Palm, K. M., Strong, D. R., Lejuez, C. W., Kahler, C. W., Zvolensky, M. J., et al. (2008). Distress tolerance treatment for early lapse smokers: Rationale, program description and preliminary findings. *Behavior Modification, 32,* 302–332.

Campbell-Sills, L., Barlow, D. H., Brown, T. A., & Hofmann, S. G. (2006). Effects of suppression and acceptance on emotional responses of individuals with anxiety and mood disorders. *Behaviour Research and Therapy, 44,* 1251–1263.

Catania, A. C., Matthews, B. A., & Shimoff, E. (1982). Instructed versus shaped human verbal behavior: Interactions with nonverbal responding. *Journal of the Experimental Analysis of Behavior, 38,* 233–248.

Chambless, D. L., & Hollon, S. D. (1998). Defining empirically supported therapies. *Journal of Consulting and Clinical Psychology, 66*(1), 7–18.

Dahl, J., Wilson, K. G., & Nilsson, A. (2004). Acceptance and commitment therapy and the treatment of persons at risk for long-term disability resulting from stress and pain symptoms: A preliminary randomized trial. *Behavior Therapy, 35*(4), 785–801.

Dalrymple, K. L., & Herbert, J. D. (2007). Acceptance and commitment therapy for generalized social anxiety disorder. *Behavior Modification, 31*(5), 543–568.

Dawes, R. M. (2000). Proper and improper linear models. In T. Connolly, H. R. Arkes, & K. R. Hammond (Eds.), *Judgment and decision making: An interdisciplinary reader* (2nd ed., pp. 378–394). New York: Cambridge University Press.

Drossel, C., Waltz, T. J., & Hayes, S. C. (2007). An introduction to principles of behavior. In D. W. Woods & J. W. Kantor (Eds.), *Understanding behavior disorders: A contemporary behavioral perspective* (pp. 21–46). Reno, NV: Context Press.

Eysenck, H. J. (1952). The effects of psychotherapy: An evaluation. *Journal of Consulting Psychology, 16*(5), 319–324.

Feldner, M. T., Zvolensky, M. J., Eifert, G. H., & Spira, A. P. (2003). Emotional avoidance: An experimental test of individual differences and response suppression using biological challenge. *Behaviour Research and Therapy, 41,* 403–411.

Flessner, C. A., Busch, A., Heidemann, P., & Woods, D. W. (2008). Acceptance-enhanced behavior therapy (AEBT) for trichotillomania and chronic skin picking: Exploring the effects of component sequencing. *Behavior Modification, 32*(5), 579–594.

Forman, E. M., Herbert, J. D., Moitra, E., Yeomans, P. D., & Geller, P. A. (2007). A randomized controlled effectiveness trial of acceptance and commitment therapy and cognitive therapy for anxiety and depression. *Behavior Modification, 31*(6), 772–799.

Forman, E. M., Hoffman, K. L., McGrath, K. B., Herbert, J. D., Brandsma, L. L., & Lowe, M. R. (2007). A comparison of acceptance- and control-based strategies for coping with food cravings: An analog study. *Behaviour Research and Therapy, 45,* 2372–2386.

Franks, C. M. (Ed.). (1964). *Conditioning techniques in clinical practice and research.* New York: Springer.

García Montes, J. M., & Perez Alvarez, M. (2001). ACT as treatment for psychotic symptoms: The case of auditory hallucinations. *Analisis y Modificacion de Conducta, 27,* 455–472.

Gaudiano, B. A., & Herbert, J. D. (2006). Acute treatment of inpatients with psychotic symptoms using acceptance and commitment therapy. *Behaviour Research and Therapy, 44*, 415–437.

Gifford, E. V. (2002). *Acceptance based treatment for nicotine dependent smokers: Altering the regulatory functions of smoking related affect, physiological symptoms, and cognition.* Doctoral dissertation, University of Nevada, Reno.

Gifford, E. V., Kohlenberg, B., Hayes, S. C., Pierson, H. M., Piasecki, M., et al. (in press). Applying acceptance and the therapeutic relationship to smoking cessation: A randomized controlled trial. *Journal of Consulting and Clinical Psychology.*

Gifford, E. V., Kohlenberg, B. S., Hayes, S. C., Antonuccio, D. O., Piasecki, M. M., Rasmussen-Hall, M. L., et al. (2004). Acceptance-based treatment for smoking cessation. *Behavior Therapy, 35*(4), 689–705.

Greenberg, L. S., Lietaer, G., & Watson, J. C. (1998). Experiential therapy: Identity and challenges. In L. S. Greenberg, J. Watson, & G. Lietaer (Eds.), *Handbook of experiential psychotherapy* (pp. 451–466). New York: Guilford Press.

Gregg, J. A., Callaghan, G. M., Hayes, S. C., & Glenn-Lawson, J. L. (2007). Improving diabetes self-management through acceptance, mindfulness, and values: A randomized controlled trial. *Journal of Consulting and Clinical Psychology, 75*(2), 336–343.

Gutiérrez, O. M., Luciano, M. C. S., Rodriguez, M., & Fink, B. C. (2004). Comparison between an acceptance-based and a cognitive-control-based protocol for coping with pain. *Behavior Therapy, 35*(4), 767–783.

Hayes, S. C. (1984). Making sense of spirituality. *Behaviorism, 12*, 99–110.

Hayes, S. C. (1986). Behavioral philosophy in the late 1980's. *Theoretical and Philosophical Psychology, 6*(1), 39–43.

Hayes, S. C. (1987). A contextual approach to therapeutic change. In N. Jacobson (Ed.), *Cognitive and behavior therapies in clinical practice* (pp. 327–387). New York: Guilford Press.

Hayes, S. C. (Ed.). (1989). *Rule-governed behavior: Cognition, contingencies, and instructional control.* New York: Plenum Press.

Hayes, S. C. (1993). Analytic goals and the varieties of scientific contextualism. In S. C. Hayes, L. J. Hayes, H. W. Reese, & T. R. Sarbin (Eds.), *Varieties of scientific contextualism* (pp. 11–27). Reno, NV: Context Press.

Hayes, S. C. (1995). Knowing selves. *The Behavior Therapist, 18*(5), 94–96.

Hayes, S. C. (1997). Behavioral epistemology includes nonverbal knowing. In L. J. Hayes & P. M. Ghezzi (Eds.), *Investigations in behavioral epistemology* (pp. 35–43). Reno, NV: Context Press.

Hayes, S. C. (2004). Falsification and the protective belt surrounding entity-postulating theories. *Applied and Preventive Psychology, 11*(1), 35–37.

Hayes, S. C., Barnes-Holmes, D., & Roche, B. (Eds.). (2001). *Relational frame theory: A post-Skinnerian account of human language and cognition.* New York: Kluwer Academic/Plenum Press.

Hayes, S. C., Bissett, R., Korn, Z., Zettle, R. D., Rosenfarb, I., Cooper, L., et al. (1999). The impact of acceptance versus control rationales on pain tolerance. *Psychological Record, 49*(1), 33–47.

Hayes, S. C., Bissett, R., Roget, N., Padilla, M., Kohlenberg, B. S., Fisher, G., et al.

(2004). The impact of acceptance and commitment training and multicultural training on the stigmatizing attitudes of professional burnout and substance abuse counselors. *Behavior Therapy, 35*(4), 821–835.

Hayes, S. C., & Brownstein, A. J. (1986). Mentalism, behavior–behavior relations, and a behavior–analytic view of the purposes of science. *The Behavior Analyst, 9*, 175–190.

Hayes, S. C., Brownstein, A. J., Haas, J. R., & Greenway, D. E. (1986). Instructions, multiple schedules, and extinction: Distinguishing rule-governed from schedule-controlled behavior. *Journal of the Experimental Analysis of Behavior, 46*, 137–147.

Hayes, S. C., Brownstein, A. J., Zettle, R. D., Rosenfarb, I., & Korn, Z. (1986). Rule-governed behavior and sensitivity to changing consequences of responding. *Journal of the Experimental Analysis of Behavior, 45*, 237–256.

Hayes, S. C., Hayes, L. J., & Reese, H. W. (1988). Finding the philosophical core: A review of Stephen C. Pepper's world hypotheses: A study in evidence. *Journal of the Experimental Analysis of Behavior, 50*(1), 97–111.

Hayes, S. C., Korn, Z., Zettle, R. D., Rosenfarb, I., & Cooper, L. (1982, November). *Rule-governed behavior and cognitive behavior therapy: The effects of comprehensive cognitive distancing on pain tolerance.* Paper presented at the 16th meeting of the Association for Advancement of Behavior Therapy, Los Angeles.

Hayes, S. C., Levin, M., Plumb, J., Boulanger, J., & Pistorello, J. (in press). Acceptance and commitment therapy and contextual behavioral science: Examining the progress of a distinctive model of behavioral and cognitive therapy. *Behavior Therapy.*

Hayes, S. C., Luoma, J. B., Bond, F. W., Masuda, A., & Lillis, J. (2006). Acceptance and commitment therapy: Model, processes and outcomes. *Behaviour Research and Therapy, 44*(1), 1–25.

Hayes, S. C., Masuda, A., Shenk, C., Yadavaia, J. E., Boulanger, J., Vilardaga, R., et al. (2007). Applied extensions of behavior principles: Applied behavioral concepts and behavioral theories. In D. W. Woods & J. W. Kantor (Eds.), *Understanding behavior disorders: A contemporary behavioral perspective* (pp. 47–80). Reno, NV: Context Press.

Hayes, S. C., Rosenfarb, I., Wulfert, E., Mint, E., Zettle, R. D., & Korn, Z. (1985). Self-reinforcement effects: An artifact of social standard setting? *Journal of Applied Behavior Analysis, 18*, 201–214.

Hayes, S. C., Strosahl, K., Bunting, K., Twohig, M., & Wilson, K. G. (2004). What is acceptance and commitment therapy? In S. C. Hayes & K. Strosahl (Eds.), *A practical guide to acceptance and commitment therapy* (pp. 1–29). New York: Springer.

Hayes, S. C., Strosahl, K., Wilson, K. G., Bissett, R., Pistorello, J., Toarmino, D., et al. (2004). Measuring experiential avoidance: A preliminary test of a working model. *Psychological Record, 54*, 553–578.

Hayes, S. C., Strosahl, K. D., & Wilson, K. G. (1999). *Acceptance and commitment therapy: An experiential approach to behavior change.* New York: Guilford Press.

Hayes, S. C., Wilson, K. G., Gifford, E. V., Bissett, R., Piasecki, M. M., Batten, S.

V., et al. (2004). A preliminary trial of twelve-step facilitation and acceptance and commitment therapy with polysubstance-abusing methadone-maintained opiate addicts. *Behavior Therapy, 35*(4), 667–688.

Hayes, S. C., Wilson, K. G., Gifford, E. V., Follette, V. M., & Strosahl, K. (1996). Experiential avoidance and behavioral disorders: A functional dimensional approach to diagnosis and treatment. *Journal of Consulting and Clinical Psychology, 64*(6), 1152–1168.

Hayes, S. C., & Wolf, M. (1984). Cues, consequences, and therapeutic talk: Effects of social context and coping statements on pain. *Behaviour Research and Therapy, 22*, 385–392.

Heffner, M., Sperry, J., & Eifert, G. H. (2002). Acceptance and commitment therapy in the treatment of an adolescent female with anorexia nervosa: A case example. *Cognitive and Behavioral Practice, 9*(3), 232–236.

Hineline, P. N. (1984). What then is Skinner's operationism? *Behavior and Brain Sciences, 7*, 560.

Hollon, S. D., & Kendall, P. C. (1980). Cognitive self-statement in depression: Development of an automatic thoughts questionnaire. *Cognitive Therapy and Research, 4*, 383–395.

Huerta, F. R., Gomez, S. M., Molina, A. M. M., & Luciano, M. C. S. (1998). Generalized anxiety: A case study. *Analisis y Modificacion de Conducta, 24*, 751–766.

John of Salisbury. (1982). *The metalogicon of John of Salisbury: A twelfth-century defense of the verbal and logical arts of the trivium* (D. D. McGarry, Trans.). Westport, CT: Greenwood Press.

Lappalainen, R., Lehtonen, T., Skarp, E., Taubert, E., Ojanen, M., & Hayes, S. C. (2007). The impact of CBT and ACT models using psychology trainee therapists: A preliminary controlled effectiveness trial. *Behavior Modification, 31*(4), 488–511.

Lazarus, A. A. (1967). In support of technical eclecticism. *Psychological Reports, 21*(2), 415–416.

Leahey, T. H. (2004). *A history of psychology: Main currents in psychological thought* (6th ed.). Upper Saddle River, NJ: Pearson Education.

Levite, J. T., Brown, T. A., Gorilla, S. M., & Barlow, D. H. (2004). The effects of acceptance versus suppression of emotion on subjective and psychophysiological response to carbon dioxide challenge in patients with panic disorder. *Behavior Therapy, 35*(4), 747–766.

Lillis, J., Hayes, S. C., Bunting, K., & Masuda, A. I. (2009). Teaching acceptance and mindfulness to improve the lives of the obese: A preliminary test if a theoretical model. *Annals of Behavioral Medicine, 37*(1), 58–69.

Lopez Ortega, S., & Arco Tirado, J. L. (2002). ACT as an alternative to patients that do not respond to traditional treatments: A case study. *Analisis y Modificacion de Conducta, 28*, 585–616.

Luciano, M. C. S., & Cabello, F. L. (2001). Bereavement and acceptance and commitment therapy (ACT). *Analisis y Modificacion de Conducta, 27*, 399–424.

Luciano, M. C. S., & Gomez, S. M. (2001). Alcoholism, experiential avoidance, and acceptance and commitment therapy (ACT). *Analisis y Modificacion de Conducta, 27*, 333–371.

Luciano, M. C. S., Visdomine, J. C. L., Gutiérrez, O. M., & Montesinos, F. M. (2001). ACT and chronic pain. *Analisis y Modificacion de Conducta, 27*, 473–501.

Lundgren, T., Dahl, J., & Hayes, S. C. (2008). Evaluation of mediators of change in the treatment of epilepsy with acceptance and commitment therapy. *Journal of Behavioral Medicine, 31*(3), 225–235.

Lundgren, T., Dahl, J., Melin, L., & Kies, B. (2006). Evaluation of acceptance and commitment therapy for drug refractory epilepsy: A randomized controlled trail in South Africa—A pilot study. *Epilepsia, 47*(12), 2173–2179.

Luoma, J. B., & Hayes, S. C. (2003). Cognitive defusion. In W. O'Donohue, J. E. Fisher, & S. C. Hayes (Eds.), *Cognitive behavior therapy: Applying empirically supported techniques in your practice* (pp. 71–78). Hoboken, NJ: Wiley.

Luoma, J. B., Twohig, M. P., Waltz, T. J., Hayes, S. C., Roget, N., Padilla, M., et al. (2007). An investigation of stigma in individuals receiving treatment for substance abuse. *Addictive Behaviors, 32*, 1331–1346.

Masuda, A. I., & Esteve, M. R. (2007). Effects of suppression, acceptance and spontaneous coping on pain tolerance, pain intensity and distress. *Behaviour Research and Therapy, 45*, 199–209.

Masuda, A., Hayes, S. C., Fletcher, L., Seignourel, P. J., Bunting, K., Herbst, S. A., et al. (2007). Impact of acceptance and commitment therapy versus education on stigma toward people with psychological disorders. *Behaviour Research and Therapy, 45*, 2764–2772.

McCracken, L. M., & Eccleston, C. (2005). A prospective study of acceptance of pain and patient functioning with chronic pain. *Pain, 118*, 164–169.

McCracken, L. M., & Eccleston, C. (2006). A comparison of the relative utility of coping and acceptance-based measures in a sample of chronic pain sufferers. *European Journal of Pain, 10*, 23–29.

McCracken, L. M., MacKichan, F., & Eccleston, C. (2007). Contextual cognitive-behavioral therapy for severely disabled chronic pain sufferers: Effectiveness and clinically meaningful change. *European Journal of Pain, 11*, 314–322.

McCracken, L. M., & Vowles, K. E. (2008). A prospective analysis of acceptance of pain and values-based action in patients with chronic pain. *Health Psychology, 27*(2), 215–220.

McCracken, L. M., Vowles, K. E., & Eccleston, C. (2004). Acceptance of chronic pain: Component analysis and a revised assessment method. *Pain, 107*, 159–166.

McCracken, L. M., Vowles, K. E., & Eccleston, C. (2005). Acceptance-based treatment for persons with complex, long standing chronic pain: A preliminary analysis of treatment outcome in comparison to a waiting phase. *Behaviour Research and Therapy, 43*, 1335–1246.

McHugh, L., Barnes-Holmes, Y., & Barnes-Holmes, D. (2004). Perspective taking as relational responding: A developmental profile. *Psychological Record, 54*(1), 115–144.

Moore, J. (2003). Explanation and description in traditional neobehaviorism, cognitive psychology, and behavior analysis. In K. A. Cattalo & P. N. Chase (Eds.), *Behavior theory and philosophy* (pp. 13–39). New York: Kluwer Academic/Plenum Press.

Ossman, W. A., Wilson, K. G., Storaasli, R. D., & McNeill, J. W. (2006). A preliminary investigation of the use of acceptance and commitment therapy in group treatment for social phobia. *International Journal of Psychology and Psychological Therapy*, 6(3), 397–416.

Öst, L. (2008). Efficacy of the third-wave behavioral therapies: A systematic review and meta-analysis. *Behaviour Research and Therapy*, 46, 296–321.

Paez, M. B., Luciano, M. C. S., & Gutiérrez, O. M. (2007). Tratamiento psicológico para el afrontamiento del cáncer de mama: Estudio comparativo entre estrategias de aceptación y de control cognitivo. [Psychological treatment for coping with breast cancer. A comparative study of acceptance and cognitive-control strategies.] *Psicooncologia*, 4, 75–95.

Pepper, S. C. (1942). *World hypotheses*. Berkeley: University of California Press.

Persons, J. B. (2003). The Association for Behavioral and Cognitive Therapies: An idea whose time has come. *The Behavior Therapist*, 26(2), 225.

Petersen, C. L., & Zettle, R. D. (2008). *Impacting depression in inpatients with comorbid alcohol use disorders: A comparison of acceptance and commitment therapy versus treatment as usual*. Manuscript submitted for publication.

Roemer, L., Orsillo, S. M., & Salters-Pedneault, K. (2008). Efficacy of an acceptance-based behavior therapy for generalized anxiety disorder: Evaluation in a randomized controlled trial. *Journal of Consulting and Clinical Psychology*, 76(6), 1083–1089.

Rosenfarb, I., & Hayes, S. C. (1984). Social standard setting: the Achilles Heel of informational accounts of therapeutic change. *Behavior Therapy*, 15, 515–528.

Shawyer, F., Ratcliff, K., Mackinnon, A., Farhall, J., Hayes, S. C., & Copolov, S. (2007). The Voices Acceptance and Action Scale (VAAS): Pilot data. *Journal of Clinical Psychology*, 63(6), 593–606.

Shimoff, E., Catania, A. C., & Matthews, B. A. (1981). Uninstructed human responding: Sensitivity of low-rate performance to schedule contingencies. *Journal of the Experimental Analysis of Behavior*, 36, 207–220.

Skinner, B. F. (1945). The operational analysis of psychological terms. *Psychological Review*, 52(5), 270–277.

Skinner, B. F. (1948). *Walden two*. New York: MacMillan.

Smith, L. D. (1986). *Behaviorism and logical positivism: A reassessment of the alliance*. Stanford, CA: Stanford University Press.

Smout, M. F., Longo, M., Krasnikow, S., Minniti, R., Wickes, W., & White, J. M. (2008). *Behavior therapy for methamphetamine abuse: An empirical comparison of cognitive behavior therapy and acceptance and commitment therapy*. Manuscript submitted for publication.

Strosahl, K., Hayes, S. C., & Bergan, J. (1998). Assessing the field effectiveness of acceptance and commitment therapy: An example of the manipulated training research method. *Behavior Therapy*, 29(1), 35–64.

Strosahl, K., Hayes, S. C., Wilson, K. G., & Gifford, E. V. (2004). An ACT primer: Core therapy processes, intervention strategies, and therapist competencies. In S. C. Hayes & K. Strosahl (Eds.), *A practical guide to acceptance and commitment therapy* (pp. 31–58). New York: Springer.

Twohig, M. P., Hayes, S. C., & Masuda, A. (2006a). Increasing willingness to experience obsessions: Acceptance and commitment therapy as a treatment for obsessive–compulsive disorder. *Behavior Therapy, 37*(1), 3–13.

Twohig, M. P., Hayes, S. C., & Masuda, A. (2006b). A preliminary investigation of acceptance and commitment therapy as a treatment for chronic skin picking. *Behaviour Research and Therapy, 44*(10), 1513–1522.

Twohig, M. P., Shoenberger, D., & Hayes, S. C. (2007). A preliminary investigation of acceptance and commitment therapy as a treatment for marijuana dependence in adults. *Journal of Applied Behavior Analysis, 40*(4), 619–632.

Twohig, M. P., & Woods, D. W. (2004). A preliminary investigation of acceptance and commitment therapy and habit reversal as a treatment for trichotillomania. *Behavior Therapy, 35*(4), 803–820.

Vilardaga, R., Hayes, S. C., Levin, M., & Muto, T. (2009). Creating a strategy for progress: A contextual behavioral science approach. *The Behavior Analyst, 32*, 105–133.

Vowles, K. E., & McCracken, L. M. (2008). Acceptance and values-based action in chronic pain: A study of effectiveness and treatment process. *Journal of Consulting and Clinical Psychology, 76*(3), 397–407.

Vowles, K. E., McCracken, L. M., & Eccleston, C. (2007). Processes of change in treatment for chronic pain: The contributions of pain, acceptance, and catastrophizing. *European Journal of Pain, 11*, 779–787.

Vowles, K. E., McCracken, L. M., & Eccleston, C. (2008). Patient functioning and catastrophizing in chronic pain: The mediating effects of acceptance. *Health Psychology, 27*(Suppl. 2), S136–S143.

Vowles, K. E., McNeil, D. W., Gross, R. T., McDaniel, M. L., Mouse, A., Bates, M., et al. (2007). Effects of pain acceptance and pain control strategies on physical impairment in individuals with chronic low back pain. *Behavior Therapy, 38*(4), 412–425.

Wegner, D. (1994). Ironic processes of mental control. *Psychological Review, 1001*, 34–52.

Weil, T. M., Hayes, S. C., & Capurro, P. (2008). *The impact of training diectic frames on perspective taking in young children.* Manuscript submitted for publication.

Wicksell, R. K., Ahlqvist, J., Bring, A., Melin, L., & Olsson, G. L. (2008). Can exposure and acceptance strategies improve functioning and life satisfaction in people with chronic pain and whiplash-associated disorders (WAD)?: A randomized controlled trial. *Cognitive Behaviour Therapy, 37*(3), 1–14.

Wicksell, R. K., Melin, L., & Olsson, G. L. (2007). Exposure and acceptance in the rehabilitation of adolescents with idiopathic chronic pain: A pilot study. *European Journal of Pain, 11*, 267–274.

Woods, D. W., Wetterneck, C. T., & Flessner, C. A. (2006). A controlled evaluation of acceptance and commitment therapy plus habit reversal for trichotillomania. *Behaviour Research and Therapy, 44*, 639–656.

Zaldivar Basurto, F., & Hernández López, M. (2001). Acceptance and commitment therapy: Application to an experiential avoidance with agoraphobic form. *Analisis y Modificacion de Conducta, 27*, 425–454.

Zettle, R. D. (2003). Acceptance and commitment therapy (ACT) vs. systematic desensitization in the treatment of mathematics anxiety. *Psychological Record, 53*, 197–215.

Zettle, R. D., & Hayes, S. C. (1982). Rule governed behavior: A potential theoretical framework for cognitive-behavioral therapy. In P. C. Kendall (Ed.), *Advances in cognitive behavioral research and therapy* (pp. 73–118). New York: Academic Press.

Zettle, R. D., & Hayes, S. C. (1983). The effect of social context on the impact of coping self-statements. *Psychological Reports, 52*, 391–401.

Zettle, R. D., & Hayes, S. C. (1986). Dysfunctional control by client verbal behavior: The context of reason-giving. *The Analysis of Verbal Behavior, 4*, 30–38.

Zettle, R. D., & Hayes, S. C. (1987). Component and process analysis of cognitive therapy. *Psychological Reports, 61*, 939–953.

Zettle, R. D., & Rains, J. C. (1989). Group cognitive and contextual therapies in treatment of depression. *Journal of Clinical Psychology, 43*(3), 436–445.

CHAPTER 6

Behavioral Activation Therapy

Christopher R. Martell
Sona Dimidjian
Peter M. Lewinsohn

INTRODUCTION AND HISTORICAL BACKGROUND

Behavioral activation therapy (BA) for depression has a history reaching back to the early behaviorists in American academic psychology, as well as to the philosophy of pragmatism. While not directly considering human psychopathology, Thorndike was the first theorist to be credited for proposing ideas that have come to be closely related to BA. As Bolles (1979) observed, "Before Thorndike, human learning had been presumed to consist simply of the gathering of experience" (p. 18). It was Thorndike who, in 1911, identified the law of effect, which maintains that learning consists of the strengthening of a connection between a stimulus and a response, and that the effect of the response on the organism either strengthens or weakens the connection (Thorndike, 1911, as cited in Bolles, 1979).

Thorndike's work was later built upon by Skinner and colleagues, and became a primary focus of radical behaviorism. The contingencies of reinforcement that maintained or extinguished a behavior provided a parsimonious explanation for various behaviors and feeling states that had previously been described primarily by theories of the mind. Like the pragmatist philosopher John Dewey, the explanations of behavior by Thorndike and, later, Skinner, broke from the mind–body dualism of a Cartesian worldview. The Cartesian distinctions between that which was physical and that which was psychic were rejected by the pragmatists and by the behaviorists. Of the distinction between living things (thus assumed to have "mind") and nonliving, material things, Dewey stated:

> Empirically speaking, the most obvious difference between living and non-living things is that the activities of the former are characterized by needs, by efforts which are active demands to satisfy need, and by satisfactions. In making this statement, the terms need, effort and satisfaction are primarily employed in a biological sense. By need is meant a condition of tensional distribution of energies such that the body is in a condition of uneasy or unstable equilibrium. By demand or effort is meant the fact that this state is manifested in movements which modify environing bodies in ways which react upon the body, so that its characteristic pattern of active equilibrium is restored. (Dewey, 1925, as cited in Hickman & Alexander, 1998, p. 136)

Skinner's theory of operant conditioning followed similar reasoning, that the behavior of an organism is determined by the transactions between the organism and the environment, such that the consequences of behavior that, in Dewey's terms, "satisfy" the "need" of the organism increase the likelihood of the behavior occurring again in similar circumstances. This overall context of the activities of a living organism in a particular environment determines conditions that are developed through classically conditioned processes, as well as operant processes. Classical or Pavlovian conditioning theory posited that paired stimuli take on similar functions. For example, the neutral stimulus of a hospital building, paired with the grief experienced by an individual being who is present through the death of a loved one in hospital, becomes associated with the grief, thus eliciting this response following the pairing, and is no longer neutral but has become a conditioned stimulus for a grief reaction. Joseph Wolpe (1958) was the first to extend classical conditioning constructs to psychopathology. Wolpe's understanding of the manner in which negative emotions serve as conditioned responses to environmental stimuli remains at the heart of a behavioral understanding of depression. Operant theory posits the way that the organism and environment operate to maintain or to extinguish particular behaviors under particular circumstances; thus, the operant includes the antecedent stimuli that elicit a particular behavior, and the behavior is then more or less likely to occur under similar stimuli in the future as a result of the consequences following the behavior.

Specifically with respect to depression, Skinner emphasized individuals' reactions to various schedules of reinforcement, stating, "When reinforcement is no longer forthcoming, behavior undergoes 'extinction' and appears rarely.... A person is then said to suffer a loss of confidence, certainty, or sense of power. Instead, his feelings range from a lack of interest ... to a possibly deep depression" (1974, p. 64). Skinner also noted the impact of punishment on decreasing the likelihood that a behavior would occur in the future and the feelings associated with the loss of reinforcement. He noted, "Excessive punishment is said to make a shortage of positive reinforcement critical and leave a person 'more vulnerable to severe depression and to giving up.' We treat what is felt not by changing the feelings but by changing the contingencies. For example, by evoking the behavior without punishing it" (1974, pp. 70–71). C. B. Ferster (1973) explained depression also in terms of radical behavioral principles. According to Ferster, the lack of behavior exhibited by depressed individuals indicated that an extinction process had occurred. Furthermore, Ferster conceptualized much of the behavior emitted by depressed individuals, including reporting on their distress, as avoidance behavior. Basing his theory on an operant model, Ferster described the reinforcement schedules and contingencies that could account for the dysphoria, inertia, and negativity observed in depressed clients. When high levels of activity are required for minimal reward, the rate of the activity diminishes. Likewise when proactive behaviors are not responded to (i.e., reinforced) or are punished, the individual may engage in behaviors that function simply to escape or avoid aversive conditions rather than actively engage the environment to obtain satisfaction of the need.

Ferster's writing was in the tradition of several others who applied behavioral principles to clinical psychology, which at that time was understood exclusively in terms of psychoanalytic concepts. Others who were working in that vein were Dollard and Miller (1950), who applied Hull's behavioral theories to the understanding and treatment of psychopathology. Hull had proposed that drive and habit together determine the strength of a behavior, and that the ultimate function of behavior was to solve biological problems, such as needs for nourishment. The strength of a behavior relied mostly on habit, and habit was the result of the number of reinforcements for a particular behavior in particular circumstances (Bolles, 1979). Dollard and Miller (1950) noted that "neurotic misery is real—not imaginary. Observers ... often belittle the suffering of neurotics and confuse neurosis with malingering.... At times the depth of the misery ... is concealed by his symptoms.... Strongly driven to approach and as strongly to flee, he is not able to act to reduce either of the conflicting drives" (pp. 12–13). While the term *neurotic* is no longer used diagnostically, much of what Dollard and Miller said about suffering of individuals that we would now classify as having a DSM Axis I disorder fits with a BA conceptualization of depression and the hopelessness that results from the realities of life suffering and conflicting goals (i.e. drives or needs).

Peter Lewinsohn is credited as the first behavior therapist to develop BA as a treatment for depression. Lewinsohn, Weinstein, and Shaw (1969) attributed low rates of response-contingent positive reinforcement (resconposre; Lewinsohn, 1974) as a critical antecedent to depression. The model considered that these low rates of resconposre occur for three possible reasons (Lewinsohn, 2004):

1. Events that are contingent on behavior may not be reinforcing; thus, the behavior is extinguished. For example, an individual may find going to a book reading at a local library boring and sleep inducing, and is, thus, less likely to attend in the future.
2. Reinforcing events may become unavailable. This is the case when a dear loved one leaves either temporarily for a job or military assignment in another state, or permanently through death.
3. The individual may be unable to elicit available reinforcers because of a lack of requisite skills. For example, a person who has been shy and reticent to interact with peers throughout childhood may find him- or herself interested in attending college social events but has not learned the repertoire of behaviors for making small talk for fluid social discourse.

Lewinsohn and colleagues also posited that depressed behaviors may furthermore be reinforced through responses in the environment such as sympathy and concern from others. It is hypothesized in the model that "depressed individuals are more sensitive, experience a greater number of aversive events, and ... are less skillful in terminating aversive events" (Lewinsohn, 2001, p. 442). This original model did not take into account cognition, and it was often considered to be at odds with approaches such as the cognitive model of Beck (Beck, Rush, Shaw, & Emery, 1979).

An integrated model developed in 1985 (Lewinsohn, Hoberman, Teri, & Hautzinger, 1985) considered depression to be a product of environmental and dispositional factors. Specifically, the model postulated that "the inability to reverse the impact of a evolving event is hypothesized to lead to a heightened state of self-awareness, ... i.e., a state in which attention is focused internally which results in individuals becoming aware of their thoughts, feelings, values, and standards. Increasing self-awareness has been shown to cause individuals to become increasingly self-critical" (Lewinsohn, 2004, p. 526). This model integrated cognition into the overall understanding of depression; however, it did not assume that cognitive change is essential to treatment. In contrast, it allowed for feedback loops wherein becoming depressed, and thinking and behaving in the depressed mode, interfere with problem solving. This further impairs the individual's ability to reverse the environmental disruption. Therefore, intervention to reverse any components of this cycle will lead to the amelioration of the depression (Lewinsohn, 2001).

Lewinsohn's model made use of ideas about self-reinforcement and self-control postulated by Lynn Rehm and Carilyn Fuchs (Fuchs & Rehm, 1977; Rehm, 1977). They emphasized the importance of instructions that assist clients in connecting antecedents and consequences of their behavior. While moving more in the direction of cognitive approaches, Rehm and Fuchs developed a model that was solidly based in theories of reinforcement.

Neil S. Jacobson was originally associated with behavioral marital therapy following the publication of a book he coauthored with Gayla Margolin, based on their respective doctoral research (Jacobson & Margolin, 1979). During the course of his career, however, Jacobson had three separate programs of research: marital therapy, domestic violence research, and treatment of depression (Rutter, 2000). His research suggested a strong relationship between marital discord and depression, and he began to conduct research on the interpersonal consequences of depression (Follette & Jacobson, 1988; Jacobson, Holtzworth-Munroe, & Schmaling, 1989; Rutter, 2000). Jacobson, Dobson, Fruzzetti, Schmaling, and Salusky (1991) compared cognitive-behavioral therapy with behavioral marital therapy and a treatment combining the two treatments. Outcome variables were alleviation of wives' depression and enhancement of marital satisfaction. Behavioral marital therapy had little impact on the wives' depression for couples who did not report significant marital distress. For those couples reporting pretreatment marital distress, behavioral marital therapy performed comparably to cognitive-behavioral therapy in alleviating wives' depression. The combined treatment was not more effective than either of the component treatments. Follow-up data showed that the couple's treatments did not produce greater reductions in relapse than cognitive-behavioral therapy (Jacobson, Fruzzetti, Dobson, Whisman, & Hops, 1993). Jacobson's research on couple therapy for depression was based on his conviction that depression was not something that exists "within" the individual. From a radical behavioral perspective, factors external to the organism influence behavior; thus, depression must be considered in the context of the person's life. *Context* includes factors such as family history, social systems, and political structures that have an impact on the individual (Jacobson, 1994). With this in mind, Jacobson began a research agenda to study the active components of cognitive therapy for depression and to examine behavior therapy, specifically, BA, as a contextual treatment for depression.

PHILOSOPHICAL AND THEORETICAL UNDERPINNINGS

Philosophical Base of the Model

BA is often included as a related therapy in lists of so-called "third generation" behaviorism (O'Donohue, 1998), BA has notably been used in the cognitive-behavioral treatment of depression for decades. The rise of cognitive-behavior therapy has been defined by O'Donohue as part of "second generation" behavior therapy, wherein social psychological literature and research on information processing was relied on more heavily than learning principles. Some have distinguished current, "third generation" behavior therapies from traditional behavior therapy in that they are more contextual than mechanistic (Hayes, Hayes, & Reese, 1988). Mechanistic approaches seek to determine what is wrong with the individual (e.g., poor social skills) and fix it. Contextual approaches look at the variables external to the individual that exert control over behavior and focus on changing contingencies. BA as a theory fits directly in the realm of contextualism. The main philosophical underpinnings of BA, are contextual, and the theory and treatment rely heavily on the pragmatic truth criterion (Pepper, 1942) as a guiding principle. As stated in Martell, Addis, and Jacobson (2001, p. 40):

> "In BA we follow the pragmatic truth criterion quite a bit. We don't, for example, assert that contextualism is *de facto* the right way to view depression. Rather, we find it useful to focus on changing actions and contexts.... The pragmatic truth criterion always leads us to ask our clients and ourselves "What are the consequences of thinking/talking/acting in this particular way?"

Theory of Psychopathology

The theory of psychopathology that underlies BA acknowledges the role of biological and temperamental variables increasing vulnerability to depression; however, the emphasis is clearly placed on increasing activity that will likely be reinforced in the environment. Biology is part of the context, and when any component changes, the context changes. Thus, changes that we consider behavioral are also having an impact at the biological level. Again, the Cartesian separation between mind and body does not apply here. Consistent with the early formulation by Lewinsohn that depression results from low rates of resconposre, high rates of punishment, or both, the theory that underlies behavioral activation heavily emphasizes reinforcement schedules and individual responses to contingencies. The approach is thus highly contextual in emphasis. In other words, depression is not something that exists exclusively inside the person. There is utility in considering depression a clinical syndrome, including the combination of decreased rates of resconposre and other variables that elicit dysphoric mood states. The resulting escape and avoidance behaviors serve to exacerbate the negative mood. Thus, as in cognitive theory, there is consideration of a downward spiral of depression consisting of life situations and client emotional reactions to the situations, and the behavioral patterns that follow.

The model of psychopathology underlying BA does not make a priori assumptions about any particular precipitating factors or behaviors that maintain depression. Any number of life events may have predisposed the individual to depression. Many classically conditioned emotional responses may have resulted in responses in which the individual is no longer aware of the original conditions under which the response developed. Furthermore, life events that have led to low rates of resconposre or high rates of punishment elicit a reaction in the individual. The individual experiences these reactions as aversive and acts in certain ways to alleviate the distress. An example of this is a client staying in bed for all or most of a day because he or she feels fatigued. According to the theory, the fatigue is a natural response to the reinforcement contingencies, and remaining in bed is a natural response to fatigue. Should the individual drift in and out of sleep and also escape other aversive experiences (e.g., feeling sad, ruminating about the miseries of life), staying in bed will be negatively reinforced and more likely to occur again when the individual feels fatigued. Depressive behaviors can also be maintained through positive reinforcement, and BA does not focus only on avoidance behaviors and negative reinforcement contingencies. A depressed client may receive a great deal of attention and comfort from concerned loved ones for behaviors that, in the long run, maintain the depression.

Translating Philosophy and Theory into an Individualized Case Conceptualization to Guide Treatment

In BA, as in other radical behavioral approaches, cognitions are viewed as behavior, albeit private behavior, observable only to the person engaged in the thinking process. Insofar as private behavior becomes public during conversation with the therapist, cognitions are assessed, but attempts are not made to restructure cognition. Cognitions are not dealt with directly in BA. Research therapists on the clinical outcome studies were prohibited from utilizing cognitive interventions. While therapists in the clinical community would not be held to such rigid prohibitions, the data suggest that BA is an efficacious treatment without the use of standard cognitive techniques, such as the use of automatic thought records or schema-focused approaches. In BA, a distinction is made between the content of thinking and the process of thinking. The content of thinking refers to what the individual reports that he or she is thinking. Thus, Beck's negative triad (Beck et al., 1979) of negative views of self, world, and future would come into play. In cognitive therapy, a shift in the tenacity of belief in a particular negative thought would, we hope, lead to a reduction in depressive symptoms.

Belief change as a precursor to either shifts in emotion or behavior change is not essential in BA. BA theory eschews the idea of the primacy of cognition. Some reactions are simply classically conditioned responses to environmental stimuli, and even under conditions when the client can identify a thought, there is no assumption that the thought is causing the emotion. For example, many people experience the evocative power of music. Someone who had distressing experiences during adolescence, when a particular song was popular and frequently played on the radio, may have a negative reaction to hearing the song many years later, when life circumstances have changed significantly from the distress of adolescence. The sad feelings may be associated with a memory of a particular event in adolescence (e.g., a breakup) or the words of the song itself, or the individual may hear the song, feel sad, and not be able to relate the two as connected at all.

When the content of a thought is not a focus for treatment, then what is? In BA, the process or the context of thinking is the focus. It is not the client's negative, self-deprecating, hopeless thoughts that matter but rather that the client spends time engaged in these negative ruminations. Although a connection between thoughts and emotions is not assumed, it is often the case that engaging in the private behavior of ruminating on misery interferes with enjoyment of public behavior. Take as an example going for a walk on a lovely sunny day, a behavior that many depressed clients attempt and report failure at enjoying. There are several potentially enjoyable components to such a walk. The intensity of sunlight enhances the colors of plants and houses; there is beauty in the blueness of the sky; the sun is warm against the skin; the air may smell fresh; physical exercise feels good; there may be a sense of well-being, or memories of other such lovely walks may be elicited. However, enjoyment of any of these potentially enjoyable components requires that one attend to them; otherwise, they pass without notice. It is possible to walk past the most vibrant colors of a field rich with flowers on the sunniest of days, while engaging in an endless stream of thoughts about how unhappy one is, how trapped, wondering whether one will ever feel good again. The ruminating is the behavior to which the individual attends. A worsening cycle of negative thinking occurs in that the lack of improvement in mood during the walk confirms the hopelessness of the individual, and there is then more about which to ruminate.

Recent Theoretical Developments

The recent developments in BA actually represent a return to the historical roots of the treatment. BA has been taken back from being one component of a larger cognitive-behavioral therapy (CBT) conceptualization and once again is applied as a stand-alone treatment. Thus, it is not that new theories have been generated, but that the component analysis study findings revitalized interest in theories that were proposed decades ago but have not been maximally utilized for clinical applications. The current theory suggests that avoidance behaviors may play a key role in the maintenance of depression; therefore, BA therapists pay close attention to behaviors that may function as avoidance for a particular client. Of course, such a conclusion about the function of a behavior is only made following a behavioral analysis. An emphasis on avoidance behaviors, once considered a factor in most behavioral disorders (Wolpe, 1958), has once again been considered a part of a unified treatment for many psychological disorders (Barlow, Allen, & Choate, 2004).

Current Challenges to the Theory

The current challenges to the theory behind BA are the same as they have been since the 1970s, and questions regarding the necessity of changing belief systems versus changing behavior for its own sake remain. Given the insufficient data regarding mechanisms of change in psychotherapy outcome, there is still room for several explanations for outcome in clinical trials. Whereas our proposal is that changing the context and assisting individuals to engage in activities that increase resconposre is the key to change, others have an equally valid hypothesis that changing behavior may in fact result in a change in beliefs or attitudes, which is necessary for improvement (Hollon, 2001). Still others can interpret the findings of outcome studies showing the efficacy of BA to suggest that changes in behavior lead to changes in biology that are, ultimately, antidepressant. Research on mechanisms of change are sorely needed before there can be certainty about the theory.

EMPIRICAL EVIDENCE
Empirical Status of the Theoretical Model

Concurrent areas of research reinforce the theories proposed in BA. Basic animal research supports the notion that extinction trials can result in behaviors that resemble depression. Schulz, Huston, Buddenberg, and Topic (2007) reported that adult and aged rats demonstrate a steady increase of immobility over extinction trials in a water maze. The authors suggest that the immobility resembles "despair" and that this behavior in the rat is analogous to depressive reactions seen in aging humans in response to the loss of reinforcement through loss of youth, bereavement, social isolation, and disability.

Others have suggested that one must look outside the individual to the larger contextual factors in depression, consistent with the model proposed in BA. Cutrona, Wallace, and Wesner (2006) suggest that poor neighborhood conditions may play a role in development of depressive symptoms above and beyond negative life events for any given individual, and they encourage psychologists to pay greater attention to the impact of contextual factors in well-being.

The current conceptualization of BA emphasizes the importance of modifying avoidance behaviors in the treatment of depression. Although Ferster (1973) hypothesized that much of the behavior exhibited by depressed individuals functions as avoidance, targeting avoidance has not been an active ingredient of CBT protocols in the treatment of depression, yet avoidance modification has played a major role in the treatment of anxiety disorders. Recent work in the evaluation of coping strategies lends credence to the impact of avoidance in depression. Vollman, LaMontagne, and Hepworth (2007) maintain that adults with a diagnosis of heart failure who use more escape/avoidance behaviors and less active problem-solving strategies have more depressive symptoms.

Evidence Supporting the Overall Effectiveness of the Therapy

While BA has enjoyed recent interest as an alternative to purely cognitive approaches, the question about mechanisms of change remains an important one for empirical investigation. There is an aspect of nonspecificity in depression. Studies of the components of treatment have long demonstrated that various components are equally effective in treating depression. Zeiss, Lewinsohn, and Muñoz (1979) randomly assigned to treatment focusing on either interpersonal skills training, cognitive restructuring, or pleasant events scheduling. The three treatment procedures were equally effective in treating depression, regardless of the specific target problem addressed. Thus the treatments had non-specific effects.

In the 1990s, Jacobson and colleagues (1996) conducted a component analysis of cognitive therapy for depression that stirred great interest in the field. Whereas cognitive-behavioral approaches demonstrated efficacy in many different trials for a variety of clinical problems, purely behavioral approaches were all but abandoned in clinical practice. By the mid-1980s, behavioral analytic approaches to clinical phenomenon had been relegated to treatment for developmentally disabled populations and to modification of specific behavioral problems such as bed-wetting, trichotillomania, and other discrete disorders. Syndromes such as depression were assumed to require a broader cognitive-behavioral approach, and cognitive therapy also appeared to be an appropriate choice for higher-functioning populations. In the component analysis study, the search for the active ingredient in CBT for depression began. Three conditions were identified in this dismantling approach. Participants were randomized into one of three conditions. The first condition utilized the full cognitive therapy (CT) condition based on Beck et al. (1979), wherein behavioral activation and a full protocol of cognitive techniques, including evaluation of underlying assumptions and core beliefs, were used. A second condition required therapists to use only behavioral activation and the evaluation of automatic thoughts to increase activity and to modify dysfunctional thinking. The third condition allowed the use of BA alone. To the surprise of many, there were no significant differences in outcome among the three conditions. Treatment gains were maintained in follow-up evaluations. This study called into question the assumption that cognitive change through rational restructuring is a necessary condition for improvement of depression and relapse prevention.

An analysis of 2-year follow-up data (Gortner, Gollan, Dobson, & Jacobson, 1998) demonstrated no significant differences in the long-term outcome between the full CT treatment, BA plus evaluation of automatic thoughts, and BA-alone. Gortner and colleagues concluded that "the inclusion of cognitive interventions did not have any additive positive effect in either acute treatment response or relapse prevention" (p. 381).

Replication was necessary following this controversial study. An obvious limitation of the component analysis study was the lack of a control condition. Jacobson and colleagues (see Dimidjian et al., 2006) designed a study that would replicate and extend the previous findings using methodology previously used in the Treatment on Depression Collaborative Research Program (TDCRP; Elkin et al., 1989). The Treatments for Depression Study (Dimidjian et al., 2006) made particular use of the medication protocols used in the TDCRP but used paroxetine as the antidepressant medication. Rather than compare CBT with interpersonal psychotherapy for depression, as was done in the TDCRP, the psychotherapy conditions compared in the Treatments for Depression Study were CT for depression using Beck and colleagues' (1979) manual, as well as the work of J. S. Beck (1995), and BA. The BA treatment had been both established in the previous study, using the behavioral components of CBT for depression, without any of the cognitive interventions, and expanded into a stand-alone treatment, with an emphasis on modifying avoidance behaviors (Martell et al., 2001).

Participants were randomized into the various conditions, and the psychotherapy conditions allowed a maximum of 16 weeks of treatment, with up to 24 sessions available during those weeks. For the first 8 weeks, participants were scheduled twice weekly, then once weekly in the following 8 weeks. Participants were allowed makeup sessions in the latter 8 weeks if they had missed sessions during the previous 8 weeks, but under no circumstances were participants allowed more than 24 sessions of either CT or BA. The results of this study were similar to those in the component analysis study. For low-severity participants there were no statistically significant differences among the three therapies. For the high-severity participants, BA and paroxetine showed no differences in outcome, and both significantly outperformed CT. All of the active treatments significantly outperformed the placebo (Dimidjian et al., 2006). Gains in both the BA and the CT conditions were maintained at 1-year follow-up, and gains in the pharmaceutical condition were maintained only for those participants who remained on medication. Participants previously treated with BA or CT remained significantly free from relapse 2 years posttreatment.

Evidence Supporting the Overall Effectiveness of the Therapy for Various Disorders

BA has mostly been evaluated as a treatment for depression. However, several small studies have shown that some version of BA may be beneficial in the treatment of other disorders. BA has shown promise as a treatment for veterans with posttraumatic stress disorder (PTSD; Jakupcak et al., 2006). Hopko and colleagues, who have examined a form of behavioral activation that makes use of activity scheduling and assisting clients in goal setting of various activities over the course of a week, found support for the treatment of suicidal behaviors among patients with borderline personality disorder (BPD) (Hopko, Sanchez, Hopko, Dvir, & Lejuez, 2003), the treatment of depression among inpatients (Hopko, Lejuez, LePage, Hopko, & McNeil, 2003), and the treatment of depression in patients with cancer (Hopko, Bell, Armento, Lejuez, & Hunt, 2005). Studies currently under way are examining BA as treatment for PTSD among recent veterans and for depression in adolescents.

Evidence Supporting the Use of Particular Processes and Interventions

While speculative regarding BA, Gray (1982), conducting animal research, proposed that there are two independent neurobiological mechanisms for appetitive and aversive motivation systems. The appetitive motivation—the behavioral activation system (BAS)—activates in response to signals of reward and punishment. The aversive motivation—the behavioral inhibition system (BIS)—inhibits behavior in response to signals of punishment, nonreward, and novelty. Gable, Reis, and Elliot (2000) found that persons with higher BIS react more strongly to negative events. Daily negative events predicted negative affect and daily positive events predicted positive affect. Events of the previous day predicted the present day's affect. This line of research may help to explain the negative impact of negative life events that interfere with the individual's ability to contact reinforcers in his or her environment. The interaction between negative life events and activation of the BIS system may make it more difficult for depressed clients to engage actively with their environment to make positive change.

Further support of the model regarding the problem of rumination comes from the research of Susan Nolen-Hoeksema. Nolen-Hoeksema, Morrow, and Fredrickson (1993) found that a passive, ruminative thinking style was associated with more severe depression of longer duration in depressed individuals than an active problem-solving style. This research has informed the BA model, suggesting that ruminating becomes a problematic behavior for depressed clients by preventing more productive problem-solving and activation. Treynor, Gonzáles, and Nolen-Hoeksema (2003) stress the importance of distinguishing between adaptive reflection and maladaptive brooding types of rumination. For some people, stressors may trigger reflection on the problem that leads to active problem-solving. Life stressors cause others to brood about the difficulty, and these individuals are less likely to engage in problem solving and take action to resolve problems.

These lines of research, though not directly related to BA, offer some external support for the use of techniques that engage the individual in active problem solving. BA therapists are expected to conduct a functional analysis of client behavior. Thus, each client is treated differently. For some, all that may be required is the use of activity charts and activity scheduling. Simply getting clients to increase activity as a treatment for depression is borne out by the literature on the beneficial effects of exercise on people with depression (e.g. Mather et al., 2002; Neidig, Smith, & Brashers, 2003).

Limitations to the Current Support and Applications

The need for replication cannot be understated in regard to BA. The Component Analysis Study of Cognitive Therapy (Jacobson et al., 1996) and the Treatments for Depression Study (Dimidjian et al., 2006) demonstrated similar findings, and the latter study was a replication and extension of the first. However, in the 1996 component analysis study, BA was taken whole cloth from the behavioral interventions outlined by Beck et al. (1979), and it was only during the later Treatments for Depression Study that BA emerged as a stand-alone treatment and the theory behind the treatment was more carefully articulated (Martell et al., 2001). Several interesting findings in the Dimidjian et al. (2006) study bear further investigation. A subset (28%) of participants treated with CT actually did worse at the end of treatment than at pretreatment. Such a finding has not been shown in other studies of CBT for depression. Coffman, Martell, Dimidjian, Gallop, and Hollon (2007) have conducted a series of post hoc analyses in an attempt to explain this phenomenon. They also suggest improvements to future research design that may account for such difficulties at the front end of a large randomized controlled treatment study that will ultimately be more informative and may lead to better understanding of mechanisms of change.

CLINICAL PRACTICE

Extension of the Theory as Principles for Practice

According to the behavioral theory of depression underlying BA, depression results from multiple factors. Certain vulnerabilities for particular individuals, biological or otherwise, are not denied, nor are they considered primary targets for treatment. Thus, BA eschews the search for constructs, such as core beliefs or maladaptive schemas, that may be triggered by negative life events. On the other hand, the theory suggests that an individual's response to negative life events brings his or her behavior under aversive control. In an attempt to escape or avoid negative affect, the individual engages in behavior that brings relief in the short run but may worsen the depressive symptoms in the long run. Rather than engage in active problem solving, many depressed patients engage in passive ruminative behaviors, often silently repeating over and over the narrative of their misery, or simply engaging in wishful thinking (i.e., "I just want to be happy"). As hopelessness increases, they are even less likely to take action that may alleviate depressive symptoms or improve life situations. Extreme attention to negative affective states leads to mood-dependent behaviors that intensify the negative feelings rather than alleviate them. BA attempts to (1) break reliance on mood-dependent behavior by encouraging clients to act according to planned activities and set goals rather than moods; (2) identify avoidance behavior, assist clients in developing a plan for approach, and reinforce carrying out such approach behaviors between therapy sessions; and (3) decrease the impact of ruminative thinking by helping clients learn skills that turn their attention to their experiences of the moment, allowing them to engage more fully in activities for which they have lost a sense of pleasure.

Distinctive Features of the Approach

Several features distinguish more fully BA from other treatments for depression. Consistent with Lewinsohn's earliest procedures, there is great reliance on activity scheduling. While most, if not all, cognitive-behavioral therapists make use of activity scheduling at some time during the course of treatment, BA therapists use activity scheduling throughout the treatment. In some cases, this may be the only technique used. Escape and avoidance behaviors were dealt with incidentally in Lewinsohn's earlier formulations of BA. Now they are explicitly defined, and the BA therapist is encouraged to look for behaviors that function as escape/avoidance behaviors and target them for modification. BA diverges from CT in that it considers the behavior of thinking rather than the content of thoughts as a treatment target. Thus, rather than concern themselves with negative evaluations of a client's ruminations, BA therapists work with the client to replace passive, ruminative behavior with more active strategies. This should not be interpreted to mean that the BA therapists ignore what the client is saying. Therapists always assess clients' thinking and inquire about what is on their minds, particularly when ruminations concern suicidal ideation. Still, the treatment is activity focused. In the case of a ruminative client who expresses suicidal ideation, the therapist not only works with the client to develop a safety plan, but also asks the client to articulate reasons to stay alive. Using the rumination as a cue for activity, the BA therapist develops with the client a plan for the implementation of alternative behaviors that counteract the rumination.

Illustration of Conceptualization and Techniques within a Specific Case Study

Dean, a 37-year-old, divorced, white male, was employed in a middle-management job. The father of three children, Dean lived with his second wife and saw his children on opposite weekends. Several significant life events were identified that may have played a role in the development of his depression. Dean believed that he had "been depressed" most of his life. Although he could not identify a particular age when he first became depressed, Dean did not remember ever feeling great joy in life, and he wondered if his problem was purely biological. This suggested to the therapist a long history of aversive conditioning that would make treatment more difficult. Dean's current episode of depression had lasted for 8 months prior to initiating treatment, and he could not identify an immediate precursor to the episode.

Dean reported that his mood had been deteriorating since his divorce. The conditions of his divorce were difficult, Dean and his ex-wife maintained contact but frequently fought about child-rearing practices, and the contacts were typically unpleasant for Dean. He had met his current wife just prior to the finalization of his divorce. They dated for 6 months and moved in together after that time. They were married within months of Dean's divorce becoming final and purchased a small house a few blocks away from Dean's ex-wife and the children. He and his current wife shared common interests in sports and several outdoor activities, and she was able to join him for mountain biking and hikes when they were dating. However, soon after they were married, she took a higher position in her company, increasing her workload. She often had to work late or on weekends. Dean lamented the fact that they had engaged in more activities together prior to getting married.

Dean met with his therapist for 20 sessions of BA. Initially sessions were conducted twice per week. This is ideal when working with depressed clients, but often limitations posed by insurance companies do not allow for this higher frequency of sessions. When Dean first began treatment, his Beck

Depression Inventory (BDI; Beck, Ward, Mendelson, Mock, & Erbaugh, 1961) score was in the low 30s. On the inventory, Dean endorsed item 9, stating that he thought about committing suicide but would not carry it out. Assessing Dean's suicidality was given priority in the early sessions of treatment prior to his mood improving, and the depth of his hopelessness was initially worrisome to the therapist.

In BA there is not a set way to conduct a functional analysis. Certainly the three-point contingency of antecedents–behaviors–consequences is considered. However, in outpatient settings, as mentioned previously, the therapist is limited to the self-report of the client in gathering an understanding of these contingencies at work. Several things became clear about Dean. Feeling tired and groggy in the morning was antecedent to a behavioral pattern of staying home from work that often left Dean feeling more depressed. Staying at home subsequently was antecedent to other behaviors, such as picking a fight with his wife, that also led to more dysphoria. Having an argument with his wife was often antecedent to ruminative behaviors that increased Dean's sense of self-loathing, hopelessness, and irritability. When developing a case conceptualization, the BA therapist can ask several questions that help in treatment planning. Asking what activities the client engages in during periods when he is not depressed can give an idea of activities that may, at times, have antidepressant qualities. It is not uncommon for clients to be able to name these behaviors and activities, yet quickly discount them as part of the treatment, because they no longer bring pleasure or satisfaction. This was the case with Dean. When asked what his life was like when he was not depressed, he said:

> "I get my work done, and go every day. I need to be doing that even now, although it is hard. I also really enjoy watching a football game and my wife and I used to enjoy that together; we'd sometimes have friends over. I don't ask friends over now. The house is not in great shape. I've had a few projects that I need to finish, and I would feel bad if my friends came over and there were holes in the wall and carpet pulled up. My wife and I get in fights about that too, and we don't really have any leisure time together because she gets on me about having started these projects and not finishing them."

In this brief answer the therapist had several clues about possible treatment targets. First, Dean had derived great satisfaction from his work, and had a sense of accomplishment when he went to work regularly. However, since becoming depressed, he had been missing work frequently. Thus, he was being deprived of possible reinforcement from his work, and staying away from work also led to punishing situations when he would get into arguments with his wife. Second, he used to take pleasure in watching football, particularly with his wife. This was another behavior in which he no longer engaged. It was possible that watching football was antecedent to rumination about his failures to complete projects around the house, or to arguments with his wife about getting these projects completed. Third, although it was not yet clear how much enjoyment Dean got from doing the projects around the house, he was clearly engaging in mood-dependent behavior wherein he lost track of his goals to complete a project and stopped because he did not feel like working on it. Finally, Dean engaged in social withdrawal, further isolating and depriving himself of possible rewards of socializing with his friends. These were not the only problems that the therapist identified for Dean, but we provide them here as an example of the wealth of information that can be obtained from a client following a brief answer to a straightforward question.

Another useful question to ask is how others have responded since the client has been depressed. In some cases, loved ones withdraw from depressed individuals or burn out, causing greater despair for the client. In other cases loved ones reinforce depressive behavior. This was the case with Dean. His wife did not enjoy it when Dean stayed home from work and picked fights with her when she returned home from work. However, she also was very worried about him. Dean stated that his wife frequently inquired about his feelings, suggested things they could do together to cheer him up, and mostly took on more responsibility for household tasks. Prior to being depressed, Dean liked to cook some of his favorite meals or barbecue in the summer months. When he was depressed, his wife prepared all the meals, even cooking those things that Dean enjoyed preparing for the family, such as steaks. She may inadvertently have been reinforcing his depression with her loving behaviors.

BA therapists can look at behavioral excesses and behavioral deficits when formulating the problem for a particular client. For Dean the behavioral deficits included decreased frequency of the following interpersonal activities: engaging in conversations with neighbors about yard work and projects; watching sports events on television or live with friends; telling jokes with people at work; calling members of his family who lived out of state; and going on planned activities outside of the home with his wife and his children on weekends. His behavioral excesses included ruminating on his problems and on things that irritated him about others; occasionally drinking wine to excess; and complaining to his wife about inconsequential irritations that resulted in arguments. The therapist worked with Dean to address these problems systematically.

There is not a session-by-session protocol for BA. The idiographic nature of the treatment demands that each therapy comprise different elements., and no BA therapist is required to utilize all of the suggested techniques to aid in treatment (cf. Martell et al., 2001). As we mentioned earlier, activity monitoring and scheduling is always used, but even in this BA thera-pists are less concerned about clients completing forms than about clients engaging in the activities and being able to report on them. The following is a breakdown of the types of interventions during the course of Dean's therapy.

Sessions 1–4

Initially the therapist used clinical interviewing to develop a working case conceptualization with Dean. They agreed on goals for therapy. Needless to say, the client's goal to "feel better" is not a useful goal for BA. That is like having the goal to "have a million dollars." Without a plan for how to attain such things, there is little chance of attainment. Thus, Dean's goals were ultimately articulated as follows: (1) to consistently go to work and stay on task throughout the day; (2) to start the day off by saying something complimentary to his wife; (3) to improve his relationship with his children by engaging in shared activities on their weekly visits; and (4) to spend less time ruminating and worrying about problems, and more time engaging in life. The last goal, admittedly, was broad, but it served to target the ruminat-ing behavior that became a focus of treatment in later sessions. Dean used activity charts to monitor his current activity, and the therapist helped Dean to see the connection between activity and mood. They then worked collab-oratively to schedule one or two activities during the week.

Activity monitoring and scheduling were utilized throughout the course of therapy. Activity scheduling was used systematically to increase Dean's general activity, as well as approach behaviors. Avoidance behaviors often became apparent when Dean scheduled activities, then did not complete them. He and his therapist discussed the barriers that interfered with the accomplishment of his goals. Both external barriers (e.g., a friend not being home to receive a scheduled telephone call) and internal barriers (e.g. feeling "too depressed" to attempt the task) were addressed.

Sessions 5–6

Dean had been showing slight improvement on his BDI scores until session 5. The weekend prior to this session Dean had gone on a trip with his wife and friends to a local campground to fulfill an obligation that had been planned prior to the onset of his depression. He felt particularly blue on the drive to the campground, and rather than join his wife and the others on a hike, he stayed alone back at the camp. When alone, he began to ruminate about how his wife would be better off without him. Although he had gone to work the second week of therapy and was showing improvement, Dean had not gone to work since the weekend of this camping trip, and he was feeling increasingly hopeless. He and his therapist agreed on a plan for Dean to go to work every day, no matter what. If he awakened in a blue mood and thought he would not go to work, Dean was to leave a message on the therapist's answering machine stating, "I know going to work is likely to make me feel better, but I have decided not to feel better and to just stay home, even though I know it will make me feel worse." Between sessions 5 and 6, Dean did in fact begin to leave such a message with the therapist, but he decided during the message that it was foolish not to go to work, and he showered, dressed, and was on his way. His mood improved slightly by session 5.

Sessions 6–10

These sessions focused on continued activities with Dean's wife and friends. He also had begun to work on some of the projects he needed to complete around his house. It is a common saying among BA therapists that "activity breeds activity," and Dean found this to be true. When he completed a project patching up a wall that had been broken away for rewiring, he felt "inspired" to paint the room. Once the room was painted, he saw no reason not to put down new carpeting. Before Dean knew it, his projects were completed, he had a place where he and his wife could sit down together with the children and enjoy television, and they were watching the occasional ball game together. His BDI scores continued to drop.

Sessions 10–17

Dean continued to have difficulty with ruminating behavior. Two notable examples include a weekend visit with his children and getting himself angry on the way home from work. In the first example, Dean had planned to spend a sunny afternoon in his yard with his children. The kids were building a tree house out of Dean's scrap lumber behind a shed. Instead of helping the kids in their construction work, however, Dean began his own project by pulling weeds in a flower garden on the opposite side of the house. During his weeding, Dean ruminated about how much he missed having his kids living with him full time, and that someday his first wife would remarry and the other man would replace him as "Dad." By the end of the evening, his children were in the house playing games and Dean remained outdoors in the dark, feeling sad and discouraged. His ruminating prevented him from getting the very thing he desired–time to interact with his children. The therapist asked Dean to do an attention-to-experience exercise in which he engaged in an activity and attended to sights, sounds, smells, and physical sensations in as much detail as possible. If Dean began to ruminate, he was to bring himself back to the moment and fully engage so that he could give a complete description to the therapist in a future session. The second example showed how Dean's ruminations got him worked up and triggered other behavior that led to interpersonal problems. One evening on the way home from work, Dean started to ruminate about how much money he spent on household bills. He had asked his wife the day before if they could start saving money to hire someone to do home renovations. This gave him more fodder for ruminating. By the time he arrived at home and saw the yard light on, Dean was irritable and ready to pick a fight. He walked into the house and rather than kiss his wife hello, he said "It's not that dark out. Do you all think we're made of money? I wish you'd be more responsible and shut lights off around here." His wife went into the den and shut the door behind her. Dean's assignment to deal with this was to use an alternative behavior. He chose listening to music. Dean did not consider himself a good singer, but he liked to sing to classic rock songs in his car. His assignment was to use the rumination as a cue for action and to put a CD into his car stereo and sing along, striving to get all of the words correct and to reach the various notes as best he could, even if he was horribly off key.

Sessions 17–20

The final sessions of Dean's treatment focused on relapse prevention. Dean's BDI scores had been an 8 or lower consistently for 3 weeks. He was afraid that he would become depressed again. The therapist worked with Dean to identify situations that would be difficult for him, such as meeting with his ex-wife to discuss issues regarding the children, and to develop a plan with dealing with the difficulty. Dean and his therapist also examined activities that Dean enjoyed, and they discovered that when Dean felt that he was needed and doing something nice for others, he felt happier. They then worked together to develop a plan to make Dean feel needed. This included helping around the house enough that his wife depended on him for certain chores, and to driving his children to various afterschool activities. He also considered volunteering to coach one of his children's soccer team. He needed to monitor his ruminating, however, and this remained a difficult behavior for Dean. Although he had achieved his goal to go to work consistently, and had improved on his goals for interpersonal interactions, Dean continued to struggle with a tendency to become passive and ruminate over problems, although, by the end of treatment, he no longer met criteria for major depressive disorder.

SUMMARY AND CONCLUSIONS

Theory, Current Status, and Challenges

The demonstrated success of BA in treatment outcome studies does not prove that CT is wrong. On the other hand, these current outcome studies do demonstrate that people like Lewinsohn have been onto something since the early 1970s, and that examination of their behavioral formulations may have been abandoned prematurely in favor of more cognitively oriented approaches. BA is a treatment in the tradition of radical behaviorism. Attempts are made to understand the variables contributing to depression and to target specific problems that may exacerbate depressive symptoms. Treatment is, admittedly, conducted as a series of experiments in collaboration with any given client. The principles of activation and the need to act "from the outside in" (Martell et al., 2001) rather than let moods dictate behavior apply throughout the treatment. Reliance on external anchors, such as scheduling times to engage in particular activities and making a public commitment to action, is a part of the treatment in all cases.

Since depression is seen as multifaceted, no single technique or explanation is sufficient in BA. In other words, within the model, therapists have the responsibility to assess contingencies that may be maintaining depression for each client. For some, this may be the disengagement triggered by their dysphoric mood, which has the consequence of depriving them of physical activity or social interactions that could, in fact, prove antidepressant, and their mood worsens. For others, engagement in private behaviors of ruminating over problems prevents engagement in proactive activities. In BA we encourage clients to be proactive rather than reactive. Planning ahead and following a plan is seen as an improvement over being battered about by moods. Clients are encouraged to recognize triggers for various avoidance behaviors and to engage in alternative behaviors that allow them to reengage in life.

BA therapists believe that changing context is necessary, however, and like nearly all outpatient psychotherapies, takes place in a therapists office and consists of verbal interactions between client and therapist. However, within that context are opportunities for many *in vivo* assessments and interventions to take place. For example, a depressed woman who slumps down in a chair, looks at the floor with a sad expression, and whose speech is barely audible may be gently encouraged by her therapist to experiment and to shift her posture, to raise her eyes and look at the therapist and to project her voice. The therapist and client would then assess the outcome of such an experiment. Did the client feel any differently when she changed her posture? Was there a different flow of information between client and therapist when they were looking at one another and speaking loudly and clearly? In some cases, clients are actually asked to engage in an avoided behavior, such as completing an application or calling a friend, during the session hour. Therapists may also take therapy out of the office and go on a walk through the neighborhood with the client, conducting an "attention to experience" exercise. Thus, some of the variables that may contribute to the depression can indeed be dealt with *in vivo*, albeit not in the typical environment in which the client lives.

Future Directions

The idiographic nature of BA does not mean that the treatment can easily become an eclectic combination of techniques and ideas. Within the model there are specific ways to deal with observable behaviors, as well as private, cognitive behaviors. Therapists in clinical settings are not prohibited from using standard cognitive techniques, yet there is no reason to do so when the theory of BA and the empirical support for the treatment suggest that clients improve without ever engaging in formal cognitive restructuring. Future research should focus on the application of BA in individuals with disorders that commonly are comorbid with depression, such as anxiety, substance use disorders, or conduct disorders. Furthermore, studies with adolescents and older adult populations and their caregivers will also be informative.

Whether BA remains a stand-alone treatment or becomes an ingredient of other comprehensive treatments, it has become clear that there is potential in a behavior analytic formulation of depression. BA, as proposed as part of Beck's CT, was conducted nearly completely in the service of changing beliefs and attitudes, and not simply for the sake of activation, and the unique behavioral formulation was lost. The resurgence of interest in behavioral approaches to treatment allows researchers and clinicians to develop a greater understanding of mechanisms of change, and to improve upon methodologies for changing behavior, thoughts, and feelings. In some ways, looking backward to the philosophy of Dewey and the formulations of Thorndike, Skinner, and Ferster can provide a means to look forward and come to a greater understanding of human problems and of the most expedient methods for intervention. The resurgence of the use of techniques developed by Lewinsohn decades ago seems an appropriate use of the scientific method to build upon theory and research.

REFERENCES

Barlow, D. H., Allen, L. B., & Choate, M. L. (2004). Toward a unified treatment of emotional disorders. *Behavior Therapy, 35,* 205–230.

Beck, A. T., Rush, A. J., Shaw, B. F., & Emery, G. (1979). *Cognitive therapy of depression.* New York: Guilford Press.

Beck, A. T., Ward, C. H., Mendelson, M., Mock, J. E., & Erbaugh, J. K. (1961). An inventory for measuring depression. *Archives of General Psychiatry, 4,* 561–571.

Beck, J. S. (1995). *Cognitive therapy basics and beyond.* New York: Guilford Press.

Bolles, R. C. (Ed.). (1979). *Learning theory* (2nd ed.). New York: Holt, Rinehart & Winston.

Coffman, S., Martell, C. R., Dimidjian, S., Gallop, R., & Hollon, S. (2007). Extreme non-response in cognitive therapy: Can behavioral activation aucceed where cognitive therapy fails? *Journal of Consulting and Clinical Psychology, 75,* 531–541.

Cutrona, C. E., Wallace, G., & Wesner, K. (2006). Neighborhood characteristics and depression: An examination of stress processes. *Current Directions in Psychological Science, 15*(4), 188–192.

Dimidjian, S., Hollon, S. D., Dobson, K. S., Schmaling, K. B., Kohlenberg, R. J., Addis, M. E., et al. (2006). Randomized trial of behavioral activation, cognitive therapy, and antidepressant medication in the acute treatment of adults with major depression. *Journal of Consulting and Clinical Psychology, 74*(4), 658–670.

Dollard, J., & Miller, N. E. (1950). *Personality and psychotherapy: An analysis in terms of learning, thinking, and culture.* New York: McGraw-Hill.

Elkin, I., Shea, T., Watkins, J. T., Imber, S. C., Sotsky, S. M., Collins, J. F., et al. (1989). NIMH Treatment of Depression Collaborative Research Program. *Archives of General Psychiatry, 46,* 971–982.

Ferster, C. B. (1973). A functional analysis of depression. *American Psychologist, 28,* 857–870.

Follette, W. C., & Jacobson, N. S. (1988). Behavioral marital therapy in the treatment of depressive disorders. In I. H. R. Falloon (Ed.), *Handbook of behavioral family therapy* (pp. 257–284). New York: Guilford Press.

Fuchs, C. Z., & Rehm, L. P. (1977). A self-control behavior therapy program for depression. *Journal of Consulting and Clinical Psychology, 45,* 206–215.

Gable, S. L., Reis, H. T., & Elliot, A. J. (2000). Behavioral activation and inhibition in everyday life. *Journal of Personality and Social Psychology, 78*(6), 1135–1149.

Gortner, E. T., Gollan, J. K., Dobson, K. S., & Jacobson, N. S. (1998). Cognitive-behavioral treatment for depression: Relapse prevention. *Journal of Consulting and Clinical Psychology, 66*(2), 377–384.

Gray, J. A. (1982). *The neuropsychology of anxiety: An enquiry into the functions of the septo-hippocampal system.* Oxford, UK: Oxford University Press.

Hayes, S. C., Hayes, L. J., & Reese, H. W. (1988). Finding the philosophical core: A review of Stephen C. Pepper's world hypotheses. *Journal of the Experimental Analysis of Behavior, 50,* 97–111.

Hickman, L. A., & Alexander, T. M. (Eds.). (1998). *The essential Dewey: Vol. 1. Pragmatism, education, democracy.* Bloomington and Indianapolis: Indiana University Press.

Hollon, S. D. (2001). Behavioral activation treatment for depression: A commentary. *Clinical Psychology: Science and Practice, 8,* 271–274.

Hopko, D. R., Bell, J. L., Armento, M. E. A., Lejuez, C. W., & Hunt, M. K. (2005). Behavior therapy for depressed cancer patients in primary care. *Psychotherapy: Research, Practice and Training, 42*(2), 236–243.

Hopko, D. R., Lejuez, C. W., LePage, J. P., Hopko, S. D., & McNeil, D. W. (2003). A brief behavioral activation treatment for depression: A randomized pilot trial within an inpatient psychiatric hospital. *Behavior Modification, 27*(4), 458–469.

Hopko, D. R., Sanchez, L., Hopko, S. D., Dvir, S., & Lejuez, C. W. (2003). Behavioral activation and the prevention of suicidal behaviors in patients with borderline personality disorder. *Journal of Personality Disorders, 17*(5), 460–478.

Jacobson, N. S. (1994). Contextualism is dead: Long live contextualism. *Family Process, 33*, 97–100.

Jacobson, N. S., Dobson, K., Fruzzetti, A. E., Schmaling, K. B., & Salusky, S. (1991). Marital therapy as a treatment for depression. *Journal of Consulting and Clinical Psychology, 59*(4), 547–557.

Jacobson, N. S., Dobson, K. S., Truax, P. A., Addis, M. E., Koerner, K., Gollan, J. K., et al. (1996). A component analysis of cognitive-behavioral therapy for depression. *Journal of Consulting and Clinical Psychology, 64*(2), 295–304.

Jacobson, N. S., Fruzzetti, A. E., Dobson, K., Whisman, M., & Hops, H. (1993). Couple therapy as a treatment for depression: II. The effects of relationship quality and therapy on depressive relapse. *Journal of Consulting and Clinical Psychology, 61*(3), 516–519.

Jacobson, N. S., Holtzworth-Munroe, A., & Schmaling, K. B. (1989). Marital therapy and spouse involvement in the treatment of depression, agoraphobia, and alcoholism. *Journal of Consulting and Clinical Psychology, 57*(1), 5–10.

Jacobson, N. S., & Margolin, G. (1979). *Marital therapy: Strategies based on social learning and behavior exchange principles.* New York: Brunner/Mazel.

Jakupcak, M., Roberts, L., Martell, C., Mulick, P., Michael, S., Reed, R., et al. (2006). A pilot study of behavioral activation for veterans with post-traumatic stress disorder. *Journal of Traumatic Stress, 19*, 387–391.

Lewinsohn, P. M. (1974). A behavioral approach to depression. In R. J. Friedman & M. M. Katz (Eds.), *The psychology of depression: Contemporary theory and research* (pp. 157–178). Washington, DC: Hemisphere.

Lewinsohn, P. M. (2004). Lewinsohn's model of depression. In W. E. Craighead & C. B. Nemeroff (Eds.), *The Corsini encyclopedia of psychology and behavioral science* (3rd ed., pp. 525–527). New York: Wiley.

Lewinsohn, P. M., Hoberman, H., Teri, L., & Hautzinger, M. (1985). An integrative theory of depression. In S. Reiss & R. Bootzin (Eds.), *Theoretical issues in behavior therapy* (pp. 331–359). New York: Academic Press.

Lewinsohn, P. M., Weinstein, M., & Shaw, D. (1969). Depression: A clinical research approach. In R. D. Rubin & C. M. Frank (Eds.), *Advances in behavior therapy* (pp. 231–240). New York: Academic Press.

Martell, C. R., Addis, M. E., & Jacobson, N. S. (2001). *Depression in context: Strategies for guided action.* New York: Norton.

Mather, A. S., Rodriguez, C., Guthrie, M. F., McHarg, A. M., Reid, I. C., & McMurdo, M. T. (2002). Effects of exercise on depressive symptoms in older adults with poor responsive depressive disorder: Randomized controlled trial. *British Journal of Psychiatry, 180*, 411–415.

Neidig, J. L., Smith, B. A., & Brashers, D. E. (2003). Aerobic exercise training for depressive symptom management in adults living with HIV infection. *Journal of the Association of Nurses in AIDS Care, 14*(2), 30–40.

Nolen-Hoeksema, S., Morrow, J., & Frederickson, G. L. (1993). Response styles and the duration of episodes of depressed mood. *Journal of Abnormal Psychology, 102*(1), 20–28.

O'Donohue, W. (1998). Conditioning and third-generation behavior therapy. In *Learning and behavior therapy* (pp. 1–14). Needham Heights, MA: Allyn & Bacon.

Pepper, S. C. (1942). *World hypothesis.* Berkeley: University of California Press.

Rehm, L. P. (1977). A self-control model of depression. *Behavior Therapy, 8,* 787–804.

Rutter, V. (2000). Accomplishments and innovations in couple and family therapy: In memory of Neil Jacobson. *Newsletter of the American Family Therapy Academy, 79,* 11–14.

Schulz, D., Huston, J. P., Buddenberg, T., & Topic, B. (2007). "Despair" induced by extinction trials in the water maze: Relationship with measures of anxiety in aged and adult rats. *Neurobiology of Learning and Memory, 87,* 309–323.

Skinner, B. F. (1974). *About behaviorism.* New York: Random House.

Treynor, W., González, R., & Nolen-Hoeksema, S. (2003). Rumination reconsidered: A psychometric analysis. *Cognitive Therapy and Research, 27*(3), 247–259.

Vollman, M. W., LaMontagne, L. L., & Hepworth, J. T. (2007). Coping and depressive symptoms in adults living with heart failure. *Journal of Cardiovascular Nursing, 22*(2), 125–135.

Wolpe, J. (1958). *Psychotherapy by reciprocal inhibition.* Stanford, CA: Stanford University Press.

Zeiss, A. M., Lewinsohn, P. M., & Muñoz, R. F. (1979). Nonspecific improvement effects in depression using interpersonal skills training, pleasant activities schedules, or cognitive training. *Journal of Consulting and Clinical Psychology, 47*(3), 427–439.

CHAPTER 7

Dialectical Behavior Therapy

Thomas R. Lynch
Prudence Cuper

INTRODUCTION AND HISTORICAL BACKGROUND

Marsha Linehan developed dialectical behavior therapy (DBT) in the 1970s, melding principles and techniques of behavior therapy with the genuineness espoused by Carl Rogers and Zen practices culled from her spiritual training, to treat clients who were chronically suicidal or self-injuring. Currently a faculty member at the University of Washington, Linehan has served as the president of the Association for the Advancement of Behavior Therapy (AABT; now called the Association for Behavioral and Cognitive Therapies [ABCT]), a fellow of the American Psychological Association and the American Psychopathology Association, a distinguished founding fellow of the Academy of Cognitive Therapy, and a Diplomate of the American Board of Behavioral Psychology. Among her numerous awards are the Louis I. Dublin Award for Lifetime Achievement in the Field of Suicide; the American Foundation of Suicide Prevention Award for Distinguished Research in Suicide; the American Association of Applied and Preventive Psychology Award for Distinguished Contributions to the Practice of Psychology; the Distinguished Scientist Award and the Distinguished Contributions to the Field of Psychology Award from the Society of Clinical Psychology of the American Psychological Association; and a Lifetime Achievement Award from Division 12, Section VII (Clinical Emergencies and Crisis) of the American Psychological Association.

Linehan, a native of Tulsa, Oklahoma, is one of six children. Her father, an oil executive, and her mother, a homemaker, were both active in their community. Linehan has described herself as "a sort of missionary person," who "wanted to help the most miserable people in the world" (Linehan, 2000, p. 190), and she decided early in life that she would do so through a career in psychiatry, psychology, or social work. While she admits that initially she found research to be too cold and inhuman for her taste, Linehan describes being won over when she realized how few effective treatments there were for the people she most wanted to help.

Her training began at Loyola University of Chicago, where she received a degree in experimental–personality psychology in 1971. She followed this training with a clinical internship at the Suicide Prevention and Crisis Clinic in Buffalo, New York, then went on to do a postdoctoral fellowship at the State University of New York at Stony Brook, where she worked with Gerald Davison. At Stony Brook, Linehan learned behavior modification. She hoped to apply the techniques of behavior therapy to a group of difficult-to-treat clients but quickly learned that behavior therapy required the cooperation and collaboration of the client and the therapist, and that her clients were not always willing or able to cooperate in these interventions. She realized that her treatment would need to engage clients in a way that pure behavior therapy did not, and she set about the task of adding acceptance and validation strategies to her therapy (Linehan, 2000).

Linehan honed the treatment throughout the following years, adding mindfulness skills derived from several spiritual disciplines, including Zen practice and Christian contemplative prayer. She has drawn similarities between behaviorism and Zen practice, noting that both are process theories that require a practitioner to assume a nonjudgmental stance (Linehan, 2000). Lack of judgment is a critical component of DBT, as is "radical genuineness," which Linehan found in the writings of Carl Rogers and those of the behaviorists. She has said that "behaviorists never see the patient as being different from anyone else. They see behavior on a continuum" (p. 186).

Linehan began work on DBT in the 1970s. According to Dimeff and Linehan (2001), standard cognitive and behavior therapy protocols of that era did not meet the needs of chronically suicidal clients for three reasons. First, many clients found the protocols' emphasis on behavior change to be invalidating, and common responses were arguing with the therapist or terminating therapy. Second, therapists found it difficult to teach new skills and simultaneously work on suicidal behaviors within an individual therapy session. Third, Linehan saw a pattern of clients unintentionally reinforcing ineffective therapist behaviors. For example, a client might be become more agreeable and talkative when the therapist steered the conversation away from difficult topics.

Keeping these challenges in mind, Linehan developed a protocol that would balance acceptance and change, provide separate venues for skills training and individual therapy, and offer support and consultation to therapists in their work with difficult-to-treat clients. In subsequent years, the intervention was tested, first against treatment as usual for borderline personality disorder (BPD; Linehan, Armstrong, Suarez, Allmon, & Heard, 1991), then later against community treatment by experts (Linehan et al., 2006). Several research groups have also tested the efficacy of DBT in treating other disorders. These studies are reviewed later in this chapter.

PHILOSOPHICAL AND THEORETICAL UNDERPINNINGS

In this section, we briefly review the biosocial theory of BPD, then focus the remainder of this section around three major influences that affected the development of the treatment package: behavioral science, dialectical philosophy, and Zen practice.

Biosocial Theory of BPD

The theoretical foundation for DBT is a biosocial theory formulated to explain the development and maintenance of BPD. As a theory, it accounts for the criterion behaviors associated with BPD by proposing that a biological/genetic predisposition for emotional vulnerability and a pervasive invalidating environment transact to produce the maladaptive styles of coping (e.g., emotional dysregulation) characteristic of BPD (Linehan, 1993). The theory is transactional, meaning that each element (biological, sociobiographical, and maladaptive coping) is seen reciprocally to influence and to be influenced by the others. The biological element (emotional vulnerability) refers to a biologically based predisposition for heightened sensitivity and reactivity (i.e., quick and strong reactions) to emotionally evocative stimuli, as well as a delayed return to baseline emotional arousal. The sociobiographical element (invalidating environment) is characterized by punishing, ignoring, or trivializing the individual's communication of thoughts and emotions, as well as self-initiated behaviors, and may involve sexual, physical, and emotional abuse (Wagner & Linehan, 1997). Intense emotional reactions on the part of the individual with BPD are hypothesized to exacerbate invalidating behavior on the part of caregivers/intimate others, resulting in greater emotional dysregulation. This transaction between an invalidating environment and an emotionally vulnerable individual leads to dysregulation across the individual's emotional system (i.e., maladaptive coping), characterized broadly by difficulty up- and down-regulating physiological arousal, as well as difficulty in turning attention away from emotional stimuli. As a result, individuals with BPD often experience considerable disruption of their cognitive, emotional, and behavioral systems when emotionally aroused.

In DBT, emotions are conceptualized as complex, brief, involuntary, full-system responses to internal and external stimuli that have an evolutionary adaptive value (Linehan, Bohus, & Lynch, 2007). Problem behaviors are seen as the inevitable sequelae of dysregulated emotions, or as maladaptive methods of altering emotional experiences. For example, impulsive or self-destructive behaviors, such as self-injury, suicide attempts, or disordered eating, may occur in direct response to or function to regulate dysregulated emotional responding. This theoretical stance has resulted in a treatment package that largely focuses on modifying various aspects of the patient's emotional system. Thus, treatment formulations are apt to target eliciting and consequential stimuli associated with emotion, and strategies focus on *reducing ineffective action tendencies linked with dysregulated emotions* (Lynch, Chapman, Rosenthal, Kuo, & Linehan, 2006).

Behavioral Science

Grounded in behavioral science, DBT is part of a recent third wave of behavioral theory that considers psychological acts to be best understood contextually and functionally, while avoiding assignment of causal primacy to one form of behavior over another (Hayes, Follette & Follette, 1995). For example, DBT would *not* consider private behaviors, such as thinking, sensations, or emotion, as qualitatively different from overt behaviors; both are subject to and can be understood by the same behavioral principles. In addition, DBT examines behavior functionally, not topographically; that is, problem behaviors may appear on the surface to be similar but functionally may be quite different. For example, ignoring one's own needs to care for another might function to maintain a relationship for one person, elicit nurturance for another, reduce aversive emotions in a third, and self-punish in a fourth, and/or these functions may all be within the behavioral repertoire of the same person. Thus, DBT interventions often focus on changing the function of a problem behavior and may not always involve altering its form or frequency. As a result, unlike standard behavior and cognitive therapies, which ordinarily focus on changing distressing emotions and events, a major emphasis in DBT is on learning to bear emotional pain skillfully. The DBT skills of mindfulness and distress tolerance encapsulate this approach and encompass the ability to experience and observe emotions without evaluation, and without necessarily attempting to change or control emotional experiencing, arousal, or distress. From this perspective, trying willfully to change, suppress, or inhibit unwanted private behavior (e.g., thoughts, sensations, emotions) may actually exacerbate the problem (e.g.,

Lynch, Robins, Morse, & Krause, 2001; Lynch et al., 2006). DBT emotion regulation skills, in contrast, target the reduction of emotional distress through exposure to the primary emotion in a nonjudgmental atmosphere and through the application of set of specific skills. In essence, mindfulness skills focus on *awareness* of distressing emotions, and distress tolerance skills focus on *tolerating* distressing emotions, whereas emotion regulation skills focus on *changing* distressing emotions, and interpersonal skills focus on *changing* the invalidating social environment that may exacerbate emotional arousal.

All of the skills in DBT can be seen to target emotion and emotion regulation in one way or another. As a result, behavioral–functional analyses tend to be emotion-focused, and problems are typically examined from a perspective that considers them to occur within a *context* of emotional experience (contextual factors), to be secondary to some type of *cue* or trigger (cue factors), and to become habitual because of *reinforcing consequences* (reinforcing factors). In addition, DBT emphasizes the importance of not only reducing emotional response tendencies once they have been initiated but also the importance of regulatory processes once an emotion is full-blown. Thus, skills are designed to target *both low-magnitude emotional response tendencies and high-magnitude emotional responses* based on the notion that regulatory processes that may have been effective in the initial stages of an emotional response may be much less effective under condition of intense emotional arousal (Linehan et al., 2007). Finally, DBT also targets *emotional aftereffects that can serve as new emotional cues,* refiring the same emotion or precipitating a secondary emotion (Linehan et al., 2007).

Contextual Factors

Contextual factors include biological vulnerabilities for increased sensitivity and reactivity to emotional cues and factors that momentarily enhance the reinforcement salience of particular emotional cues (i.e., establishing operations). The biosocial theory hypothesizes that individuals with BPD are *biologically vulnerable* to greater emotional sensitivity (low threshold for recognition of emotional stimuli), greater emotional reactivity (high amplitude of emotional responses), and a slower return to baseline arousal (long duration of emotional responses). Supporting the importance of a biological influence, research utilizing self-report methodology consistently finds that individuals with BPD report greater emotional intensity and reactivity relative to controls, and neuroimaging studies suggest that individuals with BPD can be characterized by neurological vulnerabilities, although behavioral and psychophysiological findings are inconclusive (see Rosenthal et al., 2008). *Establishing operations* are motivational factors that influence the evocative functions and reinforcement salience of certain stimuli and the probability that behaviors associated with those stimuli may be elicited (Dougher, Perkins, Greenway, Koons, & Chiasson, 2002; Michel, Valach, & Waeber, 1994). For example, food deprivation is an establishing operation that momentarily increases the salience of food as a form of reinforcement. In DBT, establishing operations are referred to as *emotion vulnerability* factors; examples include lack of sleep, a recent argument, physical fatigue, alcohol/drug use, and physical pain.

Once contextual factors are understood, it is then possible ideographically to apply DBT skills that may influence the development of problem behaviors and/or any associated unwanted consequences. Thus, DBT focuses on reducing vulnerabilities to emotional arousal. This is based on the premise that even when components of physiological reactivity are due to immutable genetic dispositions and early developmental experiences, they may still come under the control of the individual (Linehan et al., 2007). Accordingly, DBT skills were designed that target both biological homeostasis and the reinforcement salience of various stimuli known to influence emotional reactivity. For example, based on empirical evidence, the DBT PLEASE skills target treating *P*hysical i*L*lness (Anderson, Hackett, & House, 2004), balancing nutrition and *E*ating (Smith, Williamson, Bray, & Ryan, 1999; Green, Rogers, Elliman, & Gatenby, 1994), staying off nonprescribed mood-*A*ltering drugs, getting sufficient but not too much *S*leep (Brendel, Reynolds, & Jennings, 1990), and getting adequate *E*xercise (Stella et al., 2005). In addition, DBT skills target vulnerability to emotional arousal by modifying the context in which emotional cues occur (e.g., by teaching skills for accumulating positive life events and/or building a generalized sense of mastery).

Cue Factors

Cue factors include conditioned or unconditioned antecedent stimuli and ideographic discriminant stimuli (S^D) that trigger intense emotional states, urges, or other problem behaviors, or signal reinforcement potential. In DBT, emotional experiences and urges are considered to be *under the control* of the antecedent stimuli (i.e., respondent behavior), whereas the S^D for problem behaviors (e.g., dissociation) function primarily to signal the *likelihood of reinforcement*. As respondent behavior, emotions/urges can be elicited by either unconditioned antecedent stimuli (e.g., a loud bang) or conditioned antecedent stimuli (e.g., time of day signals hunger pangs, independent of the actual availability of food); stimuli may include places, persons, objects, sensations, and verbal and/or temporal events. For example, a neutral stimulus (e.g., roses) automatically elicits an emotion of shame because it has repeatedly been associated with (preceded) a negative stimulus (e.g., sexual abuse). Importantly, classically conditioned experiences (e.g., urges for self-harm) can develop without conscious awareness and thinking/appraisal is *not necessary* for the elicitation of conditioned associations (Öhman & Mineka, 2001). As such, emotional experience can be elicited by the current contingencies (e.g., dog growling) or historical antecedents (i.e., classically conditioned associations), or some combination of the two.

Cue factors also involve the presentation of stimuli that make it possible for actions to have consequences (stimulus–response–consequence relations). This is called *instrumental* or *operant conditioning* and is defined as learned behavior under the control of reinforcing or punishing consequences. *Discriminant* stimuli (S^D) are stimuli that signify the availability of reinforcement. S^D are also under contextual control, meaning that contextual stimuli influence the reinforcement potential of any given stimulus. For example, children may learn that a temper tantrum is more likely to result in their getting what they want (e.g., a piece of candy) when their parent is tired or distracted (the S^D) than on days their parent is well-rested and can give them full attention. Thus, despite the presence of a number of antecedents associated with candy (say, on a trip to the grocery store), the children have discriminated (although not necessarily consciously) that they will most likely receive candy following a temper tantrum when Mom is distracted by a call on her mobile phone.

DBT utilizes a number of strategies to alter classically conditioned responses and other cue factors (see Lynch et al., 2006; Linehan et al., 2007). For example, *behavioral chain analysis*, which is a common method used in DBT to evaluate the function of problem behavior, is hypothesized also to serve as method of informal behavioral exposure (Lynch et al., 2006). Contrary to prior suggestions, recent learning theorists have proposed that repeated nonreinforced exposure to a conditioned stimulus (CS) does not weaken the initial association formed by the pairing of the unconditioned stimulus (US) and the CS. Instead, exposure *masks* the CS–US relationship, and extinction training involves the learning of new CS associations (Robbins, 1990). In this framework, behavioral exposure entails the active learning of alternative responses to stimuli that elicit unwanted internal experiences (e.g., relative safety in the presence of conditioned fear cues). Behavioral chain analysis involves a detailed discussion of the emotional responses and their eliciting stimuli and promotes the client's nonreinforced exposure to emotions when attended to by a caring psychotherapist in session. For example, having a client talk in detail about shameful events or behaviors may lay down new, benign associations between the behavior or event and the emotional response of shame, thereby facilitating engagement in problem solving.

Reinforcing Factors

As mentioned, a functional-analytic approach such as that used in DBT accounts for not only relevant antecedents but also reinforcing consequences. For example, nonsuicidal self-injury may function as a means to escape extremely aversive emotions, either through the reduction of depersonalization that it induces (Wagner & Linehan, 1997) or physiological–psychological relief secondary to reductions in aversive arousal (Haines, Williams, Brain, & Wilson, 1995). Problem or emotional behaviors can also function to communicate or influence other people's behaviors and/or validate one's own perceptions and interpretations of events (i.e., "If I feel it, it must be true"). For example, prior research shows that distressed behavior prompts both negative and solicitous emotions but deters hostile reactions (Biglan, Rothlind, Hops, & Sherman, 1989), and across studies, displays of embarrassment (vs. nondisplay) following a transgression resulted in higher liking, greater forgiveness, and increased willingness to provide aid (for review, see Keltner & Anderson, 2000). Self-validation can be seen as reinforcing in that it stabilizes individuals' concepts of self (Izard, Libero, Putnam, & Haynes, 1993). Indeed, research shows that individuals favor information that confirms their self-view over other available reinforcers, particularly if that self-view is extreme (Giesler, Josephs, & Swann, 1996; Pelham & Swann, 1994; Swann, 1997; Swann, de la Ronde, & Hixon, 1994), and when self-constructs are disconfirmed, individuals tend to experience negative emotional arousal (Gellatly & Meyer, 1992). Thus, acts of self-depreciation or self-injury may be negatively reinforced by the reductions of arousal secondary to verification of a pathological sense of self.

Contingency management and the principles associated with changing operant behavior have a rich empirical basis, but due to space limitations in this chapter we do not review them here. However, some DBT principles related to contingency management are somewhat unique. For example, DBT recognizes that both the therapist and the client are subject to the same principles of reinforcement and, as such, the client can significantly influence therapeutic process (e.g., a client may over time shape a therapist into not asking about suicide by getting hostile each time it is discussed). This is one of the reasons DBT emphasizes the need for all therapists to participate weekly in a peer consultation team; a major function of the team is to help a therapist remain treatment adherent by observing with the therapist how their therapeutic strategies are being influenced by the client. As another example, although examples of generalization strategies abound in the child and adolescent literature and in relapse prevention-based adult treatments (e.g., Hiss, Foa, & Kozak, 1994), DBT is the only empirically supported treatment that explicitly incorporates telephone consultation as a generalization strategy. DBT telephone coaching is hypothesized to be effective in part because it functions to generalize skills across contexts, provides an avenue for shaping effective behavior *in vivo*, and may serve as cue for the retrieval of extinction memories or instrumental learning from therapy sessions (Lynch et al., 2006). Therefore, the therapist's presence in the client's real-world environment via a telephone interaction may not only prevent the renewal of dysfunctional behavior but also elicit skillful behavior.

Intensity of Emotion and Managing of Emotional Aftereffects

DBT takes into account both the *intensity* and *timing* of therapeutic responses based on observations that emotion regulation strategies that work well when deployed in advance of a stressful experience and/or at low levels of intensity may fail once the emotion is already fully evoked and/or at high magnitude (Linehan et al., 2007). For example, DBT provides a set of skills designed specifically to down-regulate the extreme physiological arousal that often accompanies intense emotions. These skills do not require a high level of cognitive processing to complete (Linehan et al., 2007). For example, one skill combines breath holding with face immersion in cold water. This method, derived from research on the human dive reflex, influences both branches of the autonomic nervous system: parasympathetic activation (bradycardia) and concurrent sympathetic activation (vasoconstriction) (Hurwitz & Furedy, 1986). As another example, intense physical exercise is also recommended as a method to influence high-magnitude emotions, based on research showing that while intensity of exercise did not differ in state anxiety immediately after exercise, a significant difference favoring greater intensity of exercise over the control condition emerged 30 minutes postexercise (Cox, Thomas, Hinton, & Donahue, 2006). The DBT skill of *opposite action* is another technique hypothesized to influence intense emotions by changing the entire range of physical responses that accompany the emotion action tendency, including visceral responses, body postures, and facial expression (Linehan et al., 2007). Both treatment research (e.g., Martell, Addis, & Jacobson, 2001) and experimental research (e.g., Philippot, Baeyens, Douilliez, & Francart, 2004; Soussignan, 2002) have consistently demonstrated that changing behavior influences emotional experiences and subsequent cognitive appraisal of the emotional experience.

DBT also examines the aftereffects of emotional experience and how emotions can be refired or precipitate a secondary emotion. Aftereffects of emotions on attention, memory, and reasoning are well established (for a review, see Dolan, 2002). A primary method taught in DBT to influence afteraffects are the *observe and describe emotions skills* based on research showing that processing emotional experience with greater specificity relative to overgeneral or nonspecific processing has advantages for improved emotion regulation (e.g., Williams, Stiles, & Shapiro, 1999).

Dialectical Philosophy

Dialectical philosophy provides not only a worldview for DBT but also a framework for the style or manner by which specific interventions are delivered. As a worldview, *dialectical philosophy* most often is associated with Marxist socioeconomic principles, but the philosophy of dialectics actually extends back thousands of years (Bopp & Weeks, 1984; Kaminstein, 1987). According to Hegel, the process by which a phenomenon, behavior, or argument is transformed is the dialectic, which involves three essential stages: (1) the beginning, in which an initial proposition or statement (*thesis*) occurs, (2) the negation of the beginning phenomenon, which involves a contradiction or *antithesis*, and (3) the negation of the negation, or the synthesis of thesis and antithesis. Essentially, tension develops between thesis and antithesis, and the synthesis between the two constitutes the next thesis, repeating the process ad infinitum. From a dialectical perspective, behavior is conceptualized as interrelated, contextually determined, and systemic. One advantage of this approach with regard to treatment interventions is that a dialectical philosophy naturally reduces polarization. For example, a client might take the position that illegal drugs are good because they help him or her feel better. Dialectics allows a therapist to give up being *right* but not lose his or her point of view, while encouraging synthesis. Thus, the therapist might validate the desire to feel better, while pointing out that an addictive use of drugs also appears to lead to unwanted suffering. From this the therapist might encourage synthesis: "Can we work together to find a way to help you feel better without necessarily taking drugs?"

In addition, a dialectical philosophy posits that reality is composed of interrelated parts that cannot be defined without reference to the system as a whole, and the parts constantly are in a state of change or flux, with changes in one influencing changes in others. Thus, a therapist can then acknowledge that the client influences the therapist while being influenced by the therapist, and that this type of transaction is a normal process of growth. This helps to facilitate a collaborative relationship.

Dialectical *strategies* include magnifying tension through the devil's advocate method or other such strategies (i.e., *entering the paradox, extending*), working for a synthesis of opposite opinions, feelings, or thoughts; the use of metaphor; the oscillation of speed and intensity in interacting with the patient; and the fluid use of movement in session. In addition, dialectical strategies in DBT are also designed to help the client stay awake and engaged in the treatment and/or slightly off-balance (e.g., the client begins to question whether maladaptive beliefs about him- or herself and the world are literally true). In terms of *style*, this involves balancing irreverent and reciprocal communication, and acceptance-based and change-based interventions. For example, irreverence may make it difficult for the client always to predict the therapist's behavior, and, as such, the behavior of the therapist becomes an *orienting response* (Lynch et al., 2006). An *orienting reflex* is an adaptive response to novel stimuli, the function of which is to tune the neural systems for sensory analysis to facilitate central processing of stimuli (Sokolov, 1963; Graham, 1979; Cook & Turpin, 1997). Research has shown that the orienting response *opens* the organism to the environment and facilitates deeper processing of stimuli (e.g., Siddle & Packer, 1987; Tulving, Markowitsch, & Kapur, 1994). As such, when reciprocal (*acceptance*) and irreverent (*change*) strategies are balanced in therapy, the client is self-confirmed/validated (which functions to keep him or her engaged in treatment) and challenged (which functions to maximize attention, cognitive processing, and learning).

Zen Practice

During the time that DBT was being developed and tested by Linehan (i.e., the 1970s) behavioral theory and interventions were based primarily on either first- or second-wave behavioral principles (Hayes et al., 1995). The first wave of behavioral therapy was influenced heavily by the techniques associated with operant and classical conditioning principles and the thinking of Watson (1924), who claimed that the "mind" did not exist (e.g., thinking was subvocal speech), and that the only relevant unit of analysis was overt behavior. The second wave of behavior therapy reacted to what was considered a lack of cognitive mediational accounts and added to the units of analysis the idea that behavior could be *caused* by private events (e.g., cognition or appraisals). Both waves emphasized the importance of changing the antecedents or consequences of problem behavior as the primary focus of treatment interventions. As such, first- and second-wave behavior therapy were focused on change and problem solving, based on rationality and logic, and were experimentally and empirically derived. However, as noted by Linehan (1993), not only did this bias not always work but at times it had iatrogenic effects (e.g., rigid adherence to change strategies can backfire; Lynch et al., 2001). Based on her own personal practice of Zen, Linehan noted that some of the approaches used in Zen offered a dialectical antithesis to the first- and second-order behavioral thesis. Specifically, Zen practice emphasized acceptance rather than change, validation rather than problem solving, intuitive rather than rational insight, paradoxical rather than logical reasoning, and an experiential rather than an empirical epistemological approach toward the study of nature. Essentially, DBT as a treatment package *is the synthesis between behaviorism and Zen practice*, and the dialectical underpinnings of DBT allow for both to exist without negating the impact of the other. The influence of Zen practice can best be observed within the context of mindfulness skills, which are viewed as "core" skills in DBT. These skills represent a behavioral translation of Zen meditation and practice, and include observing, describing, spontaneous participating, nonjudgmentalness, focused awareness in the present moment, and focusing on effectiveness rather than being "right" (Linehan, 1993).

EMPIRICAL EVIDENCE

Seven randomized controlled trials (RCTs) support the overall effectiveness DBT (for review, see Lynch, Trost, Salsman, & Linehan, 2007). In the original trial, Linehan and colleagues (1991) randomly assigned chronically suicidal women with BPD to DBT ($N = 24$) or treatment as usual in the community ($N = 23$), assessing the patients throughout their 12-month treatment period and at 6-month intervals in the following year. The patients receiving DBT were less likely to drop out of treatment, reported fewer and less severe episodes of parasuicide, and spent fewer days in inpatient psychiatric care. Patients in both conditions showed improvements in depression, hopelessness, suicidal ideation, and reasons for living.

Linehan and colleagues (1999) then investigated the efficacy of DBT in treating patients with comorbid BPD and substance use disorders. They examined the progress of 28 women who had been assigned to DBT or treatment as usual in the community. Once again, they found that the women assigned to DBT were more likely to remain in treatment. The patients receiving DBT also showed greater reductions in drug use, as well as greater gains in social and global adjustment.

More recent studies by Linehan's group aimed to show efficacy of DBT compared to more rigorous control conditions. In the first of these studies (Linehan et al., 2002), investigators compared DBT to comprehensive validation therapy with 12-step group attendance (CVT+12s) in the treatment of comorbid BPD and opiate addiction. Contrary to earlier findings, participants in the DBT group were more likely to drop out of therapy than those in the CVT+12s group. On other variables the groups performed similarly: Both showed significant overall reductions in psychopathology at posttreatment and follow-up, and reductions in opiate use in follow-up (4 months) assessments, as measured by urinalyses. Only the DBT group, however, maintained reductions in opiate use throughout the 12-month treatment period; the CVT+12s group increased use in the last 4 months of treatment.

The second study, utilizing a rigorous control condition (Linehan et al., 2006), compared DBT to community treatment by experts (CBTE) with a sample of women meeting criteria for BPD and endorsing recent suicidal and self-injurious behaviors. Compared to patients receiving CBTE, patients in the DBT group were less likely to attempt suicide or to be hospitalized for suicidal ideation, and showed lower medical risk in their suicidal attempts and self-injurious acts. Additionally, the DBT patients were less likely to drop out of treatment, and they had fewer psychiatric emergency room visits and hospitalizations. As in previous studies, patients in both conditions showed reduced symptoms of depression, more reasons for living, and less suicidal ideation.

Other support for the efficacy of DBT in treating BPD comes from independent research groups. In the Netherlands, Verheul and colleagues (2003) compared the outcomes of 58 women assigned to DBT or treatment as usual. All of the participants in this study had been diagnosed with BPD; some of the women also had comorbid substance abuse problems. The team of investigators found that the patients in DBT were more likely to remain in treatment. Additionally, DBT patients showed greater reductions in self-damaging and self-mutilating behaviors. This effect was most pronounced among those patients with the severest parasuicidal behaviors at baseline assessment.

A study of female veterans diagnosed with BPD, conducted at a Veterans Administration hospital in the United States, also provides support for the general efficacy of DBT (Koons et al., 2001). This study was of shorter duration than the other studies mentioned: The investigators treated women with DBT or treatment as usual for a period of 6 months. Additionally, the investigators did not require participants in this study to have a history of parasuicidal behavior, as did the investigators in previous studies. Results of this study include greater reductions in suicidal ideation, hopelessness, anger, and depression in the DBT group, and significant decreases in parasuicidal acts, anger experienced but not expressed, and dissociation in the DBT group only.

Support for Efficacy in Treating Other Disorders

DBT, originally intended for the treatment of chronically suicidal and self-injurious patients, is increasingly being used to treat a variety of mental disorders. Evidence from recent studies supports the utility of DBT in the treatment of depression, eating disorders, and numerous personality disorders. Some of the newer studies also expand the patient population to include both males and females, and older adults in addition to the younger patients more commonly seen in the earlier studies.

Two studies of DBT for eating disorders looked specifically at its usefulness in treating women with bulimia nervosa and binge-eating disorder. In the trial of DBT for bulimia (Safer, Telch, & Agras, 2001), 31 women were assigned to one of two conditions: DBT adapted for binge–purge behaviors or a waiting-list control. The DBT group showed zero attrition from treatment, as well as significant decreases in binge–purge behavior. In the trial of

DBT for binge-eating disorder (Telch, Agras, & Linehan, 2001), 44 women were assigned to either an adapted form of DBT or a waiting-list control group. Once again, patients in the DBT group showed significant improvements on measures of binge eating and eating pathology. Most women (89%) were abstaining from binge eating by the end of treatment, and many (56%) were still abstinent at the 6-month follow-up assessment.

Lynch, Morse, Mendelson, and Robins (2003) conducted a pilot study of DBT for depressed older adults, men and women age 60 and older. All participants in the study received antidepressant medication and clinical management; the experimental group also attended a DBT skills groups and received telephone coaching sessions. Although depression scores improved for both groups at posttreatment, a significantly higher percentage of the DBT group (75%) compared to the control group (31%) remained in remission at 6-month follow-up.

A second study compared DBT for older adults with depression plus comorbid personality disorder to medication and clinical management (Lynch et al., 2007). In this study, participants included 37 men and women, age 55 and older, with depression that had failed to respond to an 8-week open trial of antidepressant medication. In this study, significantly more patients in the DBT group experienced a remission from depression (defined as a score of 10 or less on the Hamilton Rating Scale for Depression) by the end of the psychotherapy treatment period. By the time of the follow-up assessments, most patients in both groups were in remission. Additionally, the DBT group showed greater improvement on two measures associated with personality disorder pathology: interpersonal sensitivity and interpersonal aggression.

Evidence Supporting Specific Processes and Interventions

DBT comprises several components: individual therapy, group skills training, phone coaching, and therapist consultation team. While several processes or mechanisms within each of these components could be tested, on a more basic level, one might ask which components appear to contribute to the efficacy of the treatment. This question becomes increasingly important as DBT gains in popularity and clinicians use DBT skills as an "add-on" to non-DBT individual therapy or as a stand-alone intervention.

To date, no published studies have taken on, as a primary aim, the dismantling of the treatment. However, two pilot studies of DBT for disorders other than BPD made use of skills training as the chief intervention. These studies, mentioned earlier, investigated the utility of DBT skills in treating binge-eating disorder (Telch et al., 2001) and major depression in older adults (Lynch et al., 2003). It is important to note that the Lynch study also included telephone coaching calls. These studies indicate that for less severely disordered patients, skills training without individual therapy may be effective. However, as Lynch et al. (2007) point out, an unpublished report by Linehan indicates that one early study comparing non-DBT individual therapy alone to non-DBT individual therapy plus DBT skills group found no differences in patient outcomes. This conflicting evidence suggests the need for a study designed to investigate the individual contributions of components of DBT.

In addition to studies testing the major components of DBT, studies of the therapeutic strategies prescribed in DBT would shed light on the therapy's critical elements. The strategies to be investigated might include validation, radical genuineness, irreverence, contingency management (as in phone coaching and four-miss rules), and the hierarchical ordering of treatment topics, among many others. The results of the 2002 study comparing DBT to CVT+12s (Linehan et al., 2002) suggests that at least one strategy, validation, appears to be a powerful therapeutic agent even in the absence of other DBT components.

CLINICAL PRACTICE

In this case, the client, a female in her 20s, meets criteria for BPD and comorbid substance use disorder. Her primary substance of abuse is heroin. Her treatment includes both DBT for substance use disorders (DBT-SUD) and an opiate replacement medication, Suboxone. In this session, the client's second with the DBT therapist, she learns more about the biological underpinnings of addiction, contingency management strategies, the mindfulness skills "observe" and "describe," and distress tolerance and emotion regulation skills targeting physiological factors. The therapist displays radical genuineness and irreverence, and he weaves a chain analysis throughout the session.

T: So, last week, you were able to come into therapy. That's great. And how's it going with the Suboxone?

C: Really good. I'm on 16 milligrams now, and I'm tolerating it well.

T: You're taking it every day?

C: Yeah, and I haven't been had any positive urinalyses. Well, maybe once …

T: When was this?

C: (*Shakes head, laughing.*) That was so bad. It was two Tuesdays ago.

T: Oh, was that right after our last session? I think I told you to go home and get rid of the pills that you were keeping, right? [*Therapist uses a matter-of-fact tone to highlight potential problem of noncompliance; the DBT strategies used here are targeting and irreverence.*]

C: Yes, and I did, except I didn't flush *all* of them.

T: So what did you do with the ones you didn't flush? You took them?

C: I took them when I woke up the next morning. I was having really strong cravings.

T: It's hard to have cravings in the morning, before you're completely awake, and before you've taken your Suboxone. Of course, the thing to do in that situation is to *just watch* those cravings. That's one of the mindfulness skills you've been learning: observing your own "addict mind." And doing that without despairing, because you know that it's just one part of you, it's not the entirety of you. But when you *don't* watch your "addict mind," it will take over and you'll start doing things like ... (*Therapist validates the difficulty of staying drug free, but also suggests a new strategy for dealing with cravings. "Addict mind" is a DBT-SUD skill akin to "Emotion mind" in traditional DBT.*)

C: ... like that?

T: Exactly! And you'll think, "What the heck am I doing?" Some people really start crashing and burning when that happens. They think, "I'm no good, I'm a horrible human being." Does that happen for you?

C: Sometimes. It hasn't happened lately. I'm feeling better about myself lately.

T: That's great. But that morning that you took the pills, did that get you? (*Therapist brings the focus back to the problem behavior, to begin analyzing it functionally.*)

C: Well, I think it did later on in the day. I crashed and burned after a while.

T: I'd like to hear a little more about that. But first I have to ask you: Are all the pills gone? (*Therapist highlights the importance of attending to dysfunctional thinking but keeps focus on determining first whether there are any drugs readily available.*)

C: Yeah, they're gone. I flushed most of them right after I saw you last week.

T: So you'd flushed most of them but saved the few that you took the next morning. Was part of you saying "just in case ... "? Or, did you have a plan to take them?

C: Well, I couldn't take them that day because I'd taken Suboxone, so I thought, "I'll just take them tomorrow when I first wake up."

T: When you look at your addict mind, what was your addict mind saying to convince you that that would be a good idea? (*Labeling the dysfunctional thoughts as "addict mind" gives the client a means cognitively to distance from the automatic thoughts.*)

C: "You're throwing the rest away! After all, there are 30 more down there that you could have taken! So why not just take these few?"

T: Oh, right. I remember us talking about how hard this might be. If I was in your shoes, my brain would start freaking out as soon as I started to approach the toilet. (*Therapist is using DBT validation level 3: He imag-*)

ines how the client might feel in such a situation, and communicates that in his mind-read.)

C: Absolutely! I remember just walking up to the toilet and (*makes motion of dumping and flushing them*). I don't remember when I counted out the ones that I saved. They didn't all disappear the first time I flushed, but I wasn't going to reach back in there and grab them, because that's just disgusting. So I flushed them again, and then they were gone. *Then* I freaked out! I didn't know what to do.

T: What about using something like ice (makes motion of holding ice in hands). Would that have helped? (*Therapist starts to weave solutions into the analysis of the event by suggesting a DBT skill designed to regulate emotion through physiology.*)

C: Yeah, that probably would have been good. I mean I was *so* freaked out about it.

T: Yes, it sounds like you were. Tell me, have you used the ice on your face yet?

C: No.

T: It probably seems silly. Do you have thoughts like that? (*Therapist assesses the client's degree of commitment to try out new skills and also gives her permission to have judgmental thoughts about DBT skills.*)

C: No, not really. I mean, I thought the idea of holding ice in my hand was silly before I tried it, but then it worked. I told everyone I saw that day. I said, "You have to try this ice thing. It's great!" I was really impressed by it.

T: I'm glad it's worked for you. OK, so getting back to the day that you flushed the pills: You kept some of them. What were you thinking? Were you thinking, "I'm about to make some changes here, so why not have a last little fling?" (*Therapist uses DBT validation level 3: therapeutic mind-read.*)

C: Exactly. I was thinking, "It's my last shot ... "

T: "My last shot..."

C: Yeah, truly, I didn't want to do any more of that. And I don't have any more drugs or paraphernalia. The closest ones I know about are 2,000 miles away, with my ex-boyfriend. I couldn't get to them before you guys would figure out that I was gone.

T: True, but you know, "addict mind" is really, really clever. (*Therapist uses DBT-SUD strategy of dialectical abstinence, by going to the opposite pole of the client's contention that lack of available drugs means that the problem may be over.*)

C: I know. "Addict mind" is clever, and so is my ex. He's tried bribing me already, telling me that we'd get a cat if I moved back. He also gives me guilt trips about work.

T: Oh really? How did you resist? (*Therapist pulls for the client to generate and label her own solutions.*)

C: I just told him no, and let it seep inside me for a minute, and then I said,

"You know, you live in a city with *millions* of people. I'm sure you can find someone else to work for you. Put an ad on the Internet and find someone. And, furthermore, if you're not willing to be supportive of me in what I'm doing right now, I don't want to talk to you anymore."

T: That's very bold and powerful to say that. How were you able to do that? (*Therapist validates the client's courage.*)

C: I just thought about it for a while. In the past, he's actually spent his own time and money trying to get me better. Now I'm doing it on my own, and he should be happy for me. If he's not, then I don't get it. Or maybe I don't really want to get it, because it makes me question his motives.

T: That sounds like it's coming from a pretty solid place. (*Therapist validates her growing new sense of self.*)

C: Yeah, I have friends now who will help me with this, so I feel really secure and safe. I couldn't say that to him when we lived in the same city, because he was everything to me back then.

T: What you're talking about is really common in relationships where people get addicted to drugs together. If one person gets well, and her partner's not ready to get well, the partner winds up sabotaging the efforts to get clean. It's not because he's a bad person—it just feels better to have you using with him. Let's go back a little bit, though, and talk about you taking the last of the pills. When you woke up the next day, how did you feel? (*Therapist models a nonjudgmental stance toward the ex-boyfriend's behavior, then returns to the functional analysis.*)

C: Like I really wanted to get stoned. I was kind of annoyed with myself, and I was thinking that I should have saved some more.

T: So you were thinking, "Why didn't I save more of them?" Maybe you were using your "wise mind" a little, when you flushed them. Maybe you knew that if you saved more of them, you would have gotten really stoned and thrown yourself out of recovery. Probably right now its best for us to think in terms of smaller increments of time; like 6-month increments. So we're gonna see if we can get you off it for 6 months in a row. If we can, your brain will start to change, and you will no longer respond to the cues in the same way. (*Therapist continues to use "we" language emphasizing the collaborative nature of the work and points out that even in the worst of times, "wise mind" may be active.*)

C: Cues?

T: Let me explain a little bit about classical conditioning. It's something that your brain does that's unconscious. You can learn a classically conditioned association and never even know it. For instance, did I ever tell you that I almost got mugged in a subway in New York City? I didn't get mugged, but it was enough to scare the hell out of me. (*Therapist uses personal self-disclosure to teach a behavioral principle.*)

C: You wouldn't want to hang out around subway stations.

T: True. But, you know, I hadn't thought about that for 15 or 20 years. Throughout much of that time I lived in the suburbs, and I didn't have to use mass transit. I didn't think about that incident at all. Then, a couple of years ago, I went to Boston and I had to ride the subway. All of a sudden: Whammo! I had this surge of fear. The subway tunnel was the cue for my fear, even though it was a different subway in a different city. So there's a lot of learning that you have, and that I have, that's outside of awareness.

C: You didn't realize that you'd be afraid when you got there?

T: No, I didn't. And the same thing might be happening with urges for you. Certain cues might make you want to use. When you walk into situations and all of these classically conditioned cues are around, your brain thinks that drugs are coming, and your body goes looking for them. Plus, there are all kinds of cues: time of day, old friends, *ex-boyfriends*, drug paraphernalia ... (*Therapist links behavioral principles to the client's personal situation.*)

C: Yeah, I was cleaning this house for someone who had syringes because she was diabetic. They were right there!

T: That's a great example. When you saw that, your brain probably got your body ready for the drug. Here's how it happens. Think of your brain going along, having no urges, everything's fine ...

C: Like it's on autopilot?

T: Yes, it's like that. And then all of a sudden it sees the cue. Because it knows that opiates make you fall asleep, your brain, to prevent that, activates other chemicals to keep you awake. So as soon as your brain sees a cue that says "Drugs are coming," it immediately gets activated and starts compensating for the effects of the drug—and that's what you feel as the urge or the sense of withdrawal. Withdrawal is when your body is geared up to receive the drug but its not there yet ... and this physically hurts. Of course, when the drug does come, it kicks the body back to normal, and that's why you feel OK. That's why cues might create some kind of painful ...

C: ... stomach churning ...

T: ... agitation kind of feeling. That's your body getting ready for the drug. Of course, the big question is, what do you do when you feel that? (*Therapist is pulling for the client to generate her own solutions.*)

C: I bet I use DBT skills.

T: Exactly! You can start simply using your mindfulness skills. Observing the urges or withdrawal as a sensation, that your body wants drugs. Just notice it while knowing what it is. What will happen, over time, is that you'll get around these things that in the past meant drugs were coming, and you're gonna lay down new associations. The old associations will still be there, but you'll recognize them for what they are. It's like me and the subway. I had to ride the subway over and over, and eventually my brain learned that subways don't always mean that something bad will happen. Now I can ride the subways without outrageous fear.

C: That sounds hard to do.

T: Well, you know, most subways are safe. That's how I got over my fear of subways—I rode the subway. So it's the same thing for you. Over time, we're gonna have you face those cues or situations that make you want to use drugs, and not use drugs, and after a while your brain will learn that syringes don't mean drugs are coming and it will stop torturing you. Its not that the old learning goes away, just that the longer you stay off drugs in those situations, the more the new learning grows. After about 6 months, the urges should really subside. (*Therapist cheerleads client to continue to work hard and avoid using drugs, and gives a sense of the amount of time it will take to change some of the behavior as a way to instill hope.*)

C: I hope you're right. It's still pretty hard not to yield to temptation.

T: Well, let's go back to that other incident. The morning that you took the pills: How long was it after you woke up that you took them? (*Therapist returns to functional analysis of the drug use that week.*)

C: About a half hour later. I was excited.

T: Yeah, isn't that funny about the brain? When the brain is ready for drugs, drugs become the most important thing in the world. Chocolate cake doesn't mean anything, looking at a beautiful sunset doesn't mean anything, nothing seems as pleasurable. So you thought, "I'm gonna take these pills today." Then what? (*Therapist highlights to the client how much she has missed out on by using drugs; this functions to strengthen commitment for abstinence.*)

C: Before I took them, I made some coffee, and then I went upstairs.

T: OK, and then what? (*Therapist is working link by link in the functional or behavioral chain analysis; this helps the client understand how her emotions, thoughts, sensations, and overt behaviors lead to problem behaviors.*)

C: I have a hard time remembering.

T: OK, so the day you took them, things got blurry. Well, let's talk about some tactics you can use when you get cravings, OK? One thing that helps is getting the emotion of disgust to occur before you use. I bet you've gotten kind of freaked out and disgusted by using. Try to bring up that memory. (*Therapist does not insist that she try and remember; later in treatment the therapist will work with the client on improving her ability to self-report the temporal sequence of important events in her life, but since this is the second session, the therapist moves to a solution analysis.*)

C: Oh, no. That's gonna be a hard one!

T: I know. But there are times when you probably do feel a little disgusted about it, right?

Like, weren't there times when you were using it a lot when you woke up in the morning and you were feeling sick, or you woke up and said, "Why the hell am I doing this?" Where you just felt like, "I've had it with this, I just really want to get off of this." (*Therapist encourages the client to use an "opposite emotion" from the distress tolerance skills IMPROVE to alter her experience; it is important to note that this DBT distress tolerance skill is different than the DBT skill of "opposite action," which changes the action tendency of the emotion and does not involve purposefully creating a different emotional experience.)*

C: Yeah.

T: It would make sense that you have some disgust with your drug use, or why would you be here, right? I can't imagine that you'd come here if there weren't some part of you, somewhere, that is sort of disgusted about it. (*Therapist cheerleads client to approach this uncomfortable emotion.*)

C: Yeah, that does make sense.

T: Try to bring to mind things that you've felt disgusted about. Come up with a list. It's just another way, when your "addict mind" wants to go for the drug to put up some barriers. Regret works, too. Disgust or regret should bring the urge right down, because it's difficult for those emotions to coexist with the feeling of excitement. You might want to write this down.

C: I think I will. I've got to make this cheat sheet small, so I can keep it in my purse.

T: Exactly. Because you'll want to pull that out whenever you have urges. Keep these things in your wallet: The pros and cons of using drugs, what makes you feel disgusted about it, some of the worst regrets that you've had about using. (*Therapist encourages the client to keep reminders of new skills she's learned.*)

C: I have lots of regrets. I hate this crap. But, you know, my "drug addict" mind often takes over. It says, "Just give it another try," even though I *always* get that horrific feeling whenever I take it.

T: Your "addict mind" is working hard. But with the skills, you're putting barriers in its way. It'll have to go through this door, then this door, then this door.... It has to go through all these doors that have locks on them, with all kinds of complicated codes. And don't worry if the skills aren't working right away. Many of them take practice. But after a while, you'll start to notice things that you hadn't noticed before. (*Therapist uses the dialectic strategy of metaphor to solidify learning, emphasizes the need to practice skills, and cheerleads by pointing out the positive benefits.*)

C: Yeah, that happened the other day. I was getting really frustrated because I couldn't get the cork out of this stupid wine bottle, but I noticed how angry I was getting, and I practiced mindful breathing.

T: That's great! Anger or frustration that's experienced mindfully is different than anger that's not experienced mindfully. So you just changed the experience of that emotion. And when you breathe, you're telling your body that it's OK. You're saying to your brain that all is well. Did you notice a slight difference after that? (*Therapist reinforces use of skills and teaches how breathing influences well-being.*)

The session concluded shortly after this exchange, with the therapist asking for the client's commitment to fill out her diary card for the next week, to call for coaching when needed, and to attend her skills group. The client, feeling optimistic about the intervention, complied. The session detailed here exemplifies many of the strategies and techniques that are central to DBT. Because the client is new to treatment, the therapist does quite a bit of orienting to the treatment model. He also takes a dialectical stance, showing acceptance and understanding for her maladaptive behaviors, while prompting her to consider behavioral changes that she could make. The therapist uses the analysis of a single episode of drug use to help the client see the antecedents and discriminant stimuli that are present before drug use, and he weaves potential solutions into their discussion to teach the client when and how to use specific DBT skills. Finally, the therapist is radically genuine with the client, using examples from his own life, and he validates her throughout the session.

SUMMARY AND CONCLUSIONS

Since the publication of the first treatment manual (Linehan, 1993) DBT has grown increasingly popular among clinicians, patients, and mental health advocate groups. The enthusiasm for this approach appears warranted when it comes to treating the behavioral dyscontrol associated with BPD, as DBT has garnered more empirical support then any other psychosocial or pharmacological intervention for the treatment of BPD (for review, see Lynch, Trost, Salsman, & Linehan, 2007). However, despite its strong empirical foundation, a number of gaps do remain in the DBT literature. These include lack of research that has included male or minority clients. In addition, there continues to be a need to understand what predicts treatment response via component, dismantling, or process-analytic studies, as well as large-sample effectiveness research in community settings. Although preliminary attempts to apply DBT to diagnoses other than BPD have yielded promising results, findings in these areas generally should still be considered experimental pending further evidence. In addition, there continues to be a need for the treatment to be expanded and/or modified, particularly in light of the fact that DBT has been more recently conceptualized as a treatment with utility for intervening with difficult-to-treat and often multiply-disordered clients, not just those with BPD (Linehan et al., 2007; Lynch et al., 2006). For example, Lynch and Cheavens (2008) contend that the majority of research in DBT has been understandably polarized, with a bias for focusing on treatment of emotionally dysregulated, impulsive, and dramatic–erratic disorders (e.g., BPD, bulimia nervosa, binge-eating disorder, substance abuse disorders) or populations (e.g., adolescents engaging in intentional self-injury). However, a number of complex and potentially treatment-resistant disorders (e.g., paranoid personality disorder, obsessive–compulsive personality disorder) or populations (e.g., older adults with chronic depression) represent the dialectical opposite of the more dramatic disorders; yet approaches for these types of problems in DBT are underdeveloped and the treatment must be modified to address fully a wider range of complex disorders. Finally, additional treatment development would be useful to address the historical antecedents that exacerbate the development of the disorder (Stage II treatment that targets trauma and/or sexual abuse). In summary, DBT is a principle-based treatment with a solid foundation in modern behavioral theory that has been informed by Zen practice and dialectical philosophy. The treatment has been empirically studied, such that it can be considered a standard of care for suicidal BPD clients. It continues to evolve as it is applied to new disorders or patient populations, and we recommend that the new developments in DBT continue the strong empirical tradition associated with its foundation.

REFERENCES

Anderson, C. S., Hackett, M. L., & House, A. O. (2004). Interventions for preventing depression after stroke. *Cochrane Database Syst. Rev.*, CD003689

Biglan, A., Rothlind, J., Hops, H., & Sherman, L. (1989). Impact of distressed and aggressive behavior. *Journal of Abnormal Psychology*, 98(3), 218–228.

Bopp, M. J., & Weeks, G. R. (1984). Dialectical metatheory in family therapy. *Family Process*, 23(1), 49–61.

Brendel, D. H., Reynolds, C. F., & Jennings, J. R. (1990). Sleep stage physiology, mood, and vigilance responses to total sleep deprivation in healthy 80-year-olds and 20-year-olds. *Psychophysiology*, 27(6), 677–685.

Cook, E., & Turpin, G. (1997). Differentiating orienting, startle, and defense responses: The role of affect and its implications for psychopathology. In P. J. Lang, R. F. Simons, & M. T. Balaban, *Attention and orienting: Sensory and motivational processes* (pp. 137–164). Mahwah, NJ: Erlbaum.

Cox, R. H., Thomas, T. R., Hinton, P. S., & Donahue, O. M. (2006). Effects of acute bouts of aerobic exercise of varied intensity on subjective mood experiences in women of different age groups across time. *Journal of Sport Behavior*, 29(1), 40–59.

Dimeff, L., & Linehan, M. M. (2001). Dialectical behavior therapy in a nutshell. *California Psychologist*, 34, 10–13.

Dolan, R. J. (2002). Emotion, cognition, and behavior. *Science*, 298(5596), 1191–1194.

Dougher, M., Perkins, D. R., Greenway, D., Koons, A., & Chiasson, C. (2002). Contextual control of equivalence-based transformation of functions. *Journal of the Experimental Analysis of Behavior*, 78(1), 63–93.

Gellatly, I. R., & Meyer, J. P. (1992). The effects of goal difficulty on physiological arousal, cognition, and task performance. *Journal of Applied Psychology*, *77*(5), 694–704.

Giesler, R. B., Josephs, R. A., & Swann, W. B. (1996). Self-verification in clinical depression: The desire for negative evaluation. *Journal of Abnormal Psychology*, *105*(3), 358–368.

Graham, S. E. (1979). The role of advance modality information in selective attention. *Dissertation Abstracts International*, *39*(9-B), 4615.

Green, M. W., Rogers, P. J., & Elliman, N. A. (1994). Impairment of cognitive performance associated with dieting and high levels of dietary restraint. *Physiology and Behavior*, *55*(3), 447–452.

Haines, J., Williams, C. L., Brain, K. L., & Wilson, G. V. (1995). The psychophysiology of self-mutilation. *Journal of Abnormal Psychology*, *104*(3), 471–489.

Hayes, S. C., Follette, W. C., & Follette, V. M. (1995). Behavior therapy: A contextual approach. In A. S. Gurman & S. B. Messer (Eds.), *Essential psychotherapies: Theory and practice* (pp. 128–181). New York: Guilford Press.

Hiss, H., Foa, E. B., & Kozak, M. J. (1994). Relapse prevention program for treatment of obsessive–compulsive disorder. *Journal of Consulting and Clinical Psychology*, *62*(4), 801–808.

Hurwitz, B. E., & Furedy, J. J. (1986). The human dive reflex—An experimental, topographical and physiological analysis. *Physiology and Behavior*, *36*, 287–294.

Izard, C. E., Libero, D. Z., Putnam, P., & Haynes, O. M. (1993). Stability of emotion experiences and their relations to traits of personality. *Journal of Personality and Social Psychology*, *64*(5), 847–860.

Kaminstein, D. S. (1987). Toward a dialectical metatheory for psychotherapy. *Journal of Contemporary Psychotherapy*, *17*(2), 87–101.

Keltner, D., & Anderson, C. (2000). Saving face for Darwin: The functions and uses of embarrassment. *Current Directions in Psychological Science*, *9*(6), 187–192.

Koons, C. R., Robins, C. J., Tweed, J. L., Lynch, T. R., Gonzalez, A. M., Morse, J. Q., et al. (2001). Efficacy of dialectical behavior therapy in women veterans with borderline personality disorder. *Behavior Therapy*, *32*, 371–390.

Linehan, M. M. (1993). *Cognitive-behavioral treatment of borderline personality disorder*. New York: Guilford Press.

Linehan, M. M. (2000). Marsha Linehan. In G. Hellinga, B. van Luyn, & H.-J. Dalewijk (Eds.), *Personalities: Master clinicians confront the treatment of borderline personality disorder* (pp. 179–202). Amsterdam: Boom.

Linehan, M. M., Armstrong, H. E., Suarez, A., Allmon, D., & Heard, H. L. (1991). Cognitive-behavioral treatment of chronically parasuicidal borderline patients. *Archives of General Psychiatry*, *48*, 1060–1064.

Linehan, M. M., Bohus, M., & Lynch, T. R. (2007). Dialectical behavior therapy for pervasive emotion dysregulation: Theoretical and practical underpinnings. In J. Gross (Ed.), *Handbook of emotion regulation* (pp. 581–605). New York: Guilford Press.

Linehan, M. M., Comtois, K. A., Murray, A. M., Brown, M. Z., Gallop, R. J., Heard, H. L., et al. (2006). Two-year randomized controlled trial and follow-up of dialectical behavior therapy vs. therapy by experts for suicidal behaviors and borderline personality disorder. *Archives of General Psychiatry, 63,* 757–766.

Linehan, M. M., Dimeff, L. A., Reynolds, S. K., Comtois, K. A., Shaw-Welch, S., Heagerty, P., et al. (2002). Dialectical behavior therapy versus comprehensive validation plus 12–step for the treatment of opioid dependent women meeting criteria for borderline personality disorder. *Drug and Alcohol Dependence, 67,* 13–26.

Linehan, M. M., Schmidt, H., Dimeff, L. A., Craft, J. C., Kanter, J., & Comtois, K. A. (1999). Dialectical behavior therapy for patients with borderline personality disorder and drug-dependence. *American Journal on Addictions, 8,* 279–292.

Lynch, T. R., Chapman, A. L., Rosenthal, M. Z., Kuo, J. R., & Linehan, M. M. (2006). Mechanisms of change in dialectical behavior therapy: Theoretical and empirical observations. *Journal of Clinical Psychology, 62*(4), 459–480.

Lynch, T. R., Cheavens, J. S. (2008). Dialectical Behavior Therapy for Comorbid Personality Disorders. *Journal of Clinical Psychology, 64,* 1–14.

Lynch, T. R., Cheavens, J. S., Cukrowicz, K. C., Thorp, S. R., Bronner, L., & Beyer, J. (2007). Treatment of older adults with co-morbid personality disorder and depression: A dialectical behavior therapy approach. *International Journal of Geriatric Psychiatry, 22,* 131–143.

Lynch, T. R., Morse, J. Q., Mendelson, T., & Robins, C. J. (2003). Dialectical behavior therapy for depressed older adults: A randomized pilot study. *American Journal of Geriatric Psychiatry, 11,* 33–45.

Lynch, T. R., Robins, C. J., Morse, J. Q., & Krause, E. D. (2001). A mediational model relating affect intensity, emotion inhibition, and psychological distress. *Behavior Therapy, 32*(3), 519–536.

Lynch, T. R., Trost, W. T., Salsman, N., & Linehan, M. M. (2007). Dialectical Behavior Therapy for borderline personality disorder. *Annual Review of Clinical Psychology, 3,* 181–205.

Martell, C. R., Addis, M. E., & Jacobson, N. S. (2001). *Depression in context: Strategies for guided action.* New York: Norton.

Michel, K., Valach, L., & Waeber, V. (1994). Understanding deliberate self-harm: The patients' views. *Crisis: The Journal of Crisis Intervention and Suicide Prevention, 15*(4), 172–178, 186.

Öhman, A., & Mineka, S. (2001). Fears, phobias, and preparedness: Toward an evolved module of fear and fear learning. *Psychological Review, 108*(3), 483–522.

Pelham, B. W., & Swann, W. B. (1994). The juncture of intrapersonal and interpersonal knowledge: Self-certainty and interpersonal congruence. *Personality and Social Psychology Bulletin, 20*(4), 349–357.

Philippot, P., Baeyens, C., Douilliez, C., & Francart, B. (2004). Cognitive regulation of emotion: Application to clinical disorders. In P. Philippot & R. S. Feldman (Eds.), *The regulation of emotion* (pp. 71–97). Mahwah, NJ: Erlbaum.

Robbins, S. J. (1990). Spontaneous recovery of Pavlovian conditioned responding. *Dissertation Abstracts International, 50*(9-B), 425.

Rosenthal, M. Z., Gratz, K. L., Kosson, D. S., Cheavens, J. S., Lejuez, C. W., & Lynch, T. R. (2008). Borderline personality disorder and emotional responding: A review of the research literature. *Annual Review of Clinical Psychology,* *3,* 181–205.

Safer, D. L., Telch, C. F., & Agras, W. S. (2001). Dialectical behavior therapy for bulimia nervosa. *American Journal of Psychiatry, 158,* 632–634.

Siddle, D. A., & Packer, J. S. (1987). Stimulus omission and dishabituation of the electrodermal orienting response: The allocation of processing resources. *Psychophysiology, 24*(2), 181–190.

Smith, C. F., Williamson, D. A., Bray, G. A., & Ryan, D. H. (1999). Flexible vs. rigid dieting strategies: Relationship with adverse behavioral outcomes. *Appetite, 32*(3), 295–305.

Sokolov, E. N. (1963). Orientirovochnyi refleks kak kiberneticheskaia sistema [Orienting reflex as a cybernetic system]. *Zhurnal Vysshei Nervnoi Deyatel'nosti, 13*(5), 816–830.

Soussignan, R. (2002). Duchenne smile, emotional experience, and autonomic reactivity: A test of the facial feedback hypothesis. *Emotion, 2*(1), 52–74.

Stella, S. G., Vilar, A. P., Lacroix, C., Fisberg, M., Santos, R. F., Mello, M. T., et al. (2005). Effects of type of physical exercise and leisure activities on the depression scores of obese Brazilian adolescent girls. *Brazilian Journal of Medical and Biological Research, 38*(11), 1683–1689.

Swann, W. B. (1997). The trouble with change: Self-verification and allegiance to the self. *Psychological Science, 8,* 177–180.

Swann, W. B., de la Ronde, C., & Hixon, J. G. (1994). Authenticity and positivity strivings in marriage and courtship. *Journal of Personality and Social Psychology, 66*(5), 857–869.

Telch, C. F., Agras, W. S., & Linehan, M. M. (2001). Dialectical behavior therapy for binge eating disorder. *Journal of Consulting and Clinical Psychology, 69,* 1061–1065.

Tulving, E., Markowitsch, H. J., & Kapur, S. (1994). Novelty encoding networks in the human brain: Positron emission tomography data. *NeuroReport, 5*(18), 2525–2528.

Verheul, R., van den Bosch, L. M. C., Koeter, M. W. J., de Ridder, M. A. J., Stijnen, T., & van den Brink, W. (2003). Dialectical behaviour therapy for women with borderline personality disorder: 12-month, randomised clinical trial in The Netherlands. *British Journal of Psychiatry, 182,* 135–140.

Wagner, A. W., & Linehan, M. M. (1997). Biosocial perspective on the relationship of childhood sexual abuse, suicidal behavior, and borderline personality disorder. In M. C. Zanarini (Ed.), *Role of sexual abuse in the etiology of borderline personality disorder* (pp. 203–223). Washington, DC: American Psychiatric Association.

Watson, J. B. (1924). Behaviourism: The modern note in psychology. *Psyche, 5,* 3–12.

Williams, J. M. G., Stiles, W. B., & Shapiro, D. A. (1999). Cognitive mechanisms in the avoidance of painful and dangerous thoughts: Elaborating the assimilation model. *Cognitive Therapy and Research, 23*(3), 285–306.

CHAPTER 8

Cognitive Analytic Therapy

Anthony Ryle

INTRODUCTION AND HISTORICAL BACKGROUND

Cognitive analytic therapy (CAT) is an integrated, time-limited psychotherapy based upon a theory of human psychological development that emphasizes the formation and maintenance of individual inter- and intrapersonal psychological processes through relationships with others. It originated in an attempted restatement of psychoanalytic object relations theories in terms of cognitive psychology. The approach was first presented as a defined psychotherapy model in the mid-1980s. Attention was focused on describing the reasons for the nonrevision of dysfunctional processes. In the early stages of CAT, three such general patterns were identified, representing relatively low-level "tactical" problems, namely, *traps*, in which negative assumptions lead to actions that result in the apparent confirmation of the assumptions; *dilemmas*, in which the options for behavior or for interpreting experience are narrowed down to polarized opposites; and *snags* ("subtle negative aspects of goals"), through which irrational guilt or the predicted negative responses of others leads to the abandonment of appropriate goals (Ryle, 1979). These patterns were related to a model of intentional action, the procedural sequence model, in which activity and experience are described as shaped by reiterated procedural sequences that encompass intentions, external events or situations, appraisals involving cognitions and affects, and behaviors and consequences, in the light of which the aim and/or the procedural sequence is confirmed or revised (Ryle, 1982).

244

Outcome research into dynamic psychotherapy required the early collaborative descriptive reformulation of the inter- and intrapersonal processes serving to maintain the patient's problems. This process was found to have a major therapeutic effect and early, joint descriptive reformulations recorded in writing and in sequential diagrams were the defining feature of what became CAT. Behavior and experience were seen to be shaped by complex procedural sequences involving the context, perceptions, appraisals, action, and the confirmation or revision of the aim or the procedure in light of the consequences. The procedural sequences of particular interest to therapists are those in which the aim of the action is to understand or elicit a response from another. The model, incorporating a recognition of the key importance of early relationships, was elaborated as the procedural sequence object relations model. Roles are enacted in response to, or in the attempt to elicit, a reciprocal role from the other. Reciprocal role procedures (RRPs) became a key concept in the CAT understanding of early development, self-management, and relationships with others, including the therapeutic relationship. The stability of the roles maintaining self processes, including dysfunctional ones, is maintained by the perception or elicitation of the sought for reciprocations (Ryle, 1990, 1991). Stimulus or context, cognitive and affective appraisal, action, and reflection on the consequences leading to confirmation or revision, so often described separately, are considered to be essentially related to each other as stages in the procedural sequence. Procedural sequences are hierarchical, and while therapeutic interventions may attend primarily to lower levels of individual psychopathology (e. g., behaviors, symptoms, or beliefs), they inevitably have implications for, or reflect, higher levels, such as values and assumptions. In more disturbed patients the system of RRPs may be fragmented.

While CAT grew out of a cognitive translation of some psychoanalytic ideas, the importance of the developing child's actual experiences was increasingly recognized. Introducing ideas from the Vygotskian school led to a clearer model of the role of relationships with others in the formation of higher mental processes and personality, and to a replacement of the concept of representation with one of internalization, a process involving the use of culturally derived, mediating conceptual tools.

CAT is normally delivered within a predetermined time frame of 16–24 sessions. The aims of therapy are defined as *procedural change*. Applying the fully developed theory helps the therapist describe how the patient is situated in his or her past and present web of inter- and intrapersonal procedures.

Training and supervision became formalized in the late 1980s, with the formation of the Association for Cognitive Analytic Therapy (ACAT), and is now available at numerous centers in the United Kingdom and in several other countries.

Biographical and Academic Genealogy

Psychotherapy theories reflect the times and places of their origins. Because my early development of CAT was carried out in relative isolation, the overall values and much of the form of the model bear my personal imprint, and the social attitudes it incorporates reflect my time and place of birth, and the political and ethical traditions of my family. My parents' personal experiences of the first half of the destructive 20th century had included my mother, as a child in South Africa, living across the road from the world's first concentration camp occupied by displaced Boer families. My parents married in 1914, and my father then spent over 4 years as a doctor in France, processing the casualties of the battles that, by 1918, had claimed the lives of many the young men my mother had known as a girl. These experiences were little spoken of, but recently, when reading Vera Brittain's *Testament of Youth* (1933), I was struck by the description of her prolonged mourning for her brother and his two friends, men whom she had loved, and its eventual resolution in her determination to remember their lives more than their deaths and to live a life at once personally full, and socially and politically devoted to the attempt to prevent the recurrence of such destruction. Her account resonated with my memories of the atmosphere of my childhood home, where I was made aware of the gathering threats evident in the rise of Nazism and in the Spanish Civil War and lived in expectation of the final devastation of World War II. Born in 1927, I was an observer of, not a participant in, that war and in all the wars that have occurred since, and have shared with many others a sense of powerless outrage in the face the frequent destructiveness, injustices, betrayals, complacencies, and hypocrisies of governments and of the passivity of most people most of the time. But I was proud of my countrymen's contribution to the winning of the necessary World War II and encouraged by the social reforms of the immediate postwar years. Among these reforms, the institution of the National Health Service (NHS) was of central importance. I qualified as a doctor less than 2 years after it was founded and worked in it directly or indirectly for over half a century. The NHS provided a channel through which I expressed my social and political values.

Many features of CAT are derived from this history, notably, its collaborative mode of working with patients and its economic practicability, which contrasted with the cost, elitist unconcern with social realties, and the obscurantism of the then-dominant psychotherapy models. The intellectual tradition in my family included what I would call *Darwinian humanism*, uniting ethical and scientific values with a skeptical view of authority and of established religion. My father's best known books were *The Natural History of Disease*, whose title indicates his strong belief that observation should precede experiment, and *Changing Disciplines*, which argued for the importance of studying the ultimate (genetic and environmental) causes, as well as the intimate (e. g., bacilli or neoplasms) causes of disease. Social medicine identifies many preventable social causes of disease in our unequal society and in the even more unequal developing world, but because its findings often indicate unpopular political priorities, its influence has been modest. Health service managers and professional bodies still give much more attention and money to treatment than to prevention in both general medicine and psychiatry.

Stages in the Development of the Model

My curriculum vitae has five distinct phases, each of which contributed to the development of the CAT model: (1) general practice; (2) director of the university health service; (3) part-time research fellow; (4) consultant psychotherapist; and (5) retirement.

General Practice (1952–1964)

The possibilities of offering all sections of society adequate medical care, which the NHS had established, combined with my lack of enthusiasm for the basic sciences, such as biochemistry, resulted in my decision to enter general practice rather than to pursue a more prestigious career. I and like-minded, left-wing colleagues set up a group practice in inner London, where we sought to deliver a standard of care hitherto unavailable to a largely working-class population. Alongside the clinical work I began to carry out some research. General practice in the NHS offered access to populations unselected for psychological problems, and my doctoral thesis (Ryle, 1959) was an epidemiological study recording the age and sex distribution of "neurosis" in the patients on my list. Following this, in collaboration with a psychiatrist (Dr., later Prof., D. A. Pond) and a social worker (Madge Hamilton), I carried out a detailed study of all the families on my list with children ages 5–11. This work, summarized in Ryle (1967), demonstrated the high prevalence of psychological problems in the adults and children in the practice population, their relation to past and present family relationships, and the scant therapeutic resources available. Madge Hamilton, who interviewed the parents together, persuaded me of the contribution made by her psychodynamic background. I was also struck by how many of my patients said that this was the first time they had sat down together to think about their lives. I have been impressed throughout my life by the power of attentive history taking and by the absence of empathic others in so many lives.

After a few years in practice I began to give patients presenting with psychological distress long appointments outside surgery hours, involving support, explanation, reassurance, and the discussion of current problems in the light of the life history. I also gained a little experience in the use of relaxation and conditioning methods, influenced by Wolpe (1958). Looking back, I can see that the main impact of these various approaches was derived from my curiosity and concerned attention—the latter being the factor that Frank (1961) showed to be common to most helpful interventions. After 12 years in general practice I was appointed to run the University Health Service in the new University of Sussex. This offered me a chance to concentrate on psychotherapy and related research.

Director of the University Health Service (1964–1976)

I started at the University of Sussex at the same time as its first large student intake. In the early years, the university gave full support for a service that offered easy access to psychological assessment and therapy, and contributed to the identification and mitigation of damaging institutional pressures. Before my appointment, the university had already appointed a consultant, Fred Shadforth, a Klein-influenced Freudian psychoanalyst, and he provided for me, and for the other doctors and nurses, recruited as the service grew, detailed group and individual supervision. Under his influence I extended my reading to writers in the object relations school and found, particularly in Guntrip and Winnicott, psychoanalytic texts I could read with interest and profit. But I reacted against the dominant Kleinian concentration on perverse, destructive, and largely autonomous "unconscious" forces. My reading also included behavioral and cognitive texts. Among those that contributed to the eventual formation of CAT were Kelly's (1955) presentation of personal construct theory and repertory grid techniques, the work of Bartlett (1954) on remembering, the concept of action plans from Miller, Galanter, and Pribram (1960), and Neisser's *Cognitive Psychology* (1967). Following Beck (1976), I made use of patient self-monitoring to explore the events and thoughts related to symptoms and increasingly replaced the psychoanalytic focus on conflict, with detailed attention to the sequence of thinking and acting associated with psychological problems. I identified with an overall dynamic, developmental, and whole-person approach to therapy and was spurred on to seek to evaluate it by Eysenckian behaviorists' slick attacks and by my irritation at the absence of serious psychodynamic research. I began to study the process and outcome of therapy through the use of the repertory grid. Grids are based on the personal construct theory of Kelly (1955), which I found inadequate, among other reasons, because his concept of "man as scientist" failed to explain why my patients were such bad scientists, in that they failed to revise their procedures even when the consequences were disastrous. But grid techniques offered a simple and powerful way of indirectly extracting descriptions of cognitive processes associated with the symptoms and relationship difficulties of my patients (Ryle, 1975). Over this period I also carried out a study of the records of a small series of completed therapies, aiming to identify what had been the agenda and paying particular attention to nonrevision of damaging procedures. From this I identified the three general patterns of dilemmas, traps, and snags (Ryle, 1979) described earlier. Involving patients in the task of describing these was initially intended to provide a basis for rating dynamic change, but the process of joint reformulation had such a powerful, positive impact that it altered my practice, and the joint descriptive reformulation of dysfunctional patterns replaced the interpretation of unconscious conflict. A small-scale study (Ryle, 1980) supported the value of early descriptive reformulation, and this became and remains a defining feature of the CAT model. For measuring outcome, I identified specific grid measures related to key problems before therapy. For example, a depressed, overcompliant person's grid, in which significant other people (the elements) were rated on a number of descriptions, might indicate the sources of his or her behavior in the assumptions suggested by a high correlation between the constructs dependent and submissive; successful therapy would be indicated by a reduction of this construct correlation. In the dyad grid (Ryle & Lunghi, 1970) the elements were relationships, commonly those between the subject and a range of others, and the constructs described interactions. For example, self to Mary, Mary to self, self to mother, and so forth, might be rated against constructs (e. g., is kind to or is controlling of). Principal component analysis of grids identifies the associations between the elements and constructs, and the main patterns derived from the first two components can be expressed graphically. This provides the most accessible summary of a completed grid and in the case of the dyad grid, one could draw "dyad lines" joining the reciprocal elements of a relationship (e. g., self to Mary to Mary to self). Parallel dyad lines indicated similar reciprocal roles (Ryle & Lunghi, 1970).

University of Sussex Part-Time Research Fellow (1976–1982)

In 1975 the university authorities decided that my psychotherapy role and my membership in the Senate were redundant. I accepted early retirement and a part-time research fellowship, and the ill wind in due course blew me some unintended good, for over the next few years I had more time for research and thinking. During this time I summarized what I saw then as the possibility of an integration of object relations theory and cognitive psychology (Ryle, 1985). I was invited by Prof. J. Watson to teach and supervise the emerging CAT model at Guy's Hospital. I had undergone no formal training in either psychiatry or psychotherapy, but, fortunately, when the Royal College of Psychiatry had been founded, the research I had done was recognized by my being elected to foundation membership, and a few years later I was made a fellow. I am grateful to the unknown colleagues who proposed me for these, making me eligible to be appointed to the consultant psychotherapist post at St. Thomas's Hospital.

St. Thomas's Hospital (1982–1992)

Here I spent the last 10 years of my full-time career. The consultant psychotherapist post had been unfilled and I had no staff, no colleagues, and for a time no dedicated space beyond a drawer in a filing cabinet in the waiting room. To run the service, which quickly attracted well over 100 referrals annually, I depended on recruiting people from various backgrounds inside and outside the hospital, who had been introduced to CAT in workshops and were prepared to see patients in exchange for supervision. Teaching and supervising experienced but largely untrained people was a test of the approach and contributed to its further development, and this led eventually to the publication of the first book describing CAT (Ryle, 1990). The management's general unconcern with psychotherapy fed a certain oppositional and pioneer spirit, and the service survived and continues to this day.

Retirement (1992 to the Present)

Since my retirement from the NHS my CAT-related activity has continued through a slowly diminishing involvement in teaching, supervising, and research. CAT organization and training were taken over by more competent colleagues and I had time to develop the theory. In particular, having focused on the integration of different approaches, I now became involved in the differentiation of CAT as a distinct theory and method, a process recorded in three books written with colleagues between 1990 and 2002, and in numerous papers. A number of detailed critiques of Kleinian case histories were published, exploring how far they could be formulated in terms of CAT concepts (Ryle, 1992, 1993, 1995, 1996), but neither these nor a less polemical, measured consideration of some welcome new psychoanalytic ideas (Ryle, 2003) received any comments in the psychoanalytic press.

The introduction by Leiman of ideas based on the writings of Vygotsky and Bakhtin (Leiman, 1992; Ryle, 1991) made a major contribution to the development of a comprehensive theoretical model The origins of reciprocal role patterns were seen to lie in the earliest relationships, notably, with caretakers, a position supported by the observational work of developmental psychologists (e. g., Stern, 1985; Trevarthen & Aitken, 2000) that demonstrated the infant's eager participation in relationships. Infant–caretaker interactions, involving imitation, turn taking, and joint action sequences, are the precursors of later established patterns of reciprocal role relationships.

The theory incorporated Vygotsky's model of how internal self-processes are derived from external relationships with others, how learning involves joint activity with a more experienced other, and how internalization depends on the establishment and use of shared signs. His description of the zone of proximal development (ZPD), indicating the individual's potential capacity to learn if supported by a more experienced other, had clear relevance to therapy. Bakhtin, rooted in literature and philosophy, provided eloquent descriptions of the essentially dialogical basis of higher mental functions. These influences, and their relation to evolutionary and biological factors, were developed further, and a comprehensive biological, social, and psychological model of the self was presented (Ryle & Kerr, 2002, Chapters 3 and 4).

Achievements to Date

When I became a psychotherapy consultant at St. Thomas's Hospital in 1982, I found an enormous appetite for teaching and supervision among the hospital staff and, subsequently, open workshops attracted literally hundreds of participants from outside, many of whom treated patients in return for supervision. Practitioners from various backgrounds became involved in the teaching and development of the model, bringing to it a range of previous trainings and perspectives. Within a few years, an organization—the present-day ACAT—was formed, and appropriate structures and standards of training and practice were instituted. Practitioner training is offered to those with existing professional qualifications, combining teaching seminars, study days, and the supervised therapy of eight cases over a 2-year period. Such training is now established in numerous U. K. centers, validated by ACAT and also, in many cases, as accredited university courses. Subsequently, interregional training for those seeking national registration as psychotherapists, involving a further 2 years of supervised practice, residential training weeks, and local seminars, was established. Applications for training exceed the available places and come increasingly from established practitioners, notably, clinical psychologists and general psychiatrists, who find in CAT an understanding of the interpersonal dimension of practice that is missing from their previous training. Overseas, training have been established in Greece, Finland, Spain, Ireland, and Australia.

Numerous papers in peer-reviewed journals and several books, of which the most recent is Ryle and Kerr (2002), describe the origins and development of CAT practice and theory. The application of CAT to different patient groups includes the study of adult survivors of childhood sexual abuse (Pollock, 2001), applications in work with the elderly (Hepple & Sutton, 2004), and the treatment of offenders (Pollock, Stowell-Smith, & Gopfert, 2006). CAT has proved particularly suited to the treatment of more disturbed and "hard to help" patients, and to the to the training and supervision of staff without psychotherapy experience in community mental health teams (CMHTs).

As regards research, CAT became established in association with a wide range of small studies concerning the process of change and the application of the theory in practice. The research publications are discussed below.

PHILOSOPHICAL AND THEORETICAL UNDERPINNINGS

The Theory of Psychopathology

Humans are the product of evolution. Biological evolution depends on the fact of random genetic variation and survival of the fittest, and is a slow process; today we are genetically much the same as our forebearers of a quarter of a million years ago. But there has been an accelerating process of social evolution whereby, once group living and communication are established, new ideas and skills can be immediately passed on to contemporary and future groups, initially by mimesis but increasingly by language (Donald, 1991, 2001). To a degree not approached anywhere else in the animal kingdom, the human understanding of objects and of people, including the self, and the organization of knowledge, values, feelings, and action, are imbued with socially derived meanings that together situate the individual in relation to the world; the psychology of modern humans is a cultural product. The developmental pathway can be easily disrupted. Early adversity may influence neurophysiological processes in ways that may not be reversible. Genetically determined temperamental characteristics may interfere with the social interactions through which personality is formed. The development of skills and the acquisition of knowledge during the phase of rapid physical maturation, while following a basic timetable, are influenced by the actual experiences of the child, and by the meanings applied to them.

The fundamental descriptive unit in CAT is the RRP. In the role procedures involved in relationships, the aim is to elicit the response from others who can be induced to reciprocate, or can be seen to do so. RRPs involve sequences of inner mental and outer environmental processes. Normal development leads to a more or less integrated personality that can be described verbally and diagrammatically in terms of a repertoire of RRPs, mobilized in response to events and contexts. Role procedures are hierarchically organized, so that lower-level "tactical" procedures are shaped in relation to higher-order "strategic" ones. A normal individual has a repertoire of role procedures integrated and mobilized appropriately by higher-order metaprocedures, so that transitions between them are usually smooth and understandable. Faced with deprivation and adversity, however, the developing child may internalize a limited array of negative patterns derived from critical or conditional care, excessive or deficient control, or neglect or abuse. This can lead to hypervigilance for signs of further neglect or abuse, to the seeking or acceptance of such neglect and abuse, and to the inflicting of neglect and abuse on both others and the self. In genetically vulnerable children exposed to repeated and severe abuse, the experience or anticipation of repetitions can provoke a partial or complete dissociation, creating split-off RRPs that become established as "self states" providing alternating frameworks for experience and behavior. Switches between procedures and states may be abrupt and seemingly unprovoked, and memory between states may be absent or impaired. The model is therefore essentially one of structural dissociation (see Howell, 2005).

Conceptualization of Individual Patients

The patient's dysfunctional procedures are reformulated in joint work, which initiates a working relationship. Dilemmas, traps and snags, and dysfunctional procedural sequences are identified by detailed attention to the patient's history and ongoing relationships. High-level "strategic" patterns are manifest in a range of "tactical" procedures. Once identified, the RRPs are described in writing or in a diagram; thereafter, self-monitoring can identify the situations, moods, symptoms, and dysfunctional behaviors associated with them. The main patterns are often manifest within the first clinical assessment interviews, in the patient's speech and demeanor, and in the therapist's felt reactions; thereafter, the descriptions can be modified by continuing self-observation and diary keeping.

Recent Theoretical Developments and Challenges to the Model

The development of CAT theory has been stimulated from the beginning by considering divergences from and with other models, and this process has continued hand in hand with ideas emerging in the course of clinical and research activity and the incorporation of ideas from Vygotsky and Bakhtin. The relation of CAT to other current models is reviewed below.

Constructivist and Cognitivist Ideas

Despite the early influence of personal construct theory, CAT's developed theory represented a radical divergence from cognitive and constructivist ideas. Individually constructed, rationally validated theories were seen to contribute little to the formation of self processes. Our sense of self and of the world is first learned in interaction with caretakers and others; internalization of these interactions means that the developed self is the complex, socially formed, and multivoiced result of the infant's entering into a particular cultural context and historical moment. In place of Descartes' "I think, therefore I am, " the view proposed for the growing child is "We engage and communicate, therefore I become" (Ryle, 2001). This paper also restated the CAT critique of the cognitive concepts of representation and information storage, arguing that learning about the world, others, and the self combines information with meanings acquired in the dialogue with others, a dialogue mediated by preverbal and verbal signs that provide in the conversation with the self the basis of conscious thought. The RRP repertoire summarizes how a person, in his or her context, goes on being and will go on being, unless challenged by a new reciprocation or equipped with new means of recognizing and thinking about the problematic procedure.

Evolutionary Psychology

In a critique of the overstated claims made by some authors for the relevance of evolutionary psychology to psychotherapy, Ryle (2005) challenged in particular the failure to acknowledge the evolutionary origins of social, as well as selfish genes; the failure to take account of human symbol-making and symbol-using capacities; and the underestimation of the scope and plasticity of the human brain. Donald (2001) and Tomasello (1999), among others, have demonstrated the cultural origins of human cognition.

Attachment Theory

CAT evolved before the relevance of attachment theory (AT) to psychotherapy was widely recognized. In my view the biological and behavioral paradigm of the early AT models paid too little attention to the particular human attributes of symbol use, but later research into the transmission of attachment patterns provides important evidence about the social formation of personality. My neglect of the AT classification of attachment patterns has been criticized within CAT (Jellema, 2000, 2002).

Dialogical Models

The dialogical theory of human personality put forward by Hermans (Hermans & Dimaggio, 2004) shares with CAT a debt to Horowitz's (1979) descriptions of states of mind. It proposes a model of mind in which multiple "voices" are in communication and competition with each other. The CAT critique of the model (Ryle, 2005) points to the absence of a developmental perspective, to the cognitivist focus on representations and skills, and to the absence of a clear distinction between normal and pathological multiplicity. The CAT view (Ryle & Fawkes, 2007) is distinguished from other dialogical models by its emphasis on the self–other origins and semiotic basis of internal dialogue.

Psychoanalysis

The Process of Change Study Group (Boston; Stern et al., 1998) proposed a number of theoretical revisions of psychoanalytic theory and practice, many of which were close to CAT. These included an emphasis on implicit, procedural knowledge as governing relationships, and the suggestion that the classical focus on interpretation was an inadequate basis for treatment. However, the implications for practice of the radical revisions of the theory proposed have not been developed, and my published suggestion (Ryle, 2003) that CAT practice could contribute to this did not evoke any published response.

Mentalization-Based Therapy

Bateman and Fonagy (2004) describe a number of revisions of psychoanalytic theory in their description of mentalization-based therapy (MBT). The convergences and contrasts between CAT and MBT were explored in a joint paper (Bateman, Ryle, Fonagy, & Kerr, 2007). This demonstrated parallels in the aims and, to a limited extent, in the practice of the models, but the theoretical differences were not resolvable.

EMPIRICAL EVIDENCE
The Status of the Theoretical Model

CAT grew out of clinical and research activities, and challenging existing models, either on the grounds that their fundamental assumptions were erroneous or restrictive, or not clearly stated, or that their evidence base was narrow or absent. The aim was to develop a model consistent with the better established theories of related disciplines, notably, developmental psychology and cognitive psychology, while challenging the dominant monadic emphasis of much work by emphasizing the cultural and interpersonal formation and dialogical structure of individual psychology. As regards practice, Bennett used task analysis to develop an empirically validated model of effective therapist interventions (Bennett, Parry, & Ryle, 2006) and demonstrated that adherence to the model was associated with good outcome. The model suggests that specific techniques (e. g., making links to the reformulation) are only effective if the relationship is characterized by the following: a collaborative but noncollusive stance; use of benign RRPs to achieve the work of therapy; nonreciprocation of damaging reciprocal roles; use of silence to facilitate access to affects and the develop-ment of the patient's self-observing capacity; reflective or linking statements within an empathic and respectful relationship; and being prepared to show aspects of vulnerability or self-disclosure, if this is indicated. In poor out-come cases, therapists had failed to apply many aspects of the model. Ben-nett and Parry (2004) subsequently developed a reliable method of rating audiotapes, which measures the quality of therapy in relation to both gen-eral and specific CAT principles.

The Overall Effectiveness of the Therapy

The evolved model has the characteristics shown by Luborsky (1990) to characterize effective dynamic therapies, namely, an emphasis on the ther-apeutic alliance, targeted goals, and feedback. In regard to patients with personality disorders, it offers the features identified as necessary by Bate-man and Fonagy (1999), namely, having a clear focus and structure, paying specific attention to maintaining a treatment alliance, and being comprehen-sible to both therapists and patients.

Mixed Anxiety, Depression, and Somatization

A forerunner of CAT was evaluated in two small studies of outcome (Ryle, 1979, 1980) that piloted the basic methodology of a subsequent random-ized controlled trial (RCT; Brockman, Poynton, Ryle, & Watson, 1987) of the treatment of patients referred to an outpatient psychotherapy service, excluding those with active psychosis and serious substance abuse. Change was measured using (1) standard inventories, (2) rating change in individu-ally defined problems, and (3) variations in specific repertory grid features identified before therapy as indicative of clinical issues. The experimental intervention and the control, a form of focused dynamic therapy, delivered by the same therapists and both time-limited, produced the same mean changes in inventory scores, but predicted changes in grid measures were significantly greater with the experimental treatment.

CAT has been widely used in the treatment of eating disorders, contrib-uting both an understanding of the relation of the symptoms to underlying inter- and intrapersonal procedures (see Bell, 1999) and a way of managing the often difficult feelings elicited in clinical staff by these patients. At this time no formal research has been published.

Borderline Personality Disorder

The structure of CAT was found helpful by patients with BPD and could in some cases assist integration (Ryle & Beard, 1993). The length of treatment was extended to 24 sessions, with follow-up at 1, 2, 3, and 6 months. Sequential diagrammatic reformulation was modified to describe these patients' array of dissociated RRPs as separate *self states*, a practical development that supported the theoretical development of the multiple self states model (MSSM; Ryle 1997). A series of 27 patients with BPD completed 24 sessions plus follow-up; half the sample no longer met diagnostic criteria at follow-up at 6 months (Ryle & Golynkina, 2000). Wildgoose, Clarke, and Waller (2001) described the impact of 16 sessions of CAT on five patients with BPD; the severity of BPD was reduced in all five, but other changes were inconsistent, and the authors point to the need to clarify further the relation of personal fragmentation and of dissociation to reductions in symptoms. Chanen, Jackson, McCutcheon, Jovev, Dudgeon, et al. (2008) completed a large-scale RCT in older adolescents, comparing CAT to a manualized control treatment and to a historical "treatment as usual" control group. Both treatments were superior to the "treatment as usual" control group, and CAT was more effective than the manualized control group in reducing externalizing symptoms.

Treatment of Offenders

A number of case studies describing the application of CAT to the treatment of offenders have been published. Pollock and Kear-Colwell (1994) published a repertory grid study of women with histories of early abuse who had committed violent offenses against their partners, showing that the women had great difficulty in acknowledging their own victim status, and illustrating the relevance of CAT understandings, and Pollock (1996) followed this with a study of seven cases, confirming that the women identified themselves as guilty aggressors and disavowed their own victimization, and showing that the women had experienced dissociative states before, during, and after their offenses. Clarke and Pearson (2000) found a similar pattern in male sexual abuse survivors treated with CAT. Pollock et al. (2006) edited a collection of writings on the treatment of offenders, including reports of the use of CAT in a wide range of conditions and situations.

Treating Poor Self-Care in Diabetes

Patients with poorly controlled diabetes generate a considerable proportion of the cost of running services through hospital admissions for diabetic ketosis and the treatment of their accumulating disabilities. Poor self-care in insulin-dependent diabetic patients has many different sources (Ryle, Boa, & Fosbury, 1993), and Fosbury demonstrated that these could be located with reference to general self-management and relationship procedures identified by sequential diagrammatic reformulation (SDR). A small RCT comparing 16 sessions of CAT with a similar number of sessions with an experienced specialist nurse was carried out. The main outcome measure was the blood level of hemoglobin, alpha 1 (HbA1), which gives a reliable measure of the general level of control. Between the 3- and 9-month follow-ups, mean HbA1 levels in the CAT group continued to fall, whereas levels in the control group returned to near the initial level (Fosbury, Bosley, Ryle, Sonksen, & Judd, 1997).

Poor Self-Care in Asthma

Walsh, Hagan, and Gamsu (2000), using a CAT framework, reported a qualitative study of poorly managed asthma in 35 patients. Patterns of denial, avoidance, and depression were identified, and the importance of the relationship between patients and their doctors, investigated through the CAT procedural model, was demonstrated.

Substance Abuse Problems

Leighton (1997), working in a residential setting, described how CAT reformulation provides an effective way of placing drug use in the context of the procedural system of individuals with BPD. Some CAT tools were incorporated into the general program, and individual therapy was offered to patients presenting with associated personality disorders.

CAT in Combination with Other Treatment Modes

Hughes (2007) noted that both CAT and art therapy depend on the creation and use of *transitional objects* (mediating tools), illustrating how art therapy and CAT methods are compatible, and suggesting that for some patients the practice of either may be strengthened by combining it with elements of the other. Compton Dickinson (2006) described an integration of CAT and music therapy in the treatment of offenders with severe and dangerous personality disorders. Joint musical improvisation offers a nonverbal, jointly created system of signs associated with states and state shifts.

CAT Applied to Staff Training and Supervision

The use of CAT understandings to support persons involved in the care of patients is of particular value in work with more disturbed patients. Beard described the construction of a sequential diagram with an adolescent patient who was causing serious disruption in the hostel where she was living (Beard, Marlowe, & Ryle, 1990). In staff caring for very disturbed patients with BPD, Dunn and Parry (1997) described the value of basing care plans on CAT reformulations. Kerr (2001a) described a short series of studies of inpatients with postacute manic psychosis making a similar use of the diagram with ward staff. Kerr (2000) described the value of *contextual reformulation*, in which the patient's diagram is shared with staff and extended to map out evoked staff reactions. CAT-based training for staff in CMHTs (Kerr, 2001b) has been developed (Thompson, Donnison, Warwock-Parkes, et al., in press) and is being evaluated as part of a larger trial of CAT treatments in Sheffield (Kerr, Dent-Brown, & Parry, 2007).

Support for Particular Interventions

Bennett and Parry (1998) compared a patient's Self States Sequential Diagram (SSSD) with analyses of audiotapes of early sessions using two established research tools (Luborsky & Crits-Christoph, 1989; Schacht & Henry, 1994) and demonstrated that diagrams could offer a comprehensible summary of the patterns of the patients' interpersonal relationships in ways that were validated by these research measures.

A *model of good CAT practice* was modified and validated by Bennett in a study of the audiotapes of therapy sessions with patients with BPD, focusing on operationally defined threats to the therapeutic alliance. The model was successively revised on the basis of studying further cases until no further revisions were indicated. The resulting empirically derived model provides a clear description of good CAT practice. Therapists of patients with good outcome had followed the model closely, whereas therapists treating patients whose outcomes were poor had identified a significantly smaller percentage of enactments and had resolved a much smaller percentage of these (Bennett et al., 2006).

The *ability of patients with BPD to describe their states* was confirmed in the repertory grid study of Golynkina and Ryle (1999). Further clinical and research studies made use of a method of guided self-reflection, the States Description Procedure (SDP; Bennett, Pollock, & Ryle, 2005; Bennett & Ryle, 2005) which involves patients in identifying and characterizing their states from provided lists of commonly use titles and features.

A *measure of CAT-specific and general psychotherapeutic competence* based on audiotape analysis was developed by Bennett and Parry (2004).

Limitations of Current Empirical Support

CAT has generated a relatively small volume of research, a fact partly accounted for by its rapid growth and its being taught in 25 geographically separate sites with no single academic base, at a time when research grants became scarcer and reorganizations of the Health Service were frequently disruptive. Development was, however, accompanied by small-scale studies of different patient groups and of innovative clinical practices such as diagrammatic reformulation. It was also accompanied by the creation of valuable research tools (Bennett & Perry, 2004; Pollock, Broadbent, Clarke, et al., 2000; Ryle, 2007), and one major RCT has now been published, described before (Chanen et al., 2008). Research into outcome and process accompanied all stages of development of the model, but large-scale RCTs were not undertaken until the last decade.

CLINICAL PRACTICE

The Relation of Practice to Theory and Distinctive Features of CAT

From the first session on, CAT therapists combine explaining the model, taking a history, and collecting other information with preliminary suggestions about the underlying patterns evident in this material and in the interchange. This represents an active listening and exploratory role in which patients are invited to contribute to descriptions of the thinking and actions underlying their difficulties. Individual psychology is understood in social, dialogical, and semiotic terms. It is social because it points to the way in which all role procedures, including dysfunctional ones, are formed by relationships with others. It is dialogical because patterns of relationship are repeated and are reproduced internally, and it is semiotic because dialogue depends upon the use of shared tools, including language, which are the origin of the internal dialogue of thought. Therapeutic work is initiated by the task of *reformulation*, involving a form of collaboration and offering a model of concerned attention that is unfamiliar to many patients. Most dysfunctional procedures are evident from the beginning to the trained therapist, and descriptions can usually be agreed on within the first four sessions. The aims of therapy are defined as *procedural revision* and *integration*. It is common for patients to forget much of the content of therapeutic conversations, especially when emotionally disturbing themes are explored, and for this reason, recording the key understandings in the reformulation letter and in diagrams is part of the basic technique. This phase of therapy can sometimes activate unhelpful procedures, such as idealization or superficial compliance followed by passive resistance, and therapists need to look out for these.

In practice, therapists write a reformulation letter, usually around session 4, which offers a narrative reconstruction suggesting links between past experiences, the strategies developed to deal with them, and current symptoms and maladaptive procedures. They also draft sequential diagrams over the early sessions; their exact form varies, but the aim is to demonstrate dysfunctional RRPs and to describe the consequences of their enactment. Diagrams may become too complex for easy use, and simpler working diagrams focusing on the central issues of the therapy may be devised.

An example provided by I. B. Kerr shows three stages in the development of an SSSD of a typical patient with BPD. Figure 8.1 shows the two RRPs commonly derived from the history of abuse and neglect. Figure 8.2 traces how these lead to the elaboration of dissociated self states, and traces procedural enactments and their consequences. Figure 8.3 shows how staff reactions may be polarized according to which aspect of the patient's system is activated.

Enacted sequences usually occur in relation to a series of actual or assumed reciprocating others and are not manifestations of a single procedure or of a preexisting schema; Leiman (1997) developed dialogical sequence analysis to make this apparent.

Joint work is supported by the use of various conceptual tools, as follows:

1. As part of the assessment, patients will be given the "psychotherapy file" (reproduced in Ryle & Kerr [2002] and earlier books), which describes symptom monitoring and explains the concepts of traps, dilemmas, and snags, giving typical examples. Patients note the descriptions that seem to apply to them and these are further discussed.

2. The eight-item *Personality Structure Questionnaire* (PSQ) can be usefully and rapidly completed during the assessment interview. It has good psychometric qualities (Pollock Broadbent & Clarke, 2001) and high scores identify patients with structural dissociation.

3. The identification and characterization of the patient's dissociated self states can be supported by the *States Description Procedure* (SDP), which involves patients in structured self-reflection (Bennett et al., 2005). This is of particular value in the reformulation of patients with dissociated states, some of which may be mobi-

FIGURE 8.1. SDR of a stereotypical fictionalized patient with BPD illustrating the first key reciprocal roles.

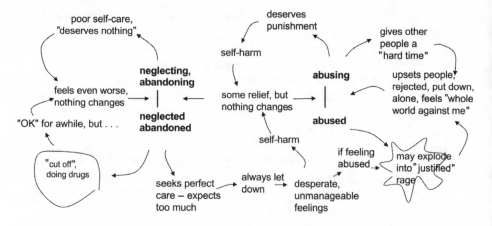

FIGURE 8.2. SDR of a stereotypical fictionalized patient with BPD illustrating key reciprocal roles, self states, and procedural enactments.

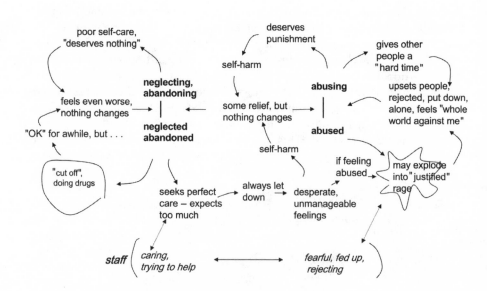

FIGURE 8.3. Rudimentary "contextual reformulation" of a stereotypical fictionalized patient with BPD showing basic staff team reciprocal reactions and splitting.

lized rapidly in response to the perception of immediate threat or of associated cues, others serving as relatively stable but dysfunctional ways of coping with a world experienced as essentially unsafe.

Ryle (2007), using a modified SDP, showed that the dissociated states experienced by a group of patients with BPD could be grouped on the basis of combining their symptoms and RRPs as follows: Patients perceiving repetitions or threats of abuse or abandonment either reenact versions of early negative relationship patterns, sometimes accompanied by dissociative symptoms, or they switch into alternative states. These may involve denial of weakness, as in the High state, fantasies of emotional safety, as in the Cloud Cuckoo Land state, the suppression of emotion, as in the Zombie state, or a combination of emotional flattening and resentful submission, as in the Soldiering On state. In the absence of threat, patients may enter the OK state or may guard against abandonment in the Powerful Caretaker state.

The reformulation letter acknowledges the patient's experiences and describes the Target Problems (TPs) and Target Problem Processes (TPPs), suggesting how they are either repetitions of early patterns or represent attempts at coping. Sequential diagrams describe the key RRPs and trace the consequences of procedural enactments. A completed reformulation therefore combines the two forms of description discussed by Bruner (1986), with the narrative offered in the letter and the paradigmatic in the diagram. Where there is a fragmented self structure, as in BPD, such diagrams trace the switches between dissociated self states.

Most patients are quick to learn how to use their diagrams to recognize their particular patterns; repeated use in the course of daily life and in the therapy sessions helps them establish a more continuous self-reflective capacity. Therapists must develop their capacity to recognize their own RRPs when they are elicited by patients. The key importance of the therapy relationship, identified by Frank (1961) as a common factor in effective therapies, is reaffirmed, but CAT emphasizes that maintaining a therapeutic relationship requires an accurate "map" of states and state shifts.

Change is anxiety arousing, and therapeutic change demands that patients feel that their experiences are accurately and empathically acknowledged. The reformulation stage in CAT establishes this, by the therapist's careful listening, acknowledging the patient's experiences, and recognizing cultural differences (class, race and gender), and by offering an understanding of how dysfunctional RRPs originated and are maintained. The patient's responsibility for what happened is explored with the aim of both challenging irrational guilt and acknowledging what harm was done. The therapist shares his or her theoretical understanding with the patient and enters into a relationship that is honest, respectful but not blandly accepting. The reformulation process usually engenders a positive relationship, but it is common for more negative attitudes to emerge later, frequently after 10 or so sessions, as hoped for magical changes do not occur, and the limits and errors of the therapist become apparent. Recognizing hostility, which is often expressed indirectly, is important for naming and surviving it, and not retaliating is often a crucial element in change. Stable therapeutic change depends on the patient's internalization of a relationship with an honest, respectful, and accurate therapist.

Case Study

This case is presented by Barbara Venning, a trainee in the CAT Advanced Psychotherapy Course. The patient gave full permission for this account to be published and read the version below. In the account, possible reciprocal roles suggested by the history are italicized.

Susie, a technical assistant in a small zoo, was referred for CAT by her general practitioner. She was an articulate, cooperative young woman living with her partner Mark. She described a life of emotional pain and chaos, and an inability to trust anyone. She had attempted suicide the year before, explaining that it was the result of being overwhelmed by desolate feelings of being dismissed and rejected.

Childhood History

Susie recalled how her father's abuse and violence had made her feel frightened and no good (*guilty, deprived in relation to abusive neglect*). Mom was weak and childlike, and Susie felt responsible, unsupported, neglected, and deprived in relation to neediness. Her parents divorced when she was 5, and she lived with her loving but barely coping mother. Her mother's family played a prominent role in Susie's early life, but a painful one, as epitomized by Susie's description of Christmas. Every year they would gather to eat together, and every year some perceived criticism would trigger a fight, verbal then physical, as they traded blows across the table and everything ended in tears.

The story suggested that the main reciprocal role Susie learned in childhood was *fearful and deprived in relation to unreliable care*, which evolved into a *deprived, caring, parental child in relation to a weak needy mother*. She told a heartbreaking childhood tale of sitting alone inside a cupboard feeling utterly desolate, defeated, and hopeless. She had scrawled "sueside" in chalk on a blackboard. The only one to see this was her brother, who laughed at her spelling. She felt criticized and dismissed. No one saw how bad she felt inside. It was clear that at home Susie's needs were not met. At school she tried to "cover up" for her perceived shame and learned ways to be "special" and win the admiration she craved. She was an "A" student, working hard to please her teachers, but it was never enough, so she feigned sickness, and told lies and fabricated stories to impress her friends (*striving, misleading/cheating to conditional acceptance*). When she was found out she was punished, this confirmed her belief that she was shamefully unworthy, undeserving, and guilty.

As an adult it remained hard for Susie to cope with ordinary, day-to-day living. She said, "I don't know how to have a close relationship, because I can't trust anyone. " Her mood would change, seemingly without warning or reason, but sometimes she would remain in a despairing state for days on end. On one occasion she packed Mark's bags, telling him to leave, then became shamefully rejecting of herself (*angry rejection in relation to perceived imperfect care, leading to self-rejection and anxious compliance*). She desperately struggled to keep everything under tight control but the effort was exhausting. (*anxiously overcontrolling to ward off feared chaos*) She took jobs that she knew were well within her capacity but she was bored and understimulated. Her very real talents went unacknowledged—by others and herself. She had little idea of what her true needs were and no idea how to get them met; Susie could not ask for anything because of her fear that she would be shamefully exposed to critical and rejecting others.

Therapy: The Early Sessions and Reformulation

On the basis of the previous account and the many other stories from her daily life, we began constructing an SDR, using the descriptions of possible RRPs I had identified. However, as pieces of paper proliferated, the situation quickly became confusingly chaotic. Looking back, I saw that I had been desperately striving to make sense of Susie's chaotic world and, while experiencing something of her feared chaos, had enacted anxious overcontrol. For Susie, my words were almost without meaning, and my supervisor recognized that the first task of therapy was for me to acknowledge the part of her derived from the neglected little girl and to give her an experience of being heard and understood. I read my provisional reformulation letter at session, using Susie's words or phrases to create a simple tool that she could understand, and I did not introduce the concept of RRPs at this stage. Part of the letter is reproduced below.

> *Dear Susie,*
>
> *You came into therapy because you have been suffering from severe depression. You say it is like being held to ransom with a gun and you live on nervous energy, all the time frightened in case you cannot cope. This letter is to set down what we know so far.*

The letter went on to reflect on Susie's early history, describing the unhealthy patterns of relating that came from her experiences at that time, and using her feeling for Mary, her small niece, to evoke empathy for herself as a child.

> *We have begun to understand together that as a child you had no secure base to operate from; no one was available to teach you about trust and safe dependency, and no one was there to help you calm your feelings and reflect a true sense of your self. You were potentially a normal little girl but you came to believe you were the bad one whom no one would want. You learned to deal with your painful feelings of rage, sadness, envy, and jealousy through patterns of misleading, concealing and by anxious overcontrol. These continue in your life today when you are overcome by difficult emotions that can take you unawares and suddenly change your mood. One of our tasks is to start to understand what triggers these overwhelming feelings and mood changes. My sense is that because you missed out on getting the secure attention and care you needed as a child, you seek unconditional care in your relationships today—to be perfectly cared for by a perfect carer. Sometimes you thought you had found what you lacked in previous therapies, but it is as if you can only get what you need in "other people's spare rooms" and it didn't last. The task of this therapy is to find a safe way of relating that avoids the old patterns. By starting to grieve for the little girl who lost out, you can begin to build up a more stable sense of your self that is not dominated by the past. We seek to recognize and change these patterns and for you to learn from our relationship more rewarding ways of being with others and of caring for yourself.*
>
> *We have begun to make a map, and with the help of the psychotherapy file we have identified that some of the unsuccessful and painful ways you go about your life come from your childhood. We need to learn to recognize these, so that alternative ways become possible. Therapy is hard work and because of your past losses, ending it is likely to be difficult, but if we can face all the mixed feelings, I believe you will be able to take away enough, and stop hoping for everything.*
>
> *With warmest good wishes,*

Therapy after Reformulation

Susie said she felt heard. I produced a tidy version of the diagram we had worked on together. Susie said it helped her to understand, and she took it home, but I had the sense that this was far too easy. In retrospect, I saw that my complicated map was crammed with too much information. Again, I had been drawn into her world and was being anxiously overcontrolling. I was also mobilizing Susie's procedure of *striving, concealing her needs in relation to conditional acceptance.*

The ensuing sessions were difficult and messy. In session 9, I started to feel Susie's rage and I needed to say that I felt there was a difficulty between us. An oppressive silence fell in the room but with help Susie told me she didn't like the map. She was angry; it was all about other people, not about her. I realized that the SDR was a false sign, not the product of joint activity I thought it was. We started again. This time it was Susie who drew a picture from which we made our first truly shared sign. She began to express herself more honestly. We had some joint understanding, and joint work was becoming a reality. I was reminded that I needed to keep it simple and take small steps at a time, working within her ZPD. From Susie's drawing, the "difficult sessions," and my countertransference, I realized how Susie had initially hoped to be perfectly cared for by a perfect carer. But when, in her eyes, I had "fallen" from that state, she angrily saw me as the "not good enough mother who wasn't getting it right"—which meant she had to do it all herself. She then became the critical, attacking one and I felt the "stab" of shame as I experienced her attack (*hurt, rejected*). But this time I was able to "step out" of the enactment and, rather than being drawn in, could make use of the shared experience in the room. We were able to talk about it and use it to draw a simplified states map, using Susie's words, so that we both understood.

We drew a square to describe ideal care or perfectly happy families. Susie said she was envious of others who had this and would strive for attention in the hope that she might have a tiny bit from others for herself. (*She could also play this role herself, but she had no insight into that at this time.*) There were two squares: the rejecting, insulting, superior one above, and the rejected, insulted inferior below. We drew two more squares and wrote *ignoring* in one and *left out, alone as if I don't exist* in the other. At the center was a square to represent *controlling (to avoid feared chaos) to controlled.* Susie experienced these reciprocal roles as totally separate states at this time. When she was in one state, all the others disappeared from her mind.

In supervision I was encouraged to recognize the importance of helping Susie to take up a more distanced position outside the existing map, where she could use what in CAT we call the "observing eye" to reflect and understand. We added this to the diagram. Susie was encouraged to take stock of her days, in particular by writing down any difficult dialogue she "heard" in her head. Later she learned to recognize and counter the negative, critical "voice" with a more positive one. Slowly things began to change. We were using our SDR to trace her states and "thinking in pictures." Susie spoke of a duck ("Woody") attacked by others, which sought refuge under her kitchen table. She cared for him. In sessions, we used "Fred, " a "prickly hedgehog" soft toy from the consulting room shelf, as a metaphor for her; she placed "Fred" under the table in the therapy room as if he were scared to come out and show himself. We put a picture of Susie as a little girl on top of the table to evoke empathy for the part of her self that was the deprived, neglected child. She wrote a powerful and insightful "not to be sent letter" from her adult-self on behalf of her child-self to her family. Susie said she wanted to be able to sit and cry, and be accepted as normal, and we both felt the emotion in the room. She added a new RRP of *nurturing to nurtured* to her previously restricted repertoire. We used a chart with stick-on smiley faces and shiny stars as rewards for things well done, and Susie stuck some on her purse to remind her that she was worthy and deserved some good things.

Susie played out all the roles of her map. She came to understand the sequence whereby, always expecting to be attacked, she would perceive it when anything made her feel uncomfortable, or when her needs were not met. She would then react by angrily attacking and rejecting others but ended up crying, out of control herself, feeling shameful and desolate. In this way she was beginning to recognize and understand what cues and misinterpretations served as triggers to her overwhelming feelings and state shifts. We worked directly on the revision of these but controlling the pace, as it was still important to proceed with Susie at her pace.

We were coming up to the final phase of therapy, and with patience and hard work (hers), it was dawning on Susie that strict control was stifling; there was no absolute right or wrong; making room to maneuver meant trusting people enough to talk openly, and asking for help was not an admission of failure and did not necessarily leave her open to attack. Asking Mark for a cuddle when she felt down meant that Susie stood a good chance of getting one and having her needs met. The states on Susie's map were connected now, and she understood them in relation to each other. In light of this understanding, we reshaped her SDR, describing the sequences of procedure that needed to be broken, a process that involved experiencing and accepting feelings that in the past she had felt to be shameful, as well as using her new understandings.

Termination

Ending our weekly sessions was traumatic and painful. We had talked about it and added an "exit" reciprocal role to our SDR of *reassuring, supportive, encouraging to reassured, encouraged* and by this time Susie's relationships at work and that between herself and Mark had begun to be characterized by this pattern. However, predictably, the end of therapy mobilized all of

Susie's dysfunctional procedures. My good-bye letter charted the progress of therapy, marked her achievements, and talked about the feelings of ending. The final paragraph read:

> I have enjoyed your insightful mind, but most importantly, I think you need to hear that you are very lovable. You deserve to be loved not only by others but also by yourself. I will not forget you as you take all you have learned out to the world, and especially to Mark. But this letter is just for you and is a very warm good-bye.

Her good-bye letter was appreciative and warm. Susie was honest about her fears, sad for the loss of our time together, but optimistic for her future. She was trying to be OK but there was a sense of avoiding the real pain of separation that was hard for both of us to face. We arranged monthly follow-ups and, because of her social isolation, I arranged an introduction to a local befriending organization for her.

Follow-Up

Ending was worse than Susie had anticipated. She felt devastated and help-less. I felt anxious and worried that I should have extended our contract, but with the help of supervision I had held to it. Susie survived, and although it was painful, it was an important learning time for her. Over the follow-up appointments we worked through her feelings and the thoughts that went with them. She was not alone and she practiced breaking the sequence on her SDR; having internalized therapy, she needed to do it for herself now. The proof that she could came one morning, when Susie woke up feeling anxious. Overwhelmed by the pressure of what she thought were unman-ageable tasks for the day and fearing shameful failure, she felt hopeless and helpless. Sobbing, she contemplated staying in bed and giving up, but then she thought about her SDR. She had stuck it on the fridge door, and now she deliberately took herself off to the kitchen. Slumped on the floor, she stared at her map, acknowledged her feelings, and traced the cascade of linking states. She understood and knew she did not want to continue on that route. She was able to revise her procedure and instead of canceling her plans she encouraged herself, "At least try, Susie—little steps, little bites. " By changing her dialogue with herself Susie managed to accomplish all the things that had felt so impossible at the beginning of the day. It was a real achievement for her. Our shared signing of the SDR had become the carrier of a gentler more encouraging voice, providing a bridge to feeling under-stood and reminding Susie of the work of therapy.

Perhaps the last word should go to Susie. When asked what she thought worked for her in this therapy, she said she thought previous therapies had contributed and that she had felt ready to move on, but the first glimmer of conscious change had come when she was allowed to express her thoughts and feelings about the first map. She felt listened to, her anger had been accepted, and, as a result, we had worked together to draw up a new diagram. Her confidence was growing as she continued to develop and to mature. We arranged just four more follow-ups, planned as seasonal touchstones—summer, winter, autumn, and spring.

SUMMARY AND CONCLUSIONS

Over the past 25 years CAT has passed through stages of integration, differentiation, incorporation of new ideas, and consolidation. It now presents the essentials of a comprehensive model of the aspects of human psychology of relevance to psychotherapy and, potentially at least, to the human interactions involved in psychiatry, medicine, and teaching. CAT practice is firmly based on a comprehensive theory drawn from a number of sources both within the psychotherapy Tower of Babel and from wider fields. The theory is *biological* in that the general potential and specific variability of humans are genetically determined. It is *social* in that personality is shaped by the historical and cultural context into which the individual is born. It is *dialogical* in that early relationships with others within the wider context are the basis of subsequent relationships with others, and of the forms of thought, care, and control of the self. It is *semiotic* in that the transmission and internalization of these influences involve the use of mediating signs that confer meaning on experience and become the basis of conscious thought. It does not isolate the cognitive, affective, and behavioral processes from each other, or from the human meanings and values they incorporate. CAT differs from most cognitive models in its emphasis on development as an essential basis for describing normal psychological structure and its pathological deviations, and on its insistence that individual processes can only be understood in relation to the social relationships and socially derived mediating tools that formed and maintain them. Even though incomplete understanding may guide some useful interventions, therapists who aim to help people with difficulties in living need a model of this complexity.

Although CAT is a relatively new and fast-growing therapy that has evolved from research into process and outcome, it has not amassed an extensive evidence base. It is becoming more widely recognized that "gold standard" RCT designs have paid inadequate attention to the particular features of psychotherapy, including the fact that each therapeutic process and conversation is the creation of the two participants, and that patients live in, and are affected by, a web of relationships with others who influence treatment response. The dominance of the RCT in psychotherapy research has meant that purchasers, who are obliged to consider the evidence base of a treatment, are persuaded more by the claim to have done an RCT than by its quality and interpretation; all is not gold that glitters. Other forms of evidence and judgment carry little weight, with the result that therapies are under pressure to focus on what is measurable, while humanly important aims and values may be disregarded. Jensen, Weersing, Hoagwood, and Goldman (2005) gave detailed consideration of 56 studies, concluding that "what is deemed 'evidence-based' or 'empirically supported' may be clearing a very low threshold indeed." Richards (2007), a past chairman of the British Association of Behavioral and Cognitive Psychotherapy, noted that "most CBT [cognitive-behavioral therapy] trials are small and poorly executed; quality thresholds for RCTs in NICE [National Institute for Clinical Excellence] guidelines are notoriously low, allowing meta-analyses of small poor quality studies to direct policy." CAT, often ignored because it has not accumulated enough evidence, does now have support from the well-designed, large-scale RCT of Chanen et al. (2008), and other such studies are under way. Research into process and specific aspects of practice, summarized earlier, has supported and modified the treatment model. The value of single-case experimental design studies, involving the repeated collection of detailed quantitative evidence from therapist and patient, has much to offer of clinical relevance, as demonstrated by Kellett (2005, 2007), and this approach is currently being used in a multisite study of CAT in BPD.

CAT will continue to develop as a theory-based treatment, in contrast to the atheoretical approach of many cognitive therapies. Comparisons between approaches need to take into account their different scope and intentions, and the values implicit in them. Simplified models of human behavior and experience may be acceptable to many patients, but they are often inadequate. Because people who experience complex failures and pains in their lives may find that the assumptions guiding CBT practice are irrelevant to their experience and diminish their human stature, these limits need not inhibit the work of gifted therapists. On the other hand, the broad perspective of CAT may be of no interest to patients with circumscribed problems, and the full approach may be overelaborate for some patients and practitioners. Specific and complex CBT techniques may be best delivered within a CAT framework that attends to the crucial role of the therapy relationship, and to the links between symptoms and more general intra- and interpsychological processes.

Over the next few years, further research may include attempts to devise useful and ethical RCTs, but other ways of assessing the effectiveness of the different components of treatment, such as multiple single-case experimental design studies, are likely to contribute more to the development of the model. Applying CAT in different treatment settings will further test and refine it. Outside formal psychotherapy, the use of the model to support teams working with BPD and other "hard to help" patients will be further extended and evaluated; this is an area of great potential importance within the public sector, and it can serve to balance the narrow psychopharmacological focus of much psychiatry. The increasing volume of academic research into early development, which is extending knowledge about the infant in relation to others, will undoubtedly contribute to refinements in the theory. The establishment of a firmer academic base for CAT is, I believe, overdue, but it is likely to take some time to establish in the face of ideological and political resistance. In the clinical field, involvement in services offering early intervention or preventive programs in families would be appropriate, and the impact of CAT on stressed pregnant women to prevent known effects on infants is currently being researched.

The ultimate aim of an integrative model should be that it absorb other influences into a generally shared understanding, such as that guiding, for example, most medical practice. But the time for that seems quite distant given that a common language for the psychotherapies is still far from achievement, and given that most writers in the field seldom refer to other models. Moreover, different schools of psychotherapy exist only in part to defend particular theories and practices; they also express different values, serve as agents in the social formation of psychotherapists, are sources of continuing education, and defend their interests in the often unsupportive world. They therefore attract loyalty for reasons that have little to do with evidence. In these respects, CAT, with its emphasis on social factors in human formation and its commitment to therapy as part of the public provision of care, attracts those who are out of tune with the dominant consumerist culture and the more technical approaches to therapy. CAT has evolved some useful techniques, but the main impact of these may well derive from the fact that they require therapists to engage at a deep human level with their patients and support the therapeutic aims of that engagement.

REFERENCES

Bartlett, F. C. (1954). *Remembering: A study in experimental and social psychology.* Cambridge, UK: Cambridge University Press.

Bateman, A. W., & Fonagy, P. (1999). The effectiveness of partial hospitalisation in the treatment of borderline personality disorder: A randomized controlled trial. *American Journal of Psychiatry, 156*, 1563–1569.

Bateman, A. W., & Fonagy, P. (2004). *Psychotherapy for borderline personality disorder: Mentalisation-based treatment.* Oxford, UK: Oxford University Press.

Bateman, A. W., Ryle, A., Fonagy, P., & Kerr, I. B. (2007). Mentalization based therapy and cognitive analytic therapy compared. *International Review of Psychiatry, 19*(1), 51–62.

Beard, H., Marlowe, M., & Ryle, A. (1990). The management and treatment of personality disordered patients: The use of sequential diagrammatic reformulation. *British Journal of Psychiatry, 156,* 541–545.

Beck, A. T. (1967). *Cognitive therapy and the emotional disorders.* New York: International Universities Press.

Bell, L. (1999). The spectrum of psychological problems in people with eating disorders, an analysis of 30 eating disordered patients treated with cognitive analytic therapy. *Clinical Psychology and Psychotherapy, 6,* 38–39.

Bennett, D., & Parry, G. (1998). The accuracy of reformulation in cognitive analytic therapy: A validation study. *Psychotherapy Research, 8,* 405–422.

Bennett, D., & Parry, P. (2004). A measure of psychotherapeutic competence derived from cognitive analytic therapy. *Psychotherapy Research, 14*(2), 176–192.

Bennett, D., Parry, G., & Ryle, A. (2006). Resolving threats to the therapeutic alliance in cognitive analytic therapy of borderline personality disorder: A task analysis. *Psychology and Psychotherapy: Theory, Research and Practice, 79,* 395–418.

Bennett, D., Pollock, P., & Ryle, A. (2005). The States Description Procedure: The use of guided self-reflection in the case formulation of patients with borderline personality disorder. *Clinical Psychology and Psychotherapy, 12,* 50–56.

Bennett, D., & Ryle, A. (2005). The characteristic features of common borderline states: A pilot study using the States Description Procedure. *Clinical Psychology and Psychotherapy, 12,* 58–66.

Brittain, V. (1933). *Testament of youth.* London: Penguin Twentieth Century Classics.

Brockman, B., Poynton, A., Ryle, A., & Watson, J. P. (1987). Effectiveness of time-limited therapy carried out by trainees: comparison of two methods. *British Journal of Psychiatry, 151,* 602–610.

Bruner, J. (1986). *Actual minds, possible worlds.* Cambridge, MA: Harvard University Press.

Chanen, A. W., Jackson, H. J., McCutcheon, L. K., Jovev, M., Dudgeon, P., et al. (2008). Early intervention for adolescents with borderline personality disorder using cognitive analytic therapy: Randomised controlled trial. *British Journal of Psychiatry, 193,* 477–484.

Clarke, S., & Pearson, C. (2000). Personal constructs of male survivors of childhood sexual abuse receiving cognitive analytic therapy. *British Journal of Medical Psychology, 73,* 169–177.

Compton Dickinson, S. (2006). Beyond body, beyond words: Cognitive analytic music therapy in forensic psychiatry—New approaches in the treatment of personality disordered offenders. *Music Therapy Today, 11*(4), 839–875.

Donald, M. (1991). *Origins of the modern mind : Three Stages in the Evolution of Culture and Cognition.* Cambridge, MA: Harvard University Press.

Donald, M. (2001). *A mind so rare: The evolution of human consciousness.* New York: Norton

Dunn, M., & Parry, G. (1997). A formulated care plan approach to caring for borderline personality disorder in a community mental health setting. *Clinical Psychology Forum, 104,* 19–22.

Fosbury, J. A., Bosley, C. M., Ryle, A., Sonksen, P. H., & Judd, J. L. (1997). A trial of cognitive analytic therapy in poorly controlled type 1 patients. *Diabetes Care,* *20,* 959–964.

Frank, I. D. (1961). *Persuasion and healing.* Baltimore: Johns Hopkins University Press.

Golynkina, K., & Ryle, A. (1999). The identification and characteristics of the partially dissociated states of patients with borderline personality disorder. *British Journal of Medical Psychology, 72,* 429–445.

Hepple, J., & Sutton, L. (Eds.). (2004). *Cognitive analytic therapy and later life.* Hove, UK: Brunner/Routledge.

Hermans, H. J. M., & Dimaggio, G. (2004). *The dialogical self.* Hove, UK: Brunner and Routledge.

Horowitz, M. J. (1979). *States of mind: Analysis of change in psychotherapy.* New York: Plenum Press.

Howell, E. F. (2005). *The dissociative mind.* London: Analytic Press.

Hughes, R. (2007). An enquiry into an integration of cognitive analytic therapy with art therapy. *International Journal of Art Therapy, 12*(1), 28–38.

Jellema, A. (2000). Insecure attachment states: Their relationship to borderline and narcissistic personality disorders and treatment process in cognitive analytic therapy. *Clinical Psychology and Psychotherapy, 7,* 138–154.

Jellema, A. (2002). Dismissing and preoccupied insecure attachment and procedures in CAT: Some implications for CAT practice. *Clinical Psychology and Psychotherapy, 9,* 225–241.

Jensen, P. S., Weersing, R., Hoagwood, K. E., & Goldman, E. (2005). What is the evidence for evidence-based treatments?: A hard look at our soft underbelly. *Mental Health Services Research, 7*(1), 53–74.

Kellett, S. (2005). The treatment of dissociative identity disorder with cognitive analytic therapy; experimental evidence of sudden gains. *Trauma and Dissociation, 6,* 55–81.

Kellett, S. (2007). A time series evaluation of the treatment of histrionic personality disorder with cognitive analytic therapy. *Psychology and Psychotherapy: Theory, Research and Practice, 80,* 389–405.

Kelly, G. A. (1955). *The psychology of personal constructs.* New York: Norton.

Kerr, I. B. (2001a). Brief cognitive analytic therapy for post-acute manic psychosis on a psychiatric intensive care unit. *Clinical Psychology and Psychotherapy, 8,* 117–129.

Kerr, I. B. (2001b). Cognitive analytic therapy for borderline personality disorder in the context of a community mental health team: Individual and organisational psychodynamic implications. *British Journal of Psychotherapy, 15,* 425–438.

Kerr, I. B. (2002). Vygotsky, activity theory and the therapeutic community: A further paradigm? *Therapeutic Communities, 21*(3), 151–163.

Kerr, I. B., Dent-Brown, K., & Parry, G. D. (2007). Psychotherapy and mental health teams. *International Review of Psychiatry, 19,* 63–80.

Leighton, T. (1997). Borderline personality and substance abuse problems. In A. Ryle (Ed.), *Cognitive analytic therapy and borderline personality disorder* (pp. 128–145). Chichester, UK: Wiley.

Leiman, M. (1992). The concept of sign in the work of Vygotsky, Winnicott and

Bakhtin: Further integration of object relations theory and activity theory. *British Journal of Medical Psychology*, 65, 209–221.

Leiman, M. (1997). Procedures as dialogical sequences: A revised version of the fundamental concept in cognitive analytic therapy. *British Journal of Medical Psychology*, 70, 193–207.

Luborsky, L. (1990). Theory and technique in dynamic psychotherapy: Curative factors and training therapists to maximise them. *Psychotherapy and Psychosomatics*, 53, 50–57.

Luborsky, L., & Crits-Christoph, P. (1990). A relationship pattern measure: The CCRT. *Psychiatry*, 52, 250–259.

Miller, G. A., Galanter, E., & Pribram, F. H. (1960). *Plans and the structure of behaviour*. New York: Holt.

Neisser, U. (1967). *Cognitive psychology*. New York: Appleton.

Pollock, P. H. (1996). Clinical issues in the cognitive analytic therapy of sexually abused women who commit violent offences against their partners. *British Journal of Medical Psychology*, 69, 117–127.

Pollock, P. H. (Ed.). (2001). *Cognitive analytic therapy for adult survivors of childhood abuse*. Chichester, UK: Wiley.

Pollock, P., Broadbent, M., & Clarke, S. (Ed.). (2000). The Personality Structure Questionnaire (PSQ): A measure of the multiple self states model of identity disturbance in cognitive analytic therapy. *Clinical Psychology and Psychotherapy*, 8, 59–72.

Pollock, P. H., Stowell-Smith, M., & Gopfert, M. (Eds.). (2006). *Cognitive analytic therapy for offenders*. London: Routledge.

Pollock, P. H., & Kear-Colwell, J. J. (1994). Women who stab: A personal construct analysis of sexual victimisation and offending behaviour. *British Journal of Medical Psychology*, 67, 13–22.

Richards, D. (2007). "Arrogant, inflexible, remote and imperious": Is this what's wrong with CBT? *BABCP Magazine*, 35, 12–13.

Ryle, A. (1959). *A general practice study of neurosis*. Dissertation submitted for the degree of Doctor of Medicine (Oxford).

Ryle, A. (1967). *Neurosis in the ordinary family*. London: Tavistock.

Ryle, A. (1975). *Frames and cages*. London: Chatto & Windus/Sussex University Press.

Ryle, A. (1979). The focus in brief interpretative psychotherapy: Dilemmas, traps and snags as target problems. *British Journal of Psychiatry*, 135, 46–64.

Ryle, A. (1980). Some measures of goal attainment in focused integrated active psychotherapy: A study of fifteen cases. *British Journal of Psychiatry*, 137, 475–486.

Ryle, A. (1982). *Psychotherapy: A cognitive integration of theory and practice*. London: Academic Press.

Ryle, A. (1985). Cognitive theory, object relations and the self. *British Journal of Medical Psychology*, 58, 1–7.

Ryle, A. (1990). *Cognitive analytic therapy: Active participation in change*. Chichester, UK: Wiley.

Ryle, A. (1991). Object relations theory and activity theory: A proposed link by way of the procedural sequence model. *British Journal of Medical Psychology*, 64, 307–316.

Ryle, A. (1992). Critique of a Kleinian case presentation. *British Journal of Medical Psychology, 65,* 309–317.

Ryle, A. (1993) Addiction to the death instinct?: A critical review of Joseph's paper "Addiction to near death." *British Journal of Psychotherapy, 10,* 88–92.

Ryle, A. (1995). Defensive organisations or collusive interpretations?: A further critique of Kleinian theory and practice. *British Journal of Psychotherapy, 12*(1), 60–68.

Ryle, A. (1996). Ogden's autistic-contiguous position and the role of interpretation in psychoanalytic theory building. *British Journal of Medical Psychology, 69*(2), 129–138.

Ryle, A. (1997). *Cognitive analytic therapy and borderline personality disorder: The model and the method.* Chichester, UK: Wiley.

Ryle, A. (2001). Constructivism and cognitive analytic therapy. *Constructivism in the Human Sciences, 6*(1–2), 51–58.

Ryle, A. (2003). Something more than "Something more than interpretation" is needed: A comment on the paper by the Process of Change Study Group. *International Journal of Psychoanalysis, 84,* 109–111.

Ryle, A. (2005). The relevance of evolutionary psychology for psychotherapy. *British Journal of Psychotherapy, 21*(3), 375–388.

Ryle, A. (2007). Investigating the phenomenology of borderline personality disorder with the States Description Procedure: Clinical implications. *Clinical Psychology and Psychotherapy, 14*(5), 329–341.

Ryle, A., & Beard, H. (1993). The integrative effect of reformulation: Cognitive analytic therapy with a patient with borderline personality disorder. *British Journal of Medical Psychology, 66,* 249–258.

Ryle, A., Boa, C., & Fosbury, J. (1993). Identifying the causes of poor self-management in insulin-dependent diabetics: The use of cognitive analytic therapy techniques. In M. Hodes & S. Moorey (Eds.), *Psychological treatment of disease and illness.* London: Gaskell.

Ryle, A., & Fawkes, L. (2007). Multiplicity of selves and others: Cognitive analytic therapy. *Journal of Clinical Psychology, 63*(2), 165–174.

Ryle, A., & Golynkina, K. (2000). Effectiveness of time-limited cognitive analytic therapy of borderline personality disorder: Factors associated with outcome. *British Journal of Medical Psychology, 73,* 197–210.

Ryle, A., & Kerr, I. B. (2002). *Introducing cognitive analytic therapy: Principles and practice.* Chichester, UK: Wiley.

Ryle, A., & Lunghi, M. (1970). The dyad grid: A modification of repertory grid technique. *British Journal of Psychiatry, 117,* 223–227.

Schacht, T. E., & Henry, W. P. (1994). Modelling recurrent relationship patterns with structural analysis of social behavior: The SASB-CMP. *Psychotherapy Research, 4,* 208–221.

Stern, D. N. (1985). *The interpersonal world of the infant: A view from psychoanalysis and developmental psychology.* New York: Basic Books.

Stern, D. N., Sander, L. S., Nahum, J. P., Harrison, A. M., Lyons-Ruth, K., Bruschweiler-Stern, N., et al. (1998). Non-interpretive mechanisms in psychoanalytic psychotherapy: The "something more" than interpretation. *International Journal of Psychoanalysis, 79,* 903–921.

Thompson, A. R., Donnison, J., Warnock-Parkes, E., Turner, J., & Kerr, I. B. (in press). Staff experience of a "skills level" training course in cognitive analytic therapy. *International Journal of Mental Health Nursing.*

Tomasello, M. (1999). *The cultural origins of human cognition.* Cambridge, MA: Harvard University Press.

Trevarthen, C., & Aitken, K. J. (2000). Intersubjective foundations in human psychological development [Annual Research Review]. *Journal of Child Psychology and Psychiatry and Allied Disciplines, 42*(1), 3–48.

Walsh, S., Hagan, T., & Gamsu, D. (2000). Rescuer and rescued: Applying a cognitive analytic perspective to explore the "mis-management" of asthma. *British Journal of Medical Psychology, 73,* 151–168.

Wildgoose, A., Clarke, S., & Waller, G. (2001). Treating personality fragmentation and dissociation in borderline personality disorder: A pilot study of the impact of cognitive analytic therapy. *British Journal of Medical Psychology, 74,* 47–55.

Wolpe, J. (1958). *Psychotherapy by reciprocal inhibition.* Stanford, CA: University of Stanford Press.

CHAPTER 9

Positive Psychology and Therapy

Nansook Park
Christopher Peterson
Steven M. Brunwasser

INTRODUCTION AND HISTORICAL BACKGROUND

Overview

Positive psychology is the scientific study of what goes right in life, from birth to death (Seligman & Csikszentmihalyi, 2000). It is the study of optimal experience, of people being their best and doing their best. Positive psychology is a newly christened approach within psychology that takes seriously as a subject matter those things that make life most worth living. Everyone's life has peaks and valleys, and positive psychology does not deny the low points. Its signature premise is more nuanced: What is good about life is as genuine as what is bad and therefore deserves equal attention from psychologists (Peterson & Park, 2003). Positive psychology assumes that life entails more than avoiding or undoing problems, and that explanations of the good life must do more than reverse accounts of problems.

History

Positive psychology has a very long past but a very short history (Peterson, 2006a). The field was named in 1998 as one of the initiatives of Martin Seligman (2002) in his role as president of the American Psychological Association. A trigger for positive psychology was Seligman's realization that psychology since World War II has focused much of its efforts on human problems and how to remedy them.

The yield of this focus on pathology has been considerable, but there has been a cost. Much of scientific psychology has neglected the study of what can go right with people and often has little to say about the psychological good life. More subtly, the underlying assumptions of psychology have shifted to embrace a disease model of human nature. People are seen as flawed and fragile, casualties of cruel environments or bad genetics. This worldview has even crept into the common culture, where many people have become self-identified victims.

PHILOSOPHICAL AND THEORETICAL UNDERPINNINGS

Positive psychology challenges the assumptions of the disease model. It calls for as much focus on strength as on weakness, as much interest in building the best things in life as in repairing the worst, and as much attention to fulfilling the lives of healthy people as to healing the wounds of the distressed. Psychologists interested in promoting human potential need to start with different assumptions and to pose different questions to their peers who assume only a disease model (Park & Peterson, 2006b). The most basic assumption of positive psychology is that human goodness and excellence are as authentic as disease, disorder, and distress. Positive psychologists argue that these topics are not secondary, derivative, or otherwise suspect.

The very long past of positive psychology stretches at least to the Athenian philosophers in the West and to Confucius and Lao-Tsu in the East. In the writings of these great thinkers can be found the same questions posed by contemporary positive psychologists. What is the good life? Is virtue its own reward? What does it mean to be happy? Is it possible to pursue happiness directly, or is fulfillment a by-product of other pursuits? What roles are played by other people and by society as a whole?

Within psychology, the premises of positive psychology were laid out long before 1998. Setting the immediate stage for positive psychology as it currently exists were humanistic psychology, as popularized by Carl Rogers (1951) and Abraham Maslow (who actually used the phrase "positive psychology" to describe his own approach; 1954); the discussion by Marie Jahoda (1958) of positive mental health; utopian visions of education, such as those of Alexander Sutherland Neill (1960); primary prevention programs based on notions of wellness, as pioneered by George Albee (1982) and Emory Cowen (1994); work by Albert Bandura (1989) and others on human agency and efficacy; studies of giftedness (Winner, 2000); conceptions of multiple intelligences (Gardner, 1983); and studies of the quality of life among medical and psychiatric patients that went beyond an exclusive focus on their symptoms and diseases (e.g., Levitt, Hogan, & Bucosky, 1990).

Today's positive psychologists do not claim to have invented notions of happiness and well-being, to have proposed their first theoretical accounts, or even to have ushered in their scientific study. Rather, the contribution of contemporary positive psychology has been twofold: (1) providing an umbrella term for what had been isolated lines of theory and research, and (2) making the self-conscious argument that what makes life worth living deserves its own field of inquiry within psychology, at least until all of psychology embraces the study of what is good along with the study of what is bad (Peterson & Park, 2003).

Topics of Concern

The framework of positive psychology provides a comprehensive scheme for describing and understanding the good life. The field can be divided into four related topics:

- Positive subjective experiences (happiness, pleasure, gratification, fulfillment, flow)
- Positive individual traits (strengths of character, talents, interests, values)
- Positive interpersonal relationships (with friends, romantic partners, family members, work colleagues)
- Positive groups and institutions (families, schools, workplaces, communities, societies)

A theory is implied here: Positive groups and institutions enable the development of positive relationships, which enable the display of positive traits, which in turn enable positive subjective experiences (Park & Peterson, 2003).

Use of the word *enable* avoids strict causal language. It is possible for people to be happy or content even in the absence of good character, and good character can operate against the interpersonal and institutional grain. But people are at their best when institutions, relationships, traits, and experiences are in alignment. Doing well in life represents a coming together of all four domains.

Questions and Criticisms

As a new field, positive psychology raises questions from the general public and the scientific community (Seligman & Pawelski, 2003). Everyday people seem to find positive psychology exciting and the sort of thing psychology should be doing. Despite the pervasiveness of a victim mentality, everyday people seem to know that the elimination or reduction of problems is not all that is involved in improving the human condition. In contrast, the scientific community is more skeptical (Cowen & Kilmer, 2002; Fineman, 2006; Hyten, 2004; Lazarus, 2003; Sugarman, 2007; Taylor, 2001). Contributing to skepticism are widespread assumptions within the social sciences about human nature as brittle and broken, notions that are more explicit among social scientists than in the general public.

Positive psychology is also criticized in some quarters for a relentless emphasis on being positive—happy and cheerful (Held, 2002, 2004; Judge & Ilies, 2004; Schumaker, 2007). We do not believe that this is a fair criticism of the field, because positive psychologists merely propose that what is positive about life is worth studying, in addition to what is negative. Happiness is a topic of interest to positive psychology, but so too are virtues such as gratitude and forgiveness, talent, perseverance, and resilience (Peterson, 2006a).

Positive psychologists do not deny the problems that people experience, and they do not ignore the negative—stress and challenge—in their attempts to understand what it means to live well (Peterson & Park, 2003). Positive psychology intends to complement business-as-usual psychology, not replace it, by expanding the topics of legitimate study to yield a full and balanced depiction of the human condition.

Indeed, what is most troubling in life can set the stage for what is most fulfilling. Consider that complex emotional experiences often blend the positive and negative; that optimism is most apparent when people confront setbacks and failures; that crisis reveals strengths of character; that ongoing challenge is a prerequisite to experiencing flow in the moment and to achieving something important in a lifetime; and so on (Peterson, 2006a). Along these lines, many positive psychologists believe that identifying and using what one does well can be an effective way to address and resolve psychological problems (Saleebey, 1992).

In fairness to the critics, positive psychology has become so popular that at least some people appropriate the label and present "positive psychology" as a dumbed-down and recycled version of the power of positive thinking. All we can do here is assert that Pollyanna is not the poster child for positive psychology, that the fortunate in life—those who are happy—deserve no special congratulations, and that the unfortunate—those who are unhappy—deserve no special blame (Ryan, 1978).

Theory of Psychopathology and Therapy

As a perspective on topics that deserve scientific study, positive psychology has no single theory. Like much of contemporary psychology, it instead relies on midrange theories that draw on a variety of larger perspectives, from evolutionary to behavioral to cognitive to sociocultural models, to make sense of specific phenomena. Different topics are explained with different theories. The eventual integration of psychology may be a worthy goal (Sternberg, 2005), but it has not yet been achieved, and neither has the goal of psychotherapy integration (Norcross & Goldfried, 2005).

At this early point in the development of positive psychology, the lack of a consensual or integrated theory is hardly a problem. The psychological good life is not yet understood, and positive psychologists are still grappling with right vocabulary to describe it (Peterson & Seligman, 2004). As we see it, the championing of a single theory at the present time would be premature, even counterproductive.

Seligman (2002) argued that positive psychology is a descriptive endeavor, not a prescriptive one. If this means that positive psychology should be an empirical science, informed by replicable facts, then this claim is a reasonable and defining feature of the entire field. If this means that positive psychology is assumption-free or value-neutral, the claim become much more difficult to defend (Martin, 2007). After all, positive psychologists make the value judgment that the "good" life is indeed good—that is, desirable, morally and otherwise—and the metatheoretical assumption that the good life can be studied with the conventional methods of psychology (Peterson, 2006a). In any event, positive psychology seems no more prescriptive than clinical psychology or psychiatry. It may even be less so given the theoretical diversity of positive psychology as it currently exists.

When Seligman (2002) first described positive psychology, he argued that its goal was not to move people from –5 to zero—the presumed goal of business-as-usual psychology—but rather from +2 to +5. This emphasis on promotion as opposed to remediation is useful in highlighting what is novel about positive psychology but does not do justice to this new field and what it might help people to achieve.

Interventions based on positive psychology can do more than help people who are doing well in life do even better. These interventions may also help people with problems lead fulfilling lives, moving them from –5 to +2 or beyond. Whatever the presenting complaints, people also bring into therapy assets and strengths that can be used to resolve their problems. A crucial task of any treatment is therefore to identify a client's resources and encourage their use, not just to solve problems. Such a balanced approach should build rapport, bolster client confidence. It will certainly make sense to clients. When asked how they can tell that treatment has been effective, individuals with DSM diagnoses of depressive disorder describe their own view of "remission" in positive psychology language, spontaneously mentioning that it would be optimistic and that they would function well (Zimmerman et al., 2006).

Positive Psychology's Vision of Psychological Health

As noted, positive psychology can be criticized for being value-infused. The offsetting virtue is that the values inherent in positive psychology are clearly stated. The real question is whether these values are idiosyncratic or culture-bound. At a certain level of abstraction, the vision of psychological well-being that emerges from positive psychology seems ubiquitous, if not universal.

If one can extrapolate from the sorts of topics that have been studied, positive psychology assumes that people are doing well when they experience more positive feelings than negative feelings, are satisfied with their lives as they have been lived, have identified what they do well and use these talents and strengths on an ongoing basis; are highly engaged in what they do, are contributing members of a social community, and have a sense of meaning and purpose in their lives. Health and safety, of course, provide an important context for psychological well-being. It is difficult to imagine a cultural group in which these components of the good life are not valued. Respect for human diversity need not entail extreme cultural relativism.

The positive psychology vision of optimal functioning provides a vision of mental health that can be used to make sense of the psychological problems that people might have. Problems (from a positive psychology perspective) represent shortcomings with respect to one or more of the components of the psychological good life. For example, people may experience more negative affect than positive affect; they may be dissatisfied with their lives and socially estranged; they may be bored, alienated, or nihilistic; and so on.

These ways of thinking about problems, of course, differ from the DSM vision of psychopathology in terms of a set of symptom-defined disorders that are either present or absent. The positive psychology vision regards so-called "symptoms" as the problem and further expects them to exist in degrees. These visions need not compete. Traditional DSM diagnostic categories are not independent of the components of well-being implied by a positive psychology perspective. For example, depression entails high negative affect and low positive affect, whereas anxiety is simply high negative affect (Dyck, Jolly, & Kramer, 1994). Indeed, a positive psychology perspective may explain *why* given DSM symptoms and diagnoses constitute problems in living by identifying the ways in which optimal personal and social functioning can be compromised by the disorders and their symptoms (Peterson, 2006b).

Besides providing a vantage point on what is considered a psychological disorder, positive psychology also speaks to other important aspects of therapy (Duckworth, Steen, & Seligman, 2005; Maddux, Snyder, & Lopez, 2004; Peterson & Park, in press-a, in press-b; Seligman & Peterson, 2003).

Even if therapeutic concern is with traditional diagnostic categories, the goals of therapy can be fleshed out with a positive psychology perspective by keeping in mind the vision of psychological health already discussed and, more generally, by taking DSM Axis V (global assessment of functioning) as seriously as Axis I and Axis II diagnoses. We emphasize again that positive psychology is intended not to replace business-as-usual psychology but to expand and complement it. The same point applies to therapy that incorporates positive psychology goals.

Positive Psychology Assessment

Assessment has long been a staple of psychology, and much of it has been tilted—understandably—toward identifying weaknesses, deficiencies, and problems. The positive psychology perspective is that business-as-usual assessment should be expanded (not replaced) by attention to areas of strength and competence. Low life satisfaction can occur in the absence of psychopathology, and it is nonetheless related to psychological and social problems (Greenspoon & Saklofske, 2001). Conversely, high life satisfaction is linked to good functioning even in the presence of symptoms (Furr & Funder, 1998; Park, 2004).

Positive psychologists have already developed an impressive set of measurement instruments that allow someone doing assessment to break through the zero point of deficiency measures (Peterson, 2000). For example, the healthiest score that one can have on a typical measure of depression is zero, but this lumps together people who are blasé with those who are filled with zest and joy. The distinction seems well worth making, and the self-report surveys and interviews developed by positive psychologists allow it.

Space does not permit a detailed presentation of positive psychology measures, but Table 9.1 provides some examples. For example, the Values in Action Inventory of Strengths (VIA-IS) is our own comprehensive survey that measures an individual's character strengths, positive traits (e.g., curiosity), social intelligence, hope, kindness, zest, and teamwork (Park & Peterson, 2006b). Positive psychology interventions are often described as strengths-based, which means that the results of this survey can provide useful information for the therapist and the client to plan and assess the effectiveness of interventions.

Fuller descriptions of the VIA-IS and other positive psychology measures can be found in Lopez and Snyder (2003), Peterson and Seligman (2004), and Peterson (2006a). Many of the popular positive self-report surveys are available online at no cost (*www.authentichappiness.org*). Upon completion of a survey, individual feedback is provided, which means that clients can be directed to this website and asked to keep a record of their scores.

TABLE 9.1. Examples of Positive Psychology Measures

Positive affect
  Positive and Negative Affect Schedule (PANAS)
  Profile of Mood States (POMS)

Happiness
  Authentic Happiness Inventory (AHI)
  Orientations to Happiness Scale (measures endorsement of pleasure, engagement, meaning)

Life satisfaction
  Satisfaction with Life Scale (SWLS)
  Marital satisfaction
  Work satisfaction
  Leisure satisfaction

Positive traits
  Values in Action Inventory of Strengths (VIA-IS) (measures positive traits)
  Ryff and Singer's Psychological Well-Being Scales
  Search Institute's Developmental Assets (for youth)

Values
  Values inventories of Rokeach, Schwartz, Scott, and others

Interests
  Strong–Campbell Vocational Interest Blank (SVIB)

Abilities
  Multiple intelligences

Social support and attachment
  Multidimensional Scale of Perceived Social Support
  Adult Attachment Style Questionnaire

Most of the existing positive psychology measures were developed for research purposes, and they are most valid when aggregated to yield conclusions about groups of people. They can also be used ipsatively, to describe the psychological characteristics of an individual and how they stay the same or change over time, but the cautious use of these descriptions is as a point of discussion and departure in treatment. They should not be used alone. None provides a strong diagnostic test, and none should be treated as if it does. Such prudence is appropriate for all psychological assessment, but it is worth emphasizing in the special case of positive psychology measures.

EMPIRICAL EVIDENCE

Although still a young field, positive psychology already has a canon of established findings that illustrate the importance of explicit attention to the positive. Here is a sampling of some of the interesting results to date.

Happiness and Positive Emotions

In contrast to stereotypes that happy people are naive, stupid, or in denial, empirical studies show that happiness and positive emotions are beneficial. Our real worry should be about people who are unhappy.

- *Happiness is causal, not epiphenomenal.* People who are successful in life's venues, of course, are happy, but the less obvious finding from experimental and longitudinal research is that happiness actually leads to success in academic, vocational, and interpersonal realms (Lyubomirsky, King, & Diener, 2005).

- *Happiness leads to physical well-being.* People who are happy recover more quickly from infectious disease (Cohen, Doyle, Turner, Alper, & Skoner, 2003) and live longer than their peers (Danner, Snowdon, & Friesen, 2001).

- *Positive emotions broaden and build people's psychological and behavioral repertoires.* Negative emotions—fear, anxiety, anger—alert people to danger. When one experiences a negative emotion, response options narrow, and the person acts with haste to avoid, escape, or undo whatever danger is signaled. In contrast, positive emotions signal safety, and the inherent response to them is not to narrow options but to broaden and build upon them (Fredrickson, 2001). The evolutionary payoff of positive emotions is therefore not in the here and now but in the future. Perhaps experiencing positive emotions is advantageous because they lead people to engage in activities that add to their behavioral and cognitive repertoires, building so-called "psychological capital."

- *Savoring produces benefits.* We try to cope with bad events, minimizing their effects. How do we respond to good events? Too often, out of a misplaced sense of modesty, we may dismiss them. In contrast, Bryant and Veroff (2006) examined the effects of savoring good events and found that people who do so are more satisfied. They also identified simple strategies for savoring, such as sharing good events with others, either in the moment or after the fact; building memories of the good events (e.g., photographs, diaries, souvenirs); congratulating the self when good things happen; sharpening perceptions during the experience of good events; and becoming fully absorbed in pleasure and not thinking about other matters.

Positive Thinking

Again, stereotypes hold that positive thinking is wishful, and if we wish to criticize people who are too optimistic and hopeful, we call them Pollyannas. But again, research shows numerous benefits of positive thinking.

- *People in trying circumstances spontaneously think of others whose circumstances are worse than their own,* thereby avoiding depression (Taylor, 1985). This downward social comparison may help explain why most people are happy most of the time (Diener & Diener, 1996).

- *A rosy view of matters is associated with physical, psychological, and social well-being* (Peterson, 2000; Peterson & Bossio, 1991; Taylor & Brown, 1988). Data showing that positive illusions are beneficial stand in sharp contrast to theoretical arguments mounted by business-as-usual clinical psychologists that realism and accuracy are the hallmarks of health.

- *Positive expectations drive analgesic placebo effects through physiological pathways.* Specifically, dopamine—implicated in the experience of positive emotions—triggers the release of endorphins (Scott et al., 2007). Optimism and hope are not only in one's head but also in one's nervous system.

Positive Traits

Our own research has focused on good character, which we approach as a family of positive traits, such as kindness, teamwork, and humor (Park & Peterson, 2006b; Peterson & Seligman, 2004). We have devised measures of these positive traits as individual differences and relate them to a variety of outcomes that matter.

- *Character strengths predict life satisfaction.* Among adults, the strengths of curiosity, gratitude, hope, love, and zest are robustly associated with happiness and well-being (Park, Peterson, & Seligman, 2004). Among youth, gratitude, hope, love, and zest are strong predictors (Park & Peterson, 2006c). And among very young children, studied with open-ended parental descriptions, hope, love, and zest figure most prominently in the descriptions of happy children (Park & Peterson, 2006a). A clear developmental trend is apparent. Perhaps because most children and youth are inherently curious, this strength does not distinguish among those who are happy or unhappy. Gratitude is a more complex strength, requiring cognitive maturation, so it is not surprising that it is absent among young children, who are necessarily egocentric.

- *Zest is associated with work satisfaction.* Across 50 different occupations that we have studied, from accountants to surgeons, in all of these groups, zest predicts the stance that work is a calling (Peterson, Park, Hall, & Seligman, 2009).

- *Eudaimonia trumps hedonism.* According to Aristotle's notion of eudaimonia, being true to one's inner self (demon), true happiness entails identifying, cultivating, and living in accordance with one's virtues. Contrast this notion with the equally venerable idea of hedonism—pursuing pleasure and avoiding pain—that is the foundation for utilitarianism, which in turn provides the underpinning of psychoanalysis and all but the most radical of the behaviorisms. Research shows that eudaimonia trumps pleasure as a predictor of life satisfaction (Peterson, Park, & Seligman, 2005). Those who pursue eudaimonic goals and activities are more satisfied than those who pursue pleasure. This is not to say that hedonism is irrelevant to life satisfaction, just that, all things being equal, hedonism contributes less to long-term happiness than does eudaimonia.

• *The "heart" matters more than the "head."* Positive psychologists have begun to study character strengths—individual differences such as curiosity, creativity, kindness, and teamwork. Measures have been devised and administered to people across the lifespan. Research consistently shows that strengths of the heart that connect people together—such as love and gratitude—are much more strongly associated with well-being than are strengths of the head that are individual in nature, such as creativity, critical thinking, and aesthetic appreciation (Park et al., 2004). Formal education, of course, stresses the latter strengths, but if one goal of education is to encourage the good life, the research results suggest that the former strengths deserve attention as well (Bacon, 2005).

Positive Relationships

Perhaps the most consistent finding in positive psychology is that good relationships with other people—friends, family members, and colleagues at work—are the single most important contributor to the psychological good life.

• *The strongest correlates of happiness are social in nature* (e.g., extraversion, social support, number of friends, leisure activities, marriage, employment [but not income]; Peterson, 2006a). Religion also confers benefits, and many of these can be attributed to the communion with others that religious worship entails (McCullough, Hoyt, Larson, Koenig, & Thoreson, 2000; Pargament, 2002).

• *Good relationships may even be a necessary condition for life satisfaction* (Diener & Seligman, 2002), a striking finding given how few necessary conditions for anything have ever been documented.

• *Viewing one's spouse in a more positive way than do others—presumably an idealization—predicts a good and lasting marriage* (Murray, Holms, Dolderman, & Griffin, 2000; Murray, Holmes, & Griffin, 1996).

• *Responding to the good news relayed by one's partner in an active and constructive way marks a good relationship* (Gable, Reis, Impett, & Asher, 2004).). Contrast "You deserve that promotion—tell me more") with "How are you going to handle those new responsibilities" or "That's nice dear—isn't Tom Brady good looking?"

- *More generally, a good relationship is one in which positive commu-nication considerably outweighs negative communication* (Fredrickson & Losada, 2005; Gottman, Coan, Carrere, & Swanson, 1998).

Positive Groups and Institutions

Positive institutions, the acknowledged weak link of positive psychology, are in need of more investigation (Peterson, Park, & Sweeney, 2008). How-ever, our own preliminary studies established some of the features of posi-tive groups.

- Members of self-identified happy families describe their families as having strengths, such as fairness, forgiveness, honesty, social intelligence, and teamwork. Notice that these are not the strengths that characterize happy individuals.

- Schools, workplaces, and communities with high morale emphasize the same organizational-level values and virtues: shared purpose, safety, fairness, kindness and decency, and the dignity of individuals (Park & Peter-son, 2003).

Taking Stock

The case has been made that attention to the positive tells us important things about the human condition that were previously unknown to a prob-lem-focused psychology. Still not well understood are the mechanisms by which positive emotions, positive thinking, positive relationships, and posi-tive groups and institutions affect people for the better. One possibility is that all of these build *psychological capital,* resources and assets that can later be deployed to good effect (Moneta & Csikszentmihalyi, 1996; Sher-noff, Csikszentmihalyi, Shneider, & Shernoff, 2003).

Indeed, happiness, strengths of character, and good social relationships are buffers against the damaging effects of stressful life events. No one goes through life without challenges and setbacks, but to the degree that people have more life satisfaction, greater character strengths, and better social support, they experience fewer psychological or physical problems in the wake of difficulties (e.g., Cobb, 1976; Peterson, Park, & Seligman, 2006; Suldo & Huebner, 2004).

Specific Techniques

Positive psychologists have demonstrated that brief interventions in the short term boost happiness, satisfaction, and fulfillment. From rigorous studies using randomization and a placebo control, there is evidence that positive psychology–based interventions increase well-being, as well as alleviate depression (Seligman, Steen, Park, & Peterson, 2005). For example, clients can be asked to count their blessings:

> "Every night for 1 week, set aside 10 minutes before you go to bed. Use that time to write down three things that went really well on that day and why they went well. You may use a journal or your computer to write about the events, but it is important that you have a physical record of what you wrote. It is not enough to do this exercise in your head. The three things you list can be relatively small or relatively large in importance. Next to each positive event in your list, answer the question 'Why did this good thing happen?' "

Clients can also be asked to use their strengths in novel ways. They take the VIA-IS online and identify their most signature strengths of character. Then they are instructed to use these strengths in their daily lives:

> "Every day for the next 7 days use one of your top five strengths in a way that you have not before. You might use your strength in a new setting or with a new person. It's your choice."

See Table 9.2 for other examples. More information about these and other interventions can be found in Linley and Joseph (2004), Park and Peterson (2006d), Peterson and Seligman (2004), and Peterson (2006a).

Some qualifications are in order if these techniques are used in the context of treatment. First, the therapist must ascertain a client's readiness to change in the particular ways requested in the exercise, as well as the client's capacity to make the change. Like any psychotherapeutic procedure, these techniques cannot be imposed on the unwilling or the unable.

Second, none of these techniques is akin to a crash diet or an antibiotic. To the degree that they have lasting effects, it is because clients integrate them into their regular behavioral routines. Counting blessings for a week will make a person happier for that week, but only if the person becomes habitually grateful will there be a more enduring effect. In our research, we found—not surprisingly—that the people who showed lasting benefits were those who continued to use the exercise.

Third, these exercises are typically presented as one size fits all, but there is no reason to think that they are equally useful for all clients. Nothing is

TABLE 9.2. Examples of Positive Psychology Techniques

Exercises to increase positive feelings
  Performing acts of kindness
  Savoring

Exercises to decrease negative feelings
  Writing about traumatic events

Exercises to increase life satisfaction
  Acting in extraverted ways
  Counting one's blessings

Exercises to develop talents and strengths
  Using talents and/or signature strengths of character in novel ways

Exercises to increase engagement
  Finding a challenging hobby

Exercises to increase social connectedness
  Being a good teammate
  Active–constructive responding

Exercises to increase meaning and purpose
  Performing secret good deeds
  Writing one's own legacy
  Working for a valued institution

Exercises to increase health and safety
  Worrying about plausible threats and dangers

known about the match of an exercise with a client's particular presenting problems or goals, or with a client's age, gender, social class, or ethnicity.

Fourth, little is known about the parameters of these interventions. For example, how many blessings should one count, and how frequently should this be done? With college students, counting blessings once a week may be more effective in increasing happiness than counting them more frequently (Sheldon & Lyubomirsky, 2004). Is this a general phenomenon or one that is specific to young adults attending college?

Fifth, all interventions run the risk of unintended harm, and whereas positive psychologists would like to believe that their techniques avoid iatrogenic effects, they cannot make this assertion with thorough confidence. For example, although optimism is related to mental and physical health, it would be simplistic and potentially hazardous to tell clients that positive expectations will solve all their difficulties. Along these lines, if a positive psychology intervention overemphasizes a client's choice and responsibility, considerable damage could be done in cases of abuse and victimization, where self-blame needs to be undone and certainly not encouraged. Once again, we point out that interventions based on positive psychology should not preclude the use of existing therapeutic strategies when indicated.

Toward Therapy Informed by Positive Psychology

Beginning to appear are so-called "positive therapies," interventions linked to positive psychology. What distinguishes these therapies from business-as-usual treatments is that their stated goal is not symptom reduction or relief but rather enhanced happiness, life satisfaction, fulfillment, productivity, and the like—one or more components of positive psychology's vision of the good life. These therapies target people with and without psychological problems.

We describe some of these therapies in the next section. Here we note the somewhat limited evidence for their effectiveness. We hasten to add that the evidence does not argue against the effectiveness of these approaches but simply that the research jury is out. The good news is that most of these therapies have been devised by research-minded psychologists, who are in the process of putting their ideas to empirical test.

The further good news is that there are decades of available lessons from the therapy outcome research literature to guide evaluation efforts (Nathan & Gorman, 1998, 2002). The need for well-characterized samples, plausible comparison groups, random assignment, treatment manuals, objective outcome measures, effect size estimates, long-term follow-ups, and analyses of process is recognized. All are readily applicable to future investigation.

We also wish to note that we regard the term *positive therapy* as misleading if it implies that these approaches are wholly new. As will be clear from our review, so-called "positive therapies" are derived from well-established conventional approaches, usually from the cognitive-behavioral arena. What is novel about them are their expanded goals and their deliberate incorporation of positive psychology interventions to achieve these goals. We therefore prefer to describe these approaches more precisely as *therapy informed by positive psychology*.

CLINICAL PRACTICE

As we discussed, *positive psychology* is an umbrella term, and no single theory defines the field. It is not clear that any of the midrange theories of positive psychology have the power or scope to frame an entire therapy. Accordingly, positive psychologists interested in therapy have turned to existing therapies (and their larger theoretical perspectives) for an overall model of treatment.

Examples

The following are sketches of some of therapies informed by (or consistent with) positive psychology and—if the information is available—what is known about their effectiveness:

1. Decades ago, Michael Fordyce (1977, 1983) developed a *Personal Happiness Program* and showed it to be effective in boosting the long-term satisfaction of college students. Fordyce surveyed the research literature on happiness and identified predictors presumably under the short-term control of ordinary people (e.g., keeping busy, socializing with others, doing meaningful work, and making the pursuit of happiness a priority). This information was conveyed to individuals along with suggested behavioral and cognitive exercises. In seven studies that included no-treatment comparison groups, Fordyce found that self-reported happiness increased and feelings of depression decreased.

2. We have already described our investigations of specific *positive psychology interventions*, such as counting one's blessings and using signature strengths in novel ways (Seligman et al., 2005). These studies were part of a deliberate program to develop and evaluate positive psychology interventions. Much like Fordyce, we surveyed the scientific and popular literature for interventions purporting to increase happiness. We identified more than 100 of these, 40 of which we were able to manualize. In work that is ongoing, we are systematically testing the effects of these manualized interventions in randomized trials against a plausible placebo control (asking individuals to write about their early memories). As described, we found that two of the interventions we have so far evaluated—counting one's blessings and using signature strengths in novel ways—increase happiness and decrease depression through 6 months of follow-up, with effect sizes as large as those of conventional psychotherapy. We also found that a third intervention—writing and delivering a letter of gratitude to another person—had a very large effect on happiness and depression, but only for 1 month. Two other interventions—writing an essay about "you at your best" and identifying one's signature strengths (without the instruction to use them in novel ways)—did not affect well-being. As noted, research continues, and it will be just as important to learn what does not work as to determine what does.

3. The *positive psychotherapy* sketched by Martin Seligman, Tayyab Rashid, and Acacia Parks (2006) is a generalization of the research program we just described. It packages together different positive psychology techniques and uses them sequentially in one-to-one therapy with depressed clients. Out-of-session homework assignments are the focus of discussion in treatment. Pilot data suggest that this form of treatment reduces depression and increases life satisfaction.

4. *Quality of life therapy* was developed by Michael Frisch (2006), who regarded it as an instance of cognitive therapy. Its goal is to increase one's quality of life (happiness) by using the sorts of techniques developed by Beck, Rush, Shaw, and Emery (1979) to decrease depression (see Scott & Freeman, Chapter 2, this volume). Like other therapies informed by positive

psychology, quality of life therapy assumes that there are multiple routes to the good life, and it describes specific techniques for achieving these, from changing one's objective situation to revising one's standards for defining personal success. Quality of life therapy can be used with individual clients or groups. Different versions of quality of life therapy have been created for clinical and nonclinical clients, and evidence is starting to accumulate that quality of life therapy is successful in its intended goal of increasing life satisfaction (e.g., Grant, Salcedo, Hynan, Frisch, & Puster, 1995; Rodrigues, Baz, Widows, & Ehlers, 2005).

5. *Positive behavioral support* is a form of behavior therapy that focuses on the environment and specifically on *problem contexts,* defined as counterproductive and unfair situations that produce or exacerbate difficulties for people (Carr, 2007). Originally devised to help people with disabilities, positive behavioral support has more general applicability. It attempts to impart to clients skills, coping strategies, and the motivation to change. It also enlists the support of family members and other key figures in the person's life. Positive behavioral support is concerned with not only what produces problems but also what promotes happiness and life satisfaction.

6. C. Rick Snyder's *hope therapy* uses cognitive-behavioral techniques to increase hope through a process of setting and monitoring explicit goals (Cheavens, Feldman, Gum, Michael, & Snyder, 2006). Lopez et al. (2004) described a number of formal and informal strategies for building and enhancing hope in children and adults. Versions of hope therapy exist for individuals and groups, and several studies demonstrate that by enhancing hope, hope therapy increases well-being and decreases symptoms of depression and anxiety (Irving et al., 2004; Klausner et al., 1998).

7. *Well-being therapy*, developed by Giovanni Fava (1997), is based on Ryff's (1989) model of psychological well-being. This model distinguishes several components of doing well—environmental mastery, personal growth, purpose in life, autonomy, self-acceptance, and positive relations with others—and overlaps considerably with the positive psychology vision of psychological health. Well-being therapy is a short-term, individual treatment that takes a thoroughly cognitive approach. In early sessions, clients are asked to identify and to situate episodes of doing well. Then they are asked to keep a diary or journal about such episodes and to identify the thoughts and beliefs that interrupt them. Finally, they are taught to challenge and to test these beliefs. Special attention is paid to components of well-being that are frequently impaired, which makes well-being therapy more remedial than other approaches mentioned here. Well-being therapy is effective in reducing anxiety and depression, and it enhances well-being (e.g., Fava, Rafanelli, & Cazzaro, 1998; Fava, Ruini, & Rafanelli, 2005).

8. *Acceptance and commitment therapy* (ACT), developed by Hayes,

Strosahl, and Wilson (1999), has unambiguously positive goals: to reduce psychological suffering of clients and to help them live a life of value (see DiGiuseppe, Chapter 4, this volume). ACT is a short-term structured therapy that has been used with individuals and groups with a variety of psychological and medical problems. It provides exercises and assignments that encourage an individual not only to accept psychological pain as normal and indeed important but also to avoid increasing it unnecessarily. ACT takes issue with the premise of typical cognitive therapies that the direct targeting of problematic ways of thinking is helpful. Indeed, the proponents of ACT argue that too much attention to thinking is counterproductive and may even exacerbate problems. ACT has a Buddhist flavor, acknowledged by its originator (Hayes, 2002), but this therapy was derived from behavior therapy and an explicit psychological theory of thought and language (Hayes, Barnes-Hohnes, & Roche, 2001). Of the therapies mentioned here, ACT has been among the most frequently tested, and it is as effective in reducing psychological problems as conventional cognitive-behavioral therapies (Hayes, Luoma, Bond, Masuda, & Lillis, 2006).

9. *Mindfulness-based cognitive therapy* (MBCT) combines techniques of cognitive therapy with the Buddhist practice of mindfulness meditation, which encourages people to be more aware of what they are thinking, to live in the moment, and to refrain from evaluating judgments about their own thoughts. Whereas typical cognitive therapy tries to change the content of thought, MBCT emphasizes nonjudgmental awareness (see Dimidjian, Kleiber, & Segal, Chapter 10, this volume). MBCT grew out of stress-reduction strategies developed by Jon Kabat-Zinn (1982) to help people with physical problems such as chronic pain and hypertension. Zindel Segal, John Teasdale, and Mark Williams (2002) adapted these strategies to help individuals with recurring depression. MBCT entails weekly group sessions and homework assignments. Outcome studies show the effectiveness of MBCT in decreasing depression and anxiety, and notable success in preventing relapse (e.g., Kenny & Williams, 2007; but see Toneatta & Nguyen, 2007). MBCT also improves the quality of life among medical patients.

10. Steven Brunwasser has created an intervention called *day rearranging*, based on the premise that people can rearrange their daily activities to decrease stress and to increase satisfaction. People may not be fully cognizant of how much time they spend doing things that make them unhappy (e.g., constantly checking e-mail) and, conversely, how little time they spend doing things that fulfill them (e.g., taking walks). They may not even be skilled at predicting what makes them happy (Gilbert, 2006). Accordingly, they are asked to keep track for 1 or 2 weeks of what they do during each day and how they feel while doing each activity (Kahneman, Kruger, Schkade, Schwarz, & Stone, 2004). Then they meet with a therapist (aka *day rear-*

ranger) who discusses with them their journal and the lessons to be learned from it. Within the constraints of common sense, can pleasant activities be increased and unpleasant activities decreased (Lewinsohn & Libet, 1972)? Can activities be rearranged so that pleasant ones reward unpleasant ones (Premack, 1959)? Can unpleasant activities be transformed into pleasant activities by using strengths and talents—the exercise of which is presumed to be fulfilling? Day rearranging resembles the strategy of *behavioral activation* used to treat depression (see Martell, Dimidjian, & Lewinsohn, Chapter 6, this volume), although day rearranging places less emphasis on adding new activities to a client's repertoire and more emphasis on rearranging or transforming those that already exist (Lewinsohn, Biglan, & Zeiss, 1976). This intervention has been used only in pilot work, and its effectiveness at present is unknown.

Case Example: Using a Signature Strength to Increase Engagement

Jason was a 20-year-old accounting major in his second year at a private university. He did well during his first year of college. He made new friends, enjoyed his classes, and was on the Dean's List. His second year of college did not go as well. To fulfill requirements for his major, Jason took three classes that he found uninteresting. In particular, his business law class was both tedious and difficult. It required extensive reading, and Jason did not see its relevance to his present or future life.

Finding the motivation to study and to complete assignments was difficult. Jason had trouble focusing on his work and often had to read passages several times before the information would stay with him. Uncharacteristically, he put off assignments until the night before they were due, and he handed in work that did not reflect his abilities. By midsemester, Jason was struggling to stay afloat in the class, scoring in the bottom 10% on the midterm and earning at best mediocre grades on class projects. He became increasingly anxious, which affected his work in other classes, as well as his social life. He stopped doing things with his friends in order to study more, although he did not find the extra study productive.

How does a positive psychologist conceptualize the case of Jason? Rather than focus on his anxiety as the primary problem or his procrastination as the symptom of this problem, a positive psychologist looks at Jason in terms of an expanded vision of well-being, asking not only what is missing but also what is present. Jason's "problem" in these terms was that his schoolwork did not engage him. His motivation for studying—intrinsic during his first year of college—had become extrinsic during his second year. At the same time, Jason had notable strengths of character.

In particular, he was humorous and playful, positive traits confirmed by the VIA-IS, as well as Jason's own self-report. Jason loved games that involved friendly competition (e.g., sports and cards), and it was during these activities that he felt most playful and alive. Despite his anxiety, this strength remained intact, although Jason rarely exercised it.

To address his problem with schoolwork, Jason met with a counselor, who identified his signature strengths of humor and playfulness early in their sessions. The counselor suggested that Jason find ways to make his courses, especially business law, more engaging by recrafting them as an opportunity to use these assets.

Two of Jason's friends were enrolled in his business law class. They, too, had similar motivation problems and in effect became coclients, although the counselor never met with them. Jason and the counselor devised a study strategy for the business law class that transformed it into a friendly competition. Each of the three students would study independently for the class 2 hours each night. At the end of the week, each would create a 10-item quiz covering class material. They would take each other's quizzes, and the two losers would buy a dessert for the winner. This strategy readily allowed therapeutic "progress" to be monitored. How much time did Jason study, and how well did he do on the quizzes?

The dessert, of course, was not the point of the competition. In one sense, it was an extrinsic reward, but Jason's progress had nothing to do with whether he won or lost at the week's end. Rather, the point was that studying had been changed into a social activity that allowed Jason to engage in banter with his friends and to be his playful self. After several weeks, studying became engaging for Jason. His procrastination ceased, for business law and for his other courses; his anxiety vanished; and friendship with his two fellow students deepened.

SUMMARY AND CONCLUSIONS

Let us discuss the therapies we just sketched (see Table 9.3). Their novel and explicit goal is to enhance well-being and to promote the good life among those with and without obvious psychological problems. As we emphasized, all are derived from established therapies such as those described in this volume. All are short-term, structured interventions for individuals or small groups. Most employ cognitive-behavioral techniques. All entail out-of-session exercises and homework assignments, the results of which are discussed in sessions. A number of these therapies ask clients to keep journals, and many of them rely on ongoing assessment.

Therapies informed by positive psychology take issue with assumptions

TABLE 9.3. Therapies Informed by Positive Psychology

	Larger model	Manualized?	Clients	Evidence?
1. Personal happiness program	Cognitive-behavioral	Yes	everyday people	Yes
2. Positive psychology interventions	Cognitive-behavioral	Yes	everyday people	Yes
3. Positive psychotherapy	Cognitive-behavioral	Yes	Depressed adults	Yes
4. Quality of life therapy	Cognitive	Yes	Everyday people and depressed adults	Yes
5. Positive behavioral support	Behavioral	Yes	Everyday people	Yes
6. Hope therapy	Cognitive-behavioral	Yes	Everyday people and those with affective disorders	Yes
7. Well-being therapy	Cognitive	Yes	Adults with affective disorders	Yes
8. Acceptance and commitment therapy	Behavioral	Yes	Adults with affective disorders	Yes
9. Mindfulness-based cognitive therapy	Cognitive–Buddhist	Yes	depressed adults and medical patients	Yes
10. Day rearranging	Behavioral	Yes	Everyday people	No

of the medical model that people in treatment are ill, and that their problems are best described as discrete (present or absent) entities à la DSM diagnoses. According to positive psychology, people's weaknesses and strengths exist in degrees (Peterson & Seligman, 2004).

As we have emphasized, research support is still accumulating. Enough outcome studies have been conducted to conclude that these therapies are more than just promising, with effect sizes in the small to moderate range, typical of psychological interventions. Not known in most cases is how these expanded therapies fare in direct comparison to business-as-usual treatments for anxiety or depression. The boundary conditions of effective therapies informed by positive psychology are completely unknown.

Many positive psychologists would like to believe that a strengths-based approach to change is superior to one that focuses on the remediation of deficiencies (Buckingham & Clifton, 2001), but this hypothesis has yet to be put to serious test. Our evenhanded suspicion is that attention to both strengths and weaknesses is critical, and that no useful purpose is served by regarding these as mutually exclusive therapeutic goals.

In the past, we thought that positive psychology interventions were inherently light-handed, meaning that they meet with little resistance and are self-sustaining (Peterson, 2004; Peterson & Seligman, 2004). Why would someone *not* want to be happier and more fulfilled, especially given the additional—presumably rewarding—benefits of being so?

Our current thinking is that positive interventions can challenge both the client and the therapist. People do not always do the "right" or "good" or "happy" thing, even when they know perfectly well what needs to be done. Experiencing flow while challenging one's skills is more exhilarating than watching television (Csikszentmihalyi, 1990). Having close friends is more fulfilling than surfing the Internet. Doing volunteer work pays more dividends than reading the tabloids. Living in accord with explicit values is more satisfying than constantly compromising. So why do people live as they do?

This question is among the most crucial for positive psychologists to answer, especially as they develop and deploy interventions (Peterson, 2006a). The not-so-good life has considerable inertia. In the case of happiness, theorists have made sense of this inertia by positing a hedonic set point (Brickman & Campbell, 1971). This set-point may reflect genetic constraints (Lykken & Tellegen, 1996); cognitive styles, such as defensive pessimism (Norem & Cantor, 1986); or habits sustained by given environments (Mischel, 1968). Although recent research shows that the hedonic set point can be changed by major life events, nothing suggests that change for the better is typical or easy (Diener, Lucas, & Scallon, 2006), which means that therapies informed by positive psychology will never take the "seven easy steps" form.

It is difficult to predict the future of these therapies except to say that their success will hinge on the relevant research. Does positive treatment work? Is it efficacious in an idealized clinical trial, as well as the fog of actual treatment? What about its efficiency? Are benefits of positive treatment evident only in comparison to no treatment, or does the positive approach represent value above and beyond existing treatments? How robust are any effects, and how long do they last? Evidence to date suggests that these therapies can increase well-being while decreasing problems; do these changes occur in lockstep or independently? Although many therapy approaches informed by positive psychology seem promising, only a few of them have been rigorously tested to date. More work need to be done.

In conclusion, positive psychology provides a valuable perspective on the human condition, as well as strategies for treatment, prevention, rehabilitation, and promotion. Positive psychology expands our view of psychological health beyond the absence of symptoms and disorders, and provides hope that a healthy, fulfilled, and productive life is possible for all.

REFERENCES

Albee, G. W. (1982). Preventing psychopathology and promoting human potential. *American Psychologist, 37,* 1043–1050.

Bacon, S. F. (2005). Positive psychology's two cultures. *Review of General Psychology, 9,* 181–192.

Bandura, A. (1989). Human agency in social cognitive theory. *American Psychologist, 14,* 175–184.

Beck, A. T., Rush, A. J., Shaw, B. F., & Emery, G. (1979). *Cognitive therapy of depression.* New York: Guilford Press.

Brickman, P., & Campbell, D. T. (1971). Hedonic relativism and planning the good society. In M. H. Appley (Ed.), *Adaptation-level theory* (pp. 287–305). New York: Academic Press.

Bryant, F. B., & Veroff, J. (2006). *The process of savoring: A new model of positive experience.* Mahwah, NJ: Erlbaum.

Buckingham, M., & Clifton, D. O. (2001). *Now, discover your strengths.* New York: Free Press.

Carr, E. G. (2007). The expanding vision of positive behavior support: Research perspectives on happiness, helpfulness, hopefulness. *Journal of Positive Behavior Interventions, 9,* 3–14.

Cheavens, J. S., Feldman, D. B., Gum, A., Michael, S. T., & Snyder, C. R. (2006). Hope therapy in a community sample: A pilot investigation. *Social Indicators Research, 77,* 61–78.

Cobb, S. (1976). Social support as a moderator of life stress. *Psychosomatic Medicine, 38,* 300–314.

Cohen, S., Doyle, W. J., Turner, R. B., Aker, C. M., & Skoner, D. P. (2003). Emotional style and susceptibility to the common cold. *Psychosomatic Medicine, 65,* 652–657.

Cowen, E. L. (1994). The enhancement of psychological wellness: Challenges and opportunities. *American Journal of Community Psychology, 22,* 149–179.

Cowen, E. L., & Kilmer, R. P. (2002). "Positive psychology": Some plusses and some open issues. *Journal of Community Psychology, 30,* 440–460.

Csikszentmihalyi, M. (1990). *Flow: The psychology of optimal experience.* New York: Harper & Row.

Danner, D. D., Snowdon, D., & Friesen, W. V. (2001). Positive emotions in early life and longevity: Findings from the nun study. *Journal of Personality and Social Psychology, 80,* 804–813.

Diener, E., & Diener, C. (1996). Most people are happy. *Psychological Science, 7,* 181–185.

Diener, E., Lucas, R. E., & Scallon, C. N. (2006). Beyond the hedonic treadmill: Revising the adaptation theory of well-being. *American Psychologist, 61*(4), 305–314.

Diener, E., & Seligman, M. E. P. (2002). Very happy people. *Psychological Science, 13,* 80–83.

Duckworth, A. L., Steen, T. A., & Seligman, M. E. P. (2005). Positive psychology in clinical practice. *Annual Review of Clinical Psychology, 1,* 629–651.

Dyck, M. J., Jolly, J. B., & Kramer, T. (1994). An evaluation of positive affectivity, negative affectivity, and hyperarousal as markers for assessing between syndrome relationships. *Personality and Individual Differences, 17,* 637–646.

Fava, G. A. (1997). Well-being therapy. *Psychotherapy and Psychosomatics, 68,* 171–178.

Fava, G. A., Rafanelli, C., & Cazzaro, M. (1998). Well-being therapy: A novel psychotherapeutic approach for residual symptoms of affective disorders. *Psychological Medicine, 28,* 475–480.

Fava, G. A., Ruini, C., & Rafanelli, C. (2005). Well-being therapy of generalized anxiety disorder. *Psychotherapy and Psychosomatics, 74,* 26–30.

Fineman, S. (2006). On being positive: Concerns and counterpoints. *Academy of Management Review, 31,* 270–291.

Fordyce, M. W. (1977). Development of a program to increase personal happiness. *Journal of Counseling Psychology, 24,* 511–520.

Fordyce, M. W. (1983). A program to increase happiness: Further studies. *Journal of Counseling Psychology, 30,* 483–498.

Fredrickson, B. L. (2001). The role of positive emotions in positive psychology: The broaden-and-build theory of positive emotions. *American Psychologist, 56,* 218–226.

Fredrickson, B. L., & Losada, M. (2005). Positive affect and the complex dynamics of human flourishing. *American Psychologist, 60,* 678–686.

Frisch, M. B. (2006). *Quality of life therapy.* New York: Wiley.

Furr, R. M., & Funder, D. C. (1998). A multimodal analysis of personal negativity. *Journal of Personality and Social Psychology, 74,* 1580–1591.

Gable, S. L., Reis, H. T., Impett, E. A., & Asher, E. R. (2004). What do you do when things go right?: The intrapersonal and interpersonal benefits of sharing good events. *Journal of Personality and Social Psychology, 87,* 228–245.

Gardner, H. (1983). *Frames of mind: The theory of multiple intelligences.* New York: Basic Books.

Gilbert, D. (2006). *Stumbling on happiness.* New York: Knopf.

Gottman, J. M., Coan, J., Carrere, S., & Swanson, C. (1998). Predicting marital happiness and stability from newlywed interactions. *Journal of Marriage and the Family, 60,* 5–22.

Grant, G. M., Salcedo, V., Hynan, L. S., Frisch, M. B., & Puster, K. (1995). Effectiveness of quality of life therapy for depression. *Psychological Reports, 76,* 1203–1208.

Greenspoon, P. J., & Saklofske, D. H. (2001). Toward an integration of subjective well-being and psychopathology. *Social Indicators Research, 54,* 81–108.

Hayes, S. C. (2002). Buddhism and acceptance and commitment therapy. *Cognitive and Behavioral Practice, 9,* 58–66.

Hayes, S. C., Barnes-Hohnes, D., & Roche, B. (Eds.). (2001). *Relational frame theory: A post-Skinnerian account of human language and cognition.* New York: Academic Press.

Hayes, S. C., Luoma, J., Bond, F., Masuda, A., & Lillis, J. (2006). Acceptance and commitment therapy: Model, processes, and outcomes. *Behaviour Research and Therapy, 44,* 1–25.

Hayes, S. C., Strosahl, K. D., & Wilson, K. G. (1999). *Acceptance and commitment therapy: An experiential approach to behavior change.* New York: Guilford Press.

Held, B. S. (2002). The tyranny of the positive attitude in America: Observation and speculation. *Journal of Clinical Psychology, 58,* 965–992.

Held, B. S. (2004). The negative side of positive psychology. *Journal of Humanistic Psychology, 44,* 9–46.

Hyten, C. (2004). Disconnecting positive psychology and OBM. *Journal of Organizational Behavior Management, 24,* 67–73.

Irving, L. M., Snyder, C. R., Cheavens, J., Gravel, L., Hanke, J., Hilberg, P., et al. (2004). The relationships between hope and outcomes at the pre-treatment, beginning, and later phases of psychotherapy. *Journal of Psychotherapy Integration, 14,* 419–443.

Jahoda, M. (1958). *Current concepts of positive mental health.* New York: Basic Books.

Judge, T. A., & Ilies, R. (2004). Is positiveness in organizations always desirable? *Academy of Management Executive, 18,* 151–155.

Kabat-Zinn, J. (1982). An out-patient program in behavioral medicine for chronic pain patients based on the practice of mindfulness meditation: Theoretical considerations and preliminary results. *General Hospital Psychiatry, 4,* 33–47.

Kahneman, D., Krueger, A. B., Schkade, D. A., Schwarz, N., & Stone, A. A. (2004). A survey method for characterizing daily life experience: The day reconstruction method. *Science, 306,* 1176–1180.

Kenny, M. A., & Williams, J. M. G. (2007). Treatment-resistant depressed patients show a good response to mindfulness-based cognitive therapy. *Behaviour Research and Therapy, 45,* 617–625.

Klausner, E. J., Clarkin, J. F., Spielman, L., Pupo, C., Abrams, R., & Alexopoulos, G. S. (1998). Late-life depression and functional disability: The role of goal-focused group psychotherapy. *International Journal of Geriatric Psychiatry, 13,* 707–716.

Lazarus, R. S. (2003). Does the positive psychology movement have legs? *Psychological Inquiry, 14,* 93–109.

Levitt, A. J., Hogan, T. P., & Bucosky, C. M. (1990). Quality of life in chronically mentally ill patients in day treatment. *Psychological Medicine, 20,* 703–710.

Lewinsohn, P. M., Biglan, A., & Zeiss, A. M. (1976). Behavioral treatment of depression. In P. O. Davidson (Ed.), *The behavioral management of anxiety, depression and pain* (pp. 91–146). New York: Brunner/Mazel.

Lewinsohn, P. M., & Libet, J. (1972). Pleasant events, activity schedules, and depressions. *Journal of Abnormal Psychology, 79,* 291–295.

Linley, P. A., & Joseph, S. (Eds.). (2004). *Positive psychology in practice.* New York: Wiley.

Lopez, S. J., & Snyder, C. R. (Eds.). (2003). *Positive psychological assessment: A handbook of models and measures.* Washington, DC: American Psychological Association.

Lopez, S. J., Snyder, C. R., Edwards, L., Pedrotti, J., Janowski, K., Turner, J., et al. (2004). Hope interventions. In P. A. Linley & S. Joseph (Eds.), *Positive psychology in practice* (pp. 388–404). New York: Wiley.

Lykken, D., & Tellegen, A. (1996). Happiness is a stochastic phenomenon. *Psychological Science, 7*, 186–189.

Lyubomirsky, S., King, L. A., & Diener, E. (2005). The benefits of frequent positive affect: Does happiness lead to success? *Psychological Bulletin, 131*, 803–855.

Maddux, J. E., Snyder, C. R., & Lopez, S. J. (2004). Toward a positive clinical psychology: Deconstructing the illness ideology and constructing an ideology of human strengths and potential. In P. A. Linley & S. Joseph (Eds.), *Positive psychology in practice* (pp. 320–334). New York: Wiley.

Martin, M. W. (2007). Happiness and virtue in positive psychology. *Journal for the Theory of Social Behaviour, 37*, 89–103.

Maslow, A. H. (1954). *Motivation and personality*. New York: Harper & Row.

McCullough, M. E., Hoyt, W. T., Larson, D. B., Koenig, H. G., & Thoreson, C. (2000). Religious involvement and mortality: A meta-analytic review. *Health Psychology, 19*, 211–222.

Mischel, W. (1968). *Personality and assessment*. New York: Wiley.

Moneta, G. B., & Csikszentmihalyi, M. (1996). The effect of perceived challenges and skills on the quality of subjective experience. *Journal of Personality, 64*, 275–310.

Murray, S. L., Holmes, J. G., Dolderman, D., & Griffin, D. W. (2000). What the motivated mind sees: Comparing friends' perspectives to married partners' views of each other. *Journal of Experimental Social Psychology, 36*, 600–620.

Murray, S. L., Holmes, J. G., & Griffin, D. W. (1996). The benefits of positive illusions: Idealization and the construction of satisfaction in close relationships. *Journal of Personality and Social Psychology, 70*, 79–98.

Nathan, P. E., & Gorman, J. M. (1998). *A guide to treatments that work*. New York: Oxford University Press.

Nathan, P. E., & Gorman, J. M. (2002). *A guide to treatments that work* (2nd ed.). New York: Oxford University Press.

Neill, A. S. (1960). *Summerhill: A radical approach to child rearing*. New York: Hart.

Norcross, J. C., & Goldfried, M. R. (Eds.). (2005). *A handbook of psychotherapy integration*. New York: Oxford University Press.

Norem, J. K., & Cantor, N. (1986). Defensive pessimism: "Harnessing" anxiety as motivation. *Journal of Personality and Social Psychology, 51*, 1208–1217.

Pargament, K. (2002). The bitter and the sweet: An evaluation of the costs and benefits of religiousness. *Psychological Inquiry, 13*, 168–181.

Park, N. (2004). The role of subjective well-being in positive youth development. *The Annals of the American Academy of Political and Social Science, 591*, 25–39.

Park, N., & Peterson, C. (2003). Virtues and organizations. In K. S. Cameron, J. E. Dutton, & R. E. Quinn (Eds.), *Positive organizational scholarship: Foundations of a new discipline* (pp. 33–47). San Francisco: Berrett-Koehler.

Park, N., & Peterson, C. (2006a). Character strengths and happiness among young children: Content analysis of parental descriptions. *Journal of Happiness Studies, 7*, 323–341.

Park, N., & Peterson, C. (2006b). Methodological issues in positive psychology and the assessment of character strengths. In A. D. Ong & M. van Dulmen (Eds.),

Handbook of methods in positive psychology (pp. 292–305). New York: Oxford University Press.

Park, N., & Peterson, C. (2006c). Moral competence and character strengths among adolescents: The development and validation of the Values in Action Inventory of Strengths for Youth. *Journal of Adolescence, 29,* 891–905.

Park, N., & Peterson, C. (2006d, November/December). Strengths of character and the family. *Family Therapy Magazine,* pp. 28–33.

Park, N., Peterson, C., & Seligman, M. E. P. (2004). Strengths of character and well-being. *Journal of Social and Clinical Psychology, 23,* 603–619.

Peterson, C. (2000). The future of optimism. *American Psychologist, 55,* 44–55.

Peterson, C. (2004). Preface. *The Annals of the American Academy of Political and Social Science, 591,* 6–12.

Peterson, C. (2006a). *A primer in positive psychology.* New York: Oxford University Press.

Peterson, C. (2006b). The Values in Action (VIA) Classification of Strengths: The un-DSM and the real DSM. In M. Csikszentmihalyi & I. Csikszentmihalyi (Eds.). *A life worth living: Contributions to positive psychology* (pp. 29–48). New York: Oxford University Press.

Peterson, C., & Bossio, L. M. (1991). *Health and optimism.* New York: Free Press.

Peterson, C., & Park, N. (2003). Positive psychology as the evenhanded positive psychologist views it. *Psychological Inquiry, 14,* 141–146.

Peterson, C., Park, N., & Sweeney, P. J. (2008). Group well-being: Morale from a positive psychology perspective. *Applied Psychology: An International Review, 57,* 19–36.

Peterson, C., & Park, N. (in press-a). Positive psychology. In B. J. Sadock, V. A. Sadock, & P. Ruiz (Eds.), *Comprehensive textbook of psychiatry* (9th ed.). Baltimore: Lippincott, Williams, & Wilkins.

Peterson, C., & Park, N. (in press-b). Positive psychology. In M. A. Strebnicki & I. Marini (Eds.), *Professional counselors' desk reference.* New York: Springer.

Peterson, C., Park, N., Hall, N., & Seligman, M. E. P. (2009). Zest and work. *Journal of Organizational Psychology, 30,* 161–172.

Peterson, C., Park, N., & Seligman, M. E. P. (2005). Orientations to happiness and life satisfaction: The full life versus the empty life. *Journal of Happiness Studies, 6,* 25–41.

Peterson, C., Park., N., & Seligman, M. E. P. (2006). Greater strengths of character and recovery from illness. *Journal of Positive Psychology, 1,* 17–26.

Peterson, C., & Seligman, M. E. P. (2004). *Character strengths and virtues: A classification and handbook.* New York: Oxford University Press.

Premack, D. (1959). Toward empirical behavioral laws: I. Positive reinforcement. *Psychological Review, 66,* 219–233.

Rodrigues, J. R., Baz, M. A., Widows, M. R., & Ehlers, S. L. (2005). A randomized evaluation of quality-of-life therapy with patients awaiting lung transplantation. *American Journal of Transplantation, 5,* 2425–2432.

Rogers, C. R. (1951). *Client-centered therapy: Its current practice, implications, and theory.* Boston: Houghton Mifflin.

Ryan, W. (1978). *Blaming the victim* (rev. ed.). New York: Random House.

Ryff, C. D. (1989). Happiness is everything, or is it?: Explorations of the meaning of psychological well-being. *Journal of Personality and Social Psychology, 57,* 1069–1081.

Saleebey, D. (Ed.). (1992). *The strengths perspective in social work practice.* New York: Longman.

Schumaker, J. F. (2007). *In search of happiness: Understanding an endangered state of mind.* Westport, CT: Praeger.

Scott, D. J., Stohler, C. S., Egnatuk, C. M., Wang, H., Koeppe, R. A., & Zubieta, J. (2007). Individual differences in reward responding explain placebo-induced expectations and effects. *Neuron, 55,* 325–336.

Segal, Z., Teasdale, J., & Williams, M. (2002). *Mindfulness-based cognitive therapy for depression.* New York: Guilford Press.

Seligman, M. E. P. (2002). *Authentic happiness.* New York: Free Press.

Seligman. M. E. P., & Csikszentmihalyi, M. (2000). Positive psychology: An introduction. *American Psychologist, 55,* 5–14.

Seligman. M. E. P., & Pawelski, J. O. (2003). Positive psychology: FAQs. *Psychological Inquiry, 14,* 159–163.

Seligman, M. E. P., & Peterson, C. (2003). Positive clinical psychology. In L. G. Aspinwall & U. M. Staudinger (Eds.), *A psychology of human strengths: Fundamental questions and future directions for a positive* (pp. 305–317). Washington, DC: American Psychological Association.

Seligman, M. E. P., Rashid, T., & Parks, A. C. (2006). Positive psychotherapy. *American Psychologist, 61,* 774–788.

Seligman, M. E. P., Steen, T. A., Park, N., & Peterson, C. (2005). Positive psychology progress: Empirical validation of interventions. *American Psychologist, 60,* 410–421.

Sheldon, K. M., & Lyubomirsky, S. (2004). Achieving sustainable new happiness: Prospects, practices, and prescriptions. In P. A. Linley & S. Joseph (Eds.), *Positive psychology in practice* (pp. 127–145). Hoboken, NJ: Wiley.

Shernoff, D. J., Csikszentmihalyi, M., Shneider, B., & Shernoff, E. S. (2003). Student engagement in high school classrooms from the perspective of flow theory. *School Psychology Quarterly, 18,* 158–176.

Sternberg, R. J. (Ed.). (2005). *Unity in psychology: Possibility or pipedream?* Washington, DC: American Psychological Association.

Sugarman, J. (2007). Practical rationality and the questionable promise of positive psychology. *Journal of Humanistic Psychology, 47,* 175–197.

Suldo, S. M., & Huebner, E. S. (2004). Does life satisfaction moderate the effects of stressful life events on psychopathological behavior during adolescence? *School Psychology Quarterly, 19,* 93–105.

Taylor, E. I. (2001). Positive psychology versus humanistic psychology: A reply to Prof. Seligman. *Journal of Humanistic Psychology, 41,* 13–29.

Taylor, S. E. (1985). Adjustments to threatening events: A theory of cognitive adaptation. *American Psychologist, 38,* 1161–1173.

Taylor, S. E., & Brown, J. D. (1988). Illusion and well-being: A social psychological perspective on mental health. *Psychological Bulletin, 103,* 193–210.

Toneatta, T., & Nguyen, L. (2007). Does mindfulness meditation improve anxiety and mood symptoms?: A review of the controlled research. *Canadian Journal of Psychiatry, 52,* 260–266.

Winner, E. (2000). The origins and ends of giftedness. *American Psychologist, 55,* 159–169.

Zimmerman, M., Clincher, J. B., Pasternak, M. A., Friedman, M., Attila, N., & Codrescu, D. (2006). How should remission from depression be defined?: The depressed patient's perspective. *American Journal of Psychiatry, 163,* 148–150.

CHAPTER 10

Mindfulness-Based Cognitive Therapy

Sona Dimidjian
Blair V. Kleiber
Zindel V. Segal

INTRODUCTION AND HISTORICAL BACKGROUND

Mindfulness-based cognitive therapy (MBCT) is an innovative brief group intervention developed for the prevention of relapse and recurrence of major depression. Using a combination of mindfulness meditation practices, psychoeducation about depression, and cognitive-behavioral strategies, MBCT has been rigorously investigated as a preventive intervention among adults with histories of recurrent depression and is being currently explored as an adjunctive treatment for major depression. This chapter describes the history of the development of MBCT, the basic theoretical model that guides MBCT, and the evidence base for the model and the clinical approach. It also describes the clinical practice of MBCT, highlighting core principles, intervention strategies, and therapist qualifications, and illustrates key components through the description of a client who participated in an 8-week MBCT group for the prevention of depressive relapse.

The development of MBCT followed an unusual course, illustrating the ways in which paying close attention to the empirical data, feedback from one's patients and colleagues, and one's own experience as a researcher and clinician can lead in unexpected and novel directions. The story began with the recognition of two major problems—the nature of depression and the limitations of extant methods to prevent depression.

Major depressive disorder (MDD) is chronic, recurrent disorder. The majority of individuals who experience one major depressive episode will go on to experience relapse or recurrence, and the risk of such future episodes increases with each episode. A history of three or more episodes is associated with a 90% chance of future episodes. It is estimated that individuals with MDD experience, on average, four depressive episodes, each of approximately 20 weeks duration (Judd, 1997). Unfortunately, despite the availability of evidence-based treatments for acute MDD, our ability to offer individuals protection against future episodes has been severely limited. Pharmacotherapy is the most commonly delivered treatment for depression, and current guidelines suggest that medication for patients with recurrent histories should be maintained indefinitely (American Psychiatric Association, 2000). Maintenance medication has been found to offer ongoing protection against future relapse; however, there is little evidence that antidepressant medication confers any enduring benefit once use is discontinued (Hollon, Thase, & Markowitz, 2002). Recent trials have compared rates of relapse among patients continued on medication following an initial treatment response and those whose medication was discontinued in a double-blind fashion. Results from these studies suggest a rapid and high rate of relapse when medication is discontinued (Dobson et al., in press; Hollon et al., 2005). Additionally, not all individuals with MDD want to take antidepressant medication (ADM), and many experience side effects. For some subgroups of depressed patients, such as pregnant and lactating women, weighing the potential benefits of ADM use relative to potential adverse effects for self and offspring is a difficult and complicated process (Wisner et al., 2000). Finally, evidence suggests that serious problems exist with both the undertreatment of patients who receive ADM (Olfson et al., 2002) and noncompliance with medication regimens (Basco & Rush, 1995).

In contrast, psychosocial treatments, such as cognitive therapy (CT) appear to provide an enduring effect (Blackburn, Eunson, & Bishop, 1986; Dobson et al., 2008; Evans et al., 1992; Hollon et al., 2005; Kovacs, Rush, Beck, & Hollon, 1981; Shea et al., 1992; Simons, Murphy, Levine, & Wetzel, 1986). These approaches, however, have not been widely studied as independent relapse prevention packages that can be delivered broadly to patients who are not currently in episode. Given the prevalence of depression and the availability of psychosocial treatments, exclusive reliance on acute-phase treatments, such as CT, is unlikely to address the risk of relapse among the majority of individuals who experience depression.

Thus, in April 1992, the codevelopers of MBCT, Zindel Segal, Mark Williams, and John Teasdale, convened to address the joint problems of the recurrent nature of MDD and the limited prevention options for patients. Initially, they planned to develop a maintenance version of CT (Beck, Rush,

Shaw, & Emery, 1979) that utilized the same principles and strategies of standard CT, but was designed for use with individuals not currently in episode. Early in the treatment development process, however, Segal, Williams, and Teasdale visited the University of Massachusetts Stress Reduction Clinic. They were invited to sit in on an initial session of the mindfulness-based stress reduction (MBSR) program developed by Kabat-Zinn (1990). MBSR is an 8-week group intervention that draws from the spiritual tradition of Buddhism to deliver core principles and practices in an explicitly secular manner. It combines mindfulness meditation, yoga, and education about mind–body relationships, with the aim of increasing the health and well-being of patients with a broad array of chronic health and stress-related disorders.

As Segal, Williams, and Teasdale learned about MBSR, their sense of excitement grew. In particular, the research team was impressed by the potential relevance of MBSR strategies to the very types of cognitive and affective processes that appeared to contribute to depressive relapse. In particular, MBSR focuses on learning to deploy one's attention in specific and intentional ways, a skill that seemed highly relevant to helping patients notice early warning signs of depression. In addition, participants in MBCT were guided in decentering from thoughts in precisely the same way that the research group had speculated was integral to the prevention of relapse in depression. Specifically, they were struck by the emphasis of Kabat-Zinn (1990) on the way in which "the simple act of recognizing your thoughts as thoughts can free you from the distorted reality they often create and allow for more clear-sightedness and a greater sense of manageability in your life" (cited in Segal, Williams, & Teasdale, 2002, p. 41).

Experts in MBSR similarly expressed excitement about these points of convergence; however, their reactions were tempered by notes of caution to the research team. They raised strong concerns about pursuing research on mindfulness and clinical practice without a solid grounding in one's own meditation practice. The research team was relatively undaunted by such cautions given that their plan was simply to add some of the MBSR practices to the traditional CT framework, which (at this point in the story) they assumed would require little modification.

Attentional control training was the team's first attempt at combining CT with mindfulness training. Structural elements of MBSR were adopted; the groups were to meet weekly for 8 weeks, and participants were to listen to 20-minute instructional mindfulness tapes recorded by Kabat-Zinn for daily homework. Attentional control training met with mixed reactions. Some participants made gains using this approach and effectively applied the skills learned in the group to their daily lives. Others, however, found that the attentional control skills were helpful for mildly negative thoughts and feelings but had limited value for intense states. These participants wanted help with difficult and intense emotions and were doubtful about the utility of the strategies offered in attentional control training. In response to such doubts, the instructors found that they frequently departed from the mindfulness framework into the traditional CT framework. They had confidence that CT would help participants to reduce or eliminate the difficult emotions by working directly with their thoughts. Unfortunately, instructors also found that in groups of 10 or more patients, it was impossible to utilize effectively the usual CT methods, such as identifying and evaluating problematic thoughts and developing behavioral experiments. Doubts began to arise within the team about the approach they were developing. Moreover, other researchers in the field seemed similarly skeptical about attentional control training. Was this just a watered down version of CT, unlikely to be effective? Did the mindfulness strategies really add anything new? What *was* the purpose of teaching mindfulness to individuals who wanted to prevent relapse of depression?

At this point, it became clear that it was necessary to go back to the drawing board if the team was to retain the mindfulness component in its nascent approach. Segal, Williams, and Teasdale traveled back to the University of Massachusetts Stress Reduction Clinic and observed several MBSR groups. In so doing, some fundamental differences between MBSR and attentional control training became evident. When faced with difficult emotions among participants, the MBSR instructors did not attempt to reduce, eliminate, or otherwise "fix" such difficulties; instead, they encouraged participants to allow negative thoughts or emotions into awareness in an open way. This approach was a complete departure from the standard CT method of working to change thoughts and solve problems to decrease difficult emotions. It was a radically different way of taking action with regard to unwanted thoughts and emotions. Participants in MBSR were actually asked to *welcome* such affective states and related thoughts into awareness. Similarly, it appeared that MBSR instructors took a very different stance in relation to participants in the groups. They embodied the very skills that they were teaching. They greeted the difficult and painful experiences that participants shared with the same gentle curiosity they were inviting participants to cultivate in the mindfulness practices they taught. The ways their own mindfulness practices allowed them to embody these core elements of the program were clear and unavoidable.

The research team returned to modify its approach to relapse prevention for depression. Armed with a more nuanced understanding of MBSR and a commitment to the importance of one's own personal practice of mindfulness, the team began to revise the intervention. The result was MBCT, a novel synthesis of cognitive therapy and mindfulness meditation practices that help to disrupt the automatic patterns of sensation, cognition, behavior, and emotion that can precipitate and maintain depressive states.

PHILOSOPHICAL AND THEORETICAL UNDERPINNINGS

Model of Depressive Relapse and Evidence for the Model

MBCT is guided by a model of the factors that increase vulnerability to depressive relapse and the ways in which intervention can help to prevent depression from returning. This conceptualization is supported by basic and clinical research, both of which are reviewed below.

The MBCT model of depressive relapse is rooted in the basic cognitive model of depression (e.g., Beck, 1967). This model suggests that when people are depressed, they interpret their experiences in a negative and biased manner. These interpretations influence how people feel in a given situation and can thus maintain depression over time. For example, if a friend fails to return a phone call promptly, then a depressed person may think, "They don't really care about me. No one has time for me." The cognitive model suggests that such interpretations influence emotion and, in this case, sadness results and depression is likely to persist. However, alternative responses, such as "I wonder what is happening. Maybe I'll give my friend a call to check it out," are likely to be associated with more positive mood states. The cognitive model suggests that when a person is depressed, thoughts are often consistent with highly negative, global, and self-critical beliefs about the self, the world, and the future. Situations are interpreted through the basic lens of such beliefs, and the contents of one's thoughts can intensify or perpetuate depression.

Given the important role of thoughts postulated by the cognitive theory of depression, what was the role of cognition and emotion in depressive relapse? The *differential activation hypothesis,* originally proposed by Teasdale (1988), extended the basic cognitive model of depression to account for the phenomenon of relapse in depression. Teasdale suggested that sad moods have the power to reactivate patterns of thinking that were present during prior depressed mood states. This model proposed that, over time, patterns of association are established between the thoughts and moods that are present during depressed states. Negative thoughts become linked to feelings of sadness, and a vulnerability to the reactivation of the link between sadness and such negative thoughts persists, even beyond the resolution of depressive episodes. Thus, specifically during times of sadness, formerly depressed people are vulnerable to the automatic reactivation of negative thinking in ways that never-depressed people are not. Unfortunately, for formerly depressed people, such negative thoughts can perpetuate the sad mood, thereby leading to a downward spiral of thought, emotion, physical sensation, and behavior, potentially initiating a depressive relapse.

Research on this model has examined the construct of *cognitive reactivity,* or the tendency of formerly depressed people to react to mild changes in mood with large changes in thinking. In a series of studies by different investigators, and with a range of clinical populations, results suggest that formerly depressed persons react differently to sad mood compared to never-depressed people (Scher, Ingram, & Segal, 2005). Specifically, when researchers induce temporary sadness by asking participants to listen to sad music, for instance, they find that formerly depressed people endorse more negative attitudes than do never-depressed people, whose cognitive styles are not as reactive to mood. In addition, studies have also suggested that following successful treatment for depression, individuals who show the greatest cognitive reactivity also show the greatest risk for relapse (Segal, Gemar, & Williams, 1999; Segal et al., 2006).

In addition to research on the content of cognition, a parallel line of research on people's styles of thinking also inform the basic model of depressive relapse in MBCT. A large body of research has suggested that a *ruminative style of thinking*, defined as the tendency to focus passively on the causes and consequences of one's problems, is associated with more severe and prolonged depressive symptoms and impaired problem solving (Nolen-Hoeksema, 1991).

Thus, the combination of patterns of cognitive reactivity to even transient mild sadness and a ruminative response style are proposed as central factors explaining vulnerability to depressive relapse. In summary, as described by Segal et al. (2002, p. 36):

> At times of lowering mood, old, habitual patterns of cognitive processing switch in relatively automatically. This has two important effects. First, thinking runs repeatedly around fairly well-worn "mental grooves," without finding an effective way forward out of depression. Second, this thinking itself intensifies depressed mood, which leads to further thoughts. In this way, through self-perpetuating vicious cycles, otherwise mild and transient mood can escalate into more severe and disabling depressed states.

Translation of Model into Conceptualization to Guide Treatment: Modes of Mind

The basic conceptualization that guides treatment in MBCT centers on the metaphor of "modes of mind." It is suggested that the mind has different methods by which it processes information that are characterized by very different ways of interacting with the world. The two modes of mind we discuss are doing mind and being mind.

Doing mind is characterized by striving toward a particular goal. It is highly oriented to processing discrepant information. In other words, when the mind senses a discrepancy between the current state and an ideal state, the person makes problem-solving efforts to reduce the discrepancy and achieve what is desired. When the mind enters this mode and action can be taken to achieve the goal, then a person may exit *doing mode*. However, if the desired end cannot be achieved, or if a solution cannot be found readily, the mind can become trapped in an endless loop of mental problem solving. Without the ability to take action to achieve the desired state, the mind mulls over possible solutions to no avail, thus putting into motion a negative, self-perpetuating cycle that limits the ability to see beyond the problem at hand. The automatic patterns of doing mind are highlighted as increasing vulnerability both to cognitive reactivity and rumination.

Being mind represents a wholly different way of interacting with experience. In this mode of mind, a person focuses on experiencing the present moment rather evaluating the present moment in relation to the past and future (as is characteristic of doing mode). Thus, a person in doing mode is thinking about or processing an event or problem. Whereas a person in being mode participates in the present moment without analyzing it. Instead of striving for a goal, being mode takes in the present moment for exactly what it is and does not try to change it. For example, being mode is experienced by an artist who becomes so engrossed in her painting that she has a moment-by-moment awareness of each brush stroke, and thoughts similarly occur without effort and pass away. Another example with which people may identify is finding a "groove" while engaging in some other athletic or creative activity.

These modes of mind both have their place in daily life. The MBCT conceptualization acknowledges that it is clearly necessary for people to use doing mind to plan strategies and to solve problems. However, doing mind can become problematic when a person is constantly engaged in attempts to find solutions to unanswerable questions or problems. It is possible to spend a lot of time in the doing mode of mind, without even realizing there is little sense of participating in the present moment. Moreover, for individuals with histories of recurrent depression, doing mind can set into motion many of the patterns of rumination and cognitive reactivity that we reviewed earlier as particular vulnerabilities to depressive relapse.

The emphasis on modes of mind serves as a framework through which MBCT instructors guide treatment. The MBCT instructor repeatedly embodies and guides the ways in which mindfulness can help one to step out of the automatic pilot mode of doing mind into a more mindful stance toward present-moment experience. Thus, the development of this ability to access being mind is presented as the foundation for skillful action, which is built throughout the 8-week program. Throughout the course, MBCT instructors help participants continually bring their focus back to the present moment through the use of in-session mindfulness practice, exercises, and assigned homework. An overall goal of the program is for participants to learn to distinguish and identify doing and being modes of mind and acquire the skills to disengage from habitual, automatic responses and engage their attention in a more direct and intentional manner.

Challenges to the Theory

There have been few direct challenges to the theory underlying MBCT. Some questions have been raised about the specific value of the mindfulness component of the intervention. For instance, Coelho, Canter, and Ernst (2007) reviewed the evidence base for MBCT, highlighting the absence of studies comparing MBCT to an active psychotherapy or placebo condition. In reply, Williams, Russell, and Russell (2008) highlighted the normative developmental trajectory of research on new interventions. Typically, as new treatments are developed, the first stage of research focuses on examining whether an effect exists, whereas later studies build on this foundation by examining whether the effects of the intervention are specifically attributed to the hypothesized mechanisms. Given data suggesting that CT may work by helping patients learn to decenter from depressive cognitions (Teasdale et al., 2002), future research is required to examine whether the mindfulness strategies offer specific benefit or add little to the standard CT strategies. Similar questions can be raised with respect to the support provided by the group context as well. Dismantling designs are required to test directly such challenges, and future research will have much to offer in this domain.

The moderation of the treatment effects for MBCT by patient depressive history represents another intriguing thread in the overall pattern of findings on MBCT. Specifically, it has been difficult to account fully for the difference in the efficacy of MBCT for those who have experienced two versus three or more episodes of depression. Does this difference challenge or support the basic theory underlying MBCT? Why would MBCT be more effective for the group with three or more depressive episodes than for those with only two prior episodes? Several possibilities have been proposed. As mentioned earlier, it is possible that the strength of associations between cognition and emotion may increase as a function of the number of episodes of depression. Whereas a person with three or more episodes may have strong associations between depressive cognition and sad mood, a person with only two prior episodes may lack the required experience with depression to build such associations. It is possible that the triggering role of life stress for individuals with less recurrent histories may help to explain the pattern of differences (Ma & Teasdale, 2004; Segal et al., 2002). On the other hand, it is also possible that patients with fewer prior episodes lack the motivation to engage in the intensive practice assigned during the 8-week program. Future research may explicate further the role of previous history in predicting the efficacy of MBCT.

EMPIRICAL EVIDENCE

Empirical Support of the Theoretical Model

There is solid support for the basic theoretical model that underlies the MBCT program. Essentially, this model postulates that the reactivation of negative thinking patterns during times of normal sad mood, coupled with ruminative response styles, can increase the vulnerability of formerly depressed individuals to depressive relapse. As reviewed in detail earlier, the large body of research on both ruminative processes in depression and cognitive reactivity provides a strong evidence base for the central theory of MBCT.

Empirical Support for the Treatment Model

The MBCT treatment model is supported by rigorous clinical research. Recently, in fact, MBCT was identified as an effective treatment for prevention of relapse in depression by the United Kingdom's National Institute of Clinical Excellence (NICE), which performed a stringent review of the evidence base. Clinical research has demonstrated that individuals with histories of multiple prior episodes can substantially reduce their risk of relapse by participation in MBCT.

Specifically, two large randomized controlled trials have been conducted. In the first clinical trial, 145 participants with histories of recurrent depression at several research sites were randomized to treatment as usual (TAU) or the MBCT program (Teasdale et al., 2000). Participants were required to have had at least two prior episodes of depression and to be in remission for at least 3 months before the start of the trial; all participants had also been previously been treated with antidepressant medication. Among participants with three or more prior episodes of depression, results suggested that participation in MBCT was associated with a significant difference in the rate of relapse compared to TAU. In fact, MBCT patients had nearly half the rate of relapse (37%) as TAU patients (66%). As described earlier, there was a nonsignificant increase in relapse rate among patients with two prior episodes who participated in MBCT. This first clinical trial was subsequently replicated by Ma and Teasdale (2004). In this study, 75 participants were randomly assigned to MBCT or TAU. Again, results suggested a significant reduction in risk for patients with three or more prior episodes who were assigned to MBCT compared to those assigned to TAU (relapse rates of 36 vs. 78%).

Recently, investigators also have begun to explore the role of MBCT in the treatment of acute depression. Kenny and Williams (2007) examined MBCT for individuals with MDD, bipolar disorder in the depressed phase, or dysthymia. All participants with MDD were required to have a prior history of three or more episodes, or to be currently experiencing depression related to ruminative thought patterns that had lasted more than 1 year. All participants could continue to take ADM while participating in the study. Results indicated that MBCT was effective in reducing Beck Depression Inventory (BDI) scores, and the effect was larger for those with more severe depression (BDI score > 25). Investigators have also begun to explore the effects of MBCT on residual symptoms of depression (Kingston, Dooley, Bates, Lawlor, & Malone, 2007). In this preliminary trial, 19 patients with residual symptoms following an acute episode were randomized to MBCT or TAU. A small subset of patients had histories of bipolar II disorder (*n* = 2), and nearly half of the patients had histories of self-harm. The majority of patients were receiving concurrent pharmacotherapy. Results were promising, indicating significant improvement in depressive symptoms as measured by the BDI among patients assigned to MBCT. Taken together, such studies reflect promising first efforts to utilize MBCT as not only a relapse prevention program but also an intervention for acute depression.

Another pilot study examined the use of MBCT for the recurrence of suicidal behavior (*n* = 16; Williams, Duggan, Crane, & Fennell, 2006). Investigators reported that participants on the whole reacted positively to the program and demonstrated an increase in mindfulness over the course of the group. The experiences of one client, "Maria," were described in detail. This client showed a decrease in drug and alcohol consumption posttreatment. She also described the ways she disengaged from automatic thought patterns and limited her experience of frustrations by tuning into her emotions. The experience of thoughts from a decentered perspective allowed this participant and others to recognize that thoughts, including thoughts about suicide, do not require action.

CLINICAL PRACTICE

Principles for Practice

Perhaps the most important guiding principle of MBCT is the instructor's own personal mindfulness practice. The theory of MBCT suggests that bringing a compassionate and curious awareness to experience, including painful emotional states, is a critical skill to develop in preventing relapse in depression. To guide participants in the development of this skill, it is important for instructors to draw upon their own experience in the development of the very same skills of awareness and compassion. In our experience, it is extremely difficult for instructors to respond effectively to participant questions and problems in the absence of their own personal practice. Instructors may instead respond with anxiety or confusion to the struggles that participants experience as they begin to practice mindfulness. In such states, instructors may be more likely to depart from the mindfulness framework into a more familiar therapeutic mode of "fixing" or "changing" the participants' experiences.

Additionally, the arousal of such reactions, without the context of a strong mindfulness practice in which to experience them, can make it difficult for instructors to attend to the range of demands in leading the group. The MBCT instructor is asked simultaneously to maintain the structure of the class (e.g., pay attention to the agenda and the time), the process of the group (e.g., who has spoken, who has not, how members are responding to one another), and the theme of the session (described in detail below), and to lead specific practices (e.g., yoga, sitting meditation), integrating mindfulness with a focus on depression or cognitive behavioral strategies, the balance between teaching experientially and didactically, and one's own moment-by-moment experience in the group. This complex interplay of activities can be extremely challenging without the presence of awareness, acceptance, and compassion.

Finally, one of the most important vehicles of teaching in MBCT is the instructor's embodiment of central aspects of the approach. As Segal et al. (2002) explain:

> The instructors' own basic understanding and orientation will be one of the most powerful influences.... Whether the instructor realizes it or not, this understanding colors the way each practice is presented, each interaction is handled ... whatever the explicit message of the instructor's words, the more powerful influences, for good or ill, will be the nature of the instructor's basic, implicit understanding. (pp. 65–66)

As instructors guide the insession practices, they are asked to guide from their own moment-to-moment experience. In this way, instructors are required to know the treatment manual well *and* to refer to it sparingly in the room, as opposed to, for instance, reading from transcripts in the manual (Segal et al., 2002). In each interaction with group participants, instructors also teach through embodying the qualities of mindfulness. Instructors are asked to bring interest, openness, and compassion to the full range of each participant's evolving experiences throughout the 8-week course. Embodying these qualities can be extremely challenging without a solid foundation of one's own personal mindfulness practice as a context for one's own learning and practice.

Relatedly, the emphasis on experiential learning is a key principle for practice. There are a number of vehicles of such experiential learning, including the role of in-session practice and inquiry, at-home practice, and poetry and metaphor. Although instructors may have information to impart in a given session, the guiding principle is to allow participants to learn from "doing." Thus, it is preferred that key "information" emerge naturally from participants' experiences in each class. The process of leading the formal practices itself provides a context for teaching, as instructors guide participants to practice with qualities such as awareness, acceptance, and kindness. In these ways, participants are encouraged to develop, for instance, compassion for themselves—not through an explicit or didactic focus on the importance or value of self-compassion, but through being guided, again and again, in a gentle and kind manner to return their awareness to the target of the practice, letting go of judgment as best they can. Compassion is thus "taught" through the experience of the compassion of the instructor and through the micromoments of compassion that arise in one's own direct moment-to-moment practice.

In addition, the process of inquiry provides a key context in which "teaching" occurs. Leading inquiry can be a challenging practice, for it asks the instructor to find ways to weave key points into live, immediate feedback from participants. In this way, optimally, teaching points emerge organically from the experiences of participants as opposed to being delivered in a didactic fashion by the instructor. In this context, there is also a strong emphasis on asking for the full range of feedback from participants (including negative or critical feedback), using open-ended questions and encouraging participants' own curiosity about their experience.

The emphasis on homework is a key part of experiential learning, and between sessions, participants are asked to engage in different experiential practices. The value of homework is highlighted with participants' first contact in the initial interview, before the commencement of the group. In this interview, the instructor emphasizes the importance of at-home practice to learning, and the important qualities of patience and perseverance over the course of the program. The instructor explains that the primary "work" of MBCT occurs not in the classes but between the classes at home. The classes provide an opportunity to experience new practices with the guidance of the instructor and to discuss experiences with the at-home practice, including struggles that arise, ways to work skillfully with such difficulties, and the relevance of such practices to preventing depression from recurring.

The experiential emphasis is also present in the frequent use of metaphor and poetry to convey core themes of the program. The use of poetry is expected to evoke a direct experience with core themes of the program, such as staying present, accepting, and taking skillful action. Poetry has the potential to help participants engage with these themes in novel and immediate ways that may be less accessible with more didactic methods of teaching.

Thus, the key principles for practice in MBCT relate specifically to the paramount importance of practice itself, both for the instructor in leading and embodying the core teachings, and for the participant in engaging directly and experientially with all aspects of the program.

Distinctive Features of the Approach

In addition to the emphasis on the experiential practice of instructor and participant, as discussed earlier, there are two distinguishing characteristics of MBCT. First, the specific integration of mindfulness and cognitive behavioral strategies distinguishes MBCT from other cognitive-behavioral and other mindfulness-based modalities. Second, the role of the instructor is distinct.

Within the MBCT program, mindfulness practice is taught within the direct and specific context of learning to work skillfully with the thoughts, emotions, and bodily sensations that create vulnerability to depressive relapse. The first half of the MBCT program focuses heavily on the development of participants' mindfulness practice as an essential foundation; the second half of the program focuses on taking skillful action to prevent depression. Thus, the structure of the program intertwines the traditions of mindfulness and cognitive-behavioral therapy for depression. Toward this end, each class is organized around a specific theme that is conveyed both through the particular practices that are taught and the inquiry with group members following each practice.

The first session begins with a focus on the theme of automatic pilot. The first mindfulness practice, eating a raisin with awareness, is intended to allow participants to experience a new way of engaging with a habitual activity, such as eating. The practice begins with the instructor giving a raisin to each person and inviting participants to focus their attention on the raisin, as if they have never seen a raisin before. The instructor then guides the group through the process of observing the raisin with each of the senses (e.g., sight, touch, smell, taste), bringing awareness systematically to the direct and immediate sensations arising through contact with the raisin. Following this practice, the instructor leads a process of "inquiry," which is a core feature of the MBCT model. Through inquiry, the instructor explores participants' direct experiences of the practice and weaves into this discussion a focus on the key theme of the session. In session 1 inquiry allows for an exploration of the ways participants experienced a new way of "being" in relation to the familiar activity of eating, and the differences between this mode and the experience of "automatic pilot" that typically is involved in activities such as eating a raisin. From this basis of exploring direct experience, there is a seamless movement to exploring the ways "automatic pilot" can be especially dangerous for individuals with histories of depression, and the ways mindfulness may be relevant for staying well.

Session 2 addresses the theme of "dealing with the barriers" that arise frequently as participants begin to engage with formal mindfulness practices, such as the body scan. This session provides a critical opportunity for the instructor to embody the qualities of mindfulness in responding to the challenges that most participants experience. The instructor welcomes the full range of experiences, bringing curiosity, acceptance, and openness to the feedback that each participant provides. In addition, participants are invited to begin to bring mindfulness into their everyday experiences, with practices such as noticing pleasant events (to be followed by noticing unpleasant events in session 3), and to bring awareness to daily activities, such as eating, showering, driving, and so forth.

Session 3 continues to build the foundation of mindful awareness, with a focus on the theme "mindfulness of the breath." In this session, a number of formal mindfulness practices are taught, including sitting meditation, yoga stretching, and mindful walking. Each provides a way to engage with the breath as an anchor into the present moment and to begin to connect with sensations in the body. Each practice provides a context in which to begin to notice the workings of one's mind and to engage the practice of returning one's awareness, again and again, to the focus of the mindfulness practice (e.g., breath or body sensations).

Session 4 builds on the formal practices taught in session 3 by exploring the theme of "staying present." In this session, participants are also guided in a more direct awareness of thoughts arising and practice with experiencing thoughts as mental events that arise and pass away in the larger spaciousness of awareness. Participants are guided in an exploration of this theme during the formal sitting practice at the outset of the session, through inquiry, and through identifying directly the typical thoughts and experiences that characterize the territory of depression for them. In addition, in this session, participants begin to explore the ways it is possible to move from an experience of depression that is most often experienced as highly private, personal, and isolating, toward the recognition of the universal themes present in such experiences. Participants may experience this as they realize that thoughts that were a source of personal shame (e.g., "I'm a failure") are also experienced by others. The recognition of such universal experiences may help participants decenter from such thoughts as they gain awareness. In addition, in this session, participants also begin to watch the video, *Healing from Within,* which discusses the MBSR program in detail and provides a sense of shared experience with respect to the mindfulness practices themselves.

Session 5 explores the theme of "allowing and letting be." Extending the theme of the previous session, this class focuses on greeting all experiences, including difficult emotions, with a sense of allowing and letting be. Accepting experience as is, without judgment or efforts to control or alter it, is a key element of the practice in the MBCT program. The skill of acceptance is taught through experiential practice. During the formal sitting practice, participants are invited to be "open to the difficult," bringing a gentle and curious attention to the experiences of difficulty and how they relate to such experiences in the body.

Sessions 6–8 move into a more direct focus on how participants can learn to take care of themselves skillfully in ways that will help to protect them from future relapse. These sessions build direction from the foundation of awareness and kindness that has been cultivated through formal practice and inquiry of sessions 1–5. At this point, opportunities are created to bring those qualities of mindfulness directly to the process of caring for oneself skillfully.

Specifically, session 6 explores the theme "Thoughts are not facts." Although this theme has been woven into many of the prior sessions, in this session participants practice seeing the ways that interpretations color responses to situations and experiencing thoughts as mental events as opposed to "truth." Sessions 7 and 8 explore the themes "How can I best take care of myself?" and "Using what's been learned to deal with future moods," respectively. These sessions focus on identifying early warning signs of depression and defining a relapse prevention plan. The importance of bringing a kind and gentle awareness to the task of self-care and identifying the links between activities and mood are discussed. Participants are asked to identify events that bring pleasure and mastery and to explore ways that such activities may comprise a "relapse prevention kit." In the final session, there is a weaving together of all the prior strands of the program, highlighting what participants have learned over the past 2 months that they can bring to bear on taking care of themselves to prevent future depressive relapse. Instructors also help participants explore how they will continue to integrate mindfulness into their daily lives, including a discussion of both formal and informal practices. In addition, this session provides an opportunity for participants to come full circle, returning again to the practice of the body scan in session, and creating time as the group ends for reflections and feedback about the experience and what they learned.

The Role of the Instructor

MBCT is distinguished by the unique role of the instructor. The MBCT instructor is asked to develop expertise in a wide range of clinical skills, including (1) teaching mindfulness meditation practice, yoga, and cognitive-behavioral models and strategies; (2) facilitating groups; and (3) understanding the psychopathology of depression adequately enough to be informed by the theoretical model underpinning MBCT and to be equipped to recognize when a participant is relapsing, and to help him or her access the help that may be required. More importantly, each of the competencies must be held within the context of the instructor's own mindfulness practice and his or her skill in bringing that practice into each class session. Thus, the most important aspect of the instructor's role is embodying the core teachings of the program: moment-to-moment awareness, decentering, kindness, and openness to all experience. These qualities inform both leading the specific mindfulness practices and each interaction with participants during inquiry, discussion of homework, assigning of homework, and so forth.

Case Illustration

Rachel, a 34-year-old woman referred by her general practitioner for participation in MBCT, had two prior episodes of depression, one of which occurred during college and the other when she was 30 years old. The episode during college lasted for approximately 6 months, during which time Rachel was required to take a leave of absence from school. Her second episode of depression was precipitated by a move to a new state, shortly after she was married. She was treated during both episodes with ADM, which she maintained in both cases for approximately 1 year following the resolution of the depressive episode. Two years prior to starting the MBCT group, Rachel gave birth to a son and left her job as a software designer to stay home and care for him. She had recently started to work again on a part-time basis and had reported to her general practitioner that she was concerned about managing the stress of work and family, and its potential impact on her mood. Her physician recommended the MBCT group as a preventive intervention for Rachel to consider. Rachel participated in a group with six other members, all of whom had prior histories of major depression and were currently in remission or experiencing substantial progress in another primary concurrent treatment.

Individual Interview

Prior to initiating the 8-week group sequence, it is recommended that the instructor conduct individual interviews with each potential group member. This allows the instructor to learn more detail about the potential participant's interests and background, to describe the MBCT model and approach, to underscore and discuss the importance of the daily homework practices that are a key component of the intervention, and to discuss any concerns the potential participant may have. In this interview, Rachel was enthusiastic about the MBCT model and its potential relevance to her life history and experience. She reported some concerns about her ability to devote adequate time for homework but said she was motivated to give it her best effort. She expressed more skepticism about the group format. She said she was concerned that talking about depression each week with a group of people with similar histories would be "depressing" and might itself induce relapse.

Week 1

Rachel was an active member of the group in the first week and reported connecting strongly to the metaphor of "automatic pilot," discussed following the mindfulness of eating practice. Rachel reported that since she had returned to work, she believed that the only way she could function was to be on automatic pilot, yet she quickly grasped the ways this same pattern might place her at increased risk for relapse. The instructor posed a question central to the MBCT program, asking, "How might learning to pay attention in this kind of intentional, present-focused, and accepting way help us to take care of ourselves differently and prevent depression from returning?" Rachel and the other group members talked about the parts of their lives that they "missed" by not paying attention, and Rachel talked at length about patterns of thought that "leave me stuck in just them, like it's impossible to notice much else." These conversations provided an important foundation to move into the body scan mindfulness practice as a way of exploring this new way to pay attention. Rachel left the first group feeling optimistic about its value and with the intention to practice the body scan and mindfully to prepare her son's breakfast each day for homework prior to week 2.

Week 2

The second week begins with the practice of the body scan, followed by inquiry about participants' direct experience of the practice, and reflections on "how this is different from the way you normally pay attention to experience" and on the relevance of such practice to preventing depression. Compared to the first session, Rachel was more reserved as this session began, as many group members expressed finding the practice to be very relaxing. Her participation shifted, however, following another group member's report that he "hated" the body scan.

The instructor welcomed this feedback from the group member. She expressed appreciation for the opportunity to discuss the wide range of experiences that are possible with the body scan practice and to clarify the intention of the practice in bringing awareness to any experience, relaxing or not. In her response, the instructor embodied for the group members how to approach difficulty with a spirit of kindness, curiosity, and patience. She asked a number of important questions about the group member's experience. She inquired about the ways in which he had hated the practice, when such feelings arose in the practice, how long they lasted, and whether thoughts or body sensations accompanied the fluctuating range of such feelings. These questions, posed in a gentle and curious manner, expressed genuine interest in exploring the difficulties he experienced. At this point, Rachel stated that she too had great difficulty with the body scan. She said that she felt like she was never "doing it right." She was sleepy during the practice in the group and reported that although she tried hard to do the practice at home, she regularly fell asleep and found herself discouraged by her "failure."

Rachel's description of her experiences provided an important context in which to explore common early misperceptions about mindfulness practice. In particular, the instructor examined with group members the range of ways people can think that they are doing the practice "wrong," including drowsiness or sleepiness, boredom, wandering attention, or physical discomfort. By emphasizing the commonality of such experiences among group members, the instructor invited participants to experience such difficulties not as personal failings but as inherent to the nature of the practice itself. Rachel described how this was a great relief to her, as she had assumed that everyone else was "doing it right."

During the second session, the instructor also introduced the cognitive model of depression and the ways automatic thought patterns can influence emotional responses. Rachel connected this discussion immediately to her experience of the body scan, noticing the ways in which the thought "I can't do this" was connected to her sense of frustration and discouragement. The second week ended with assigned homework, including the pleasant events calendar on which group members were asked to report their experiences of pleasant events as they occurred each day.

Weeks 3–5

Following the second session, group members are asked to practice with a sitting meditation focused on mindfulness of breathing; this same practice is then used to start the third session. In addition, the instructor leads practices of mindful yoga and walking, both of which provide a way to practice mindful movement. Rachel experienced considerable self-judgment in the context of these practices, reporting thoughts such as, "I used to be in such better shape. I can barely do these simple poses now." The instructor embodied for Rachel an attitude of acceptance and curiosity, inviting Rachel to return to what she experienced in her body during these practices and encouraging her to move gradually into the practice of noticing and letting go of judgmental thoughts as they arose. The instructor emphasized the importance of noticing when the mind wanders, including to self-critical and judgmental thoughts, and returning again and again to the focus of the practice. As is often repeated in MBCT, the instructor highlighted an essential maxim of mindfulness practice: "If your mind wanders a hundred times, then simply bring it back a hundred times." Rachel began to practice the yoga postures for a few minutes each morning and, over time, began to report the importance of this practice as a way of taking care of her body and approaching her experience in a more open and allowing manner.

During week 4, the instructor led a mindfulness practice in which Rachel and other group members were invited to notice the experience of thinking itself. During the practice, the instructor guided group members to experience thoughts as events arising in the mind, to notice them like clouds passing in an open sky of awareness. This was a radically new notion for Rachel, who seemed intrigued. At the end of the practice, she asked, "You were asking us to notice our thoughts coming and going, isn't that right? Are you saying that I can notice any thoughts, like even when I think 'I can't do this,' I just notice that as a thought?"

Identifying and discussing the automatic thoughts common to depression provided an important context in which to continue this inquiry with Rachel. She identified the thought "I hate myself" as the most characteristic thought when she was depressed. As the instructor asked for others' feedback, three other members of the group identified the same thought. Rachel shared that this was a very important source of understanding for her. She explained,

"I've been to a lot of psychiatrists who have given me medication and told me that those thoughts are just thoughts and I shouldn't listen to them or put much stock in them when I'm depressed, but I never really believed that. There is something about hearing that all these other people have the same thought. It's like, if they all have this thought, then maybe it's not just about me, maybe it is just a thought."

The instructor wove into the inquiry an emphasis on ways the automatic patterns of depression can create an isolation that strengthens one's perception of the power and reality of the thoughts that arise. This was then contrasted with the opportunity that mindfulness practice offers to observe the ways the mind works that are not necessarily true or personal. Although this was the aspect of the group that Rachel had feared would be "depressing," in contrast, she found this inquiry to be very beneficial. Explaining the ways she had previously believed her struggles with self-judgment and depression were specific to her, she reported feeling a great sense of relief in learning how many other people in the group had struggled with similar challenges and difficulties.

Rachel returned to session 5, reporting with some delight, "I did it! I was practicing this week and I noticed myself thinking, 'If my boss could only see me now, sitting on this cushion. He would think this was ridiculous.' It was so strange, though, it really didn't bother me. I noticed the thought and it just kind of came and went." The instructor asked about ways that Rachel might have "automatically" responded to such thoughts in the past. Rachel explained that typically she tried to ignore such thoughts, or she would tell herself that they were "silly." She explained, "I can feel kind of ashamed of having to do this whole program here, and of my whole history really. So I tell myself not to think that way, which sometimes just leaves me feeling worse." In this way, Rachel began to notice the way her automatic patterns of attempting to avoid such thought patterns with additional self-criticism could actually initiate a cycle in which she ended up feeling down. Bringing awareness to the thought patterns, without reacting with judgment, was an important alternative way of responding that Rachel began to explore.

During this time, Rachel also began to practice the 3-minute breathing space, which is intended to help members bring mindfulness in a structured way into daily life routines. It is, in a sense, a bridge between the formal practices of the body scan, sitting meditation, and mindful stretching or walking, and the informal practices of everyday life. Rachel learned to bring her attention to her present-moment experience, to anchor her attention in her breathing, and to bring a centered and spacious attention to the next moments of her day. She practiced the 3-minute breathing space during regular daily transitions, including after she dropped her son off at child care, before starting her car, and when she left work. She then began to use the breathing space during stressful times and reported it to be an extremely beneficial way of approaching such challenges with a mindful as opposed to reactive presence. She explained, "It's like my mind goes through these chain of reactions so quickly. One second, I'm feeling fine and then in the next, I'm anxious and miserable. The breathing space is helping me learn to watch it happen. It's like I can watch the spiral happen instead of getting sucked down by it."

Rachel also found that viewing the videotape *Healing from Within,* presented in sessions 4 and 5, was a powerful experience, particularly combined with reviewing the symptoms and common thought patterns of depression with other group members, as described earlier. Watching the videotape also enhanced Rachel's motivation to learn and practice. She explained,

> "I can see all of these thoughts and symptoms in my history. I don't want to experience this again, especially now that I have my son to care for. And I see how other people have kept at this with really challenging lives too. I feel like there is so much at stake for me and my family to not do this. I realize what we are learning is so important."

Weeks 6–8

The foundation of the first five sessions provided for Rachel's group a springboard from which to move into the focus on how to bring mindfulness to the task of taking care of oneself in a different way to help prevent depressive relapse. Rachel described this eloquently in one class, explaining,

"In the past, it has been more of a pattern in which I think I'm just in a bad mood. It's just a bad mood. Then—and I don't see this happening—all of a sudden, I can't get out of bed. I just don't want to do anything. I think what I've been learning here is helping me realize when it's more than just a bad mood. I can see it coming *and* I can do something differently very early on in the process. I'm developing this awareness of what's happening and knowing that I can change how I respond to it. That's really new for me."

In this context of awareness, group members begin to examine their regular daily activities and the degree to which such activities provide a sense of nourishment or depletion of energy. In addition, they examine activities that provide a sense of mastery or pleasure, and the ways in which such activities can help to provide protection against depressive relapse.

These practices allowed Rachel to develop an action plan to implement should early warning signs of depression arise in the future. She wrote a letter to herself that summarized the ways she could take action, including talking to her husband, talking walks in the park near her house, calling a friend, taking a warm bath, listening to a favorite CD, monitoring how much sleep she was getting and making increased sleep a priority, regular practice of the 3-minute breathing space, and calling her doctor if symptoms persisted.

At the conclusion of the group, Rachel reported that she had developed a detailed awareness of her patterns of "automatic pilot" and the ways they placed her at risk for relapse of depression. In particular, she was aware of the ways she tended to respond to feelings of sadness and shame by attempting to eradicate them with self-judgment and critical thought. She had also developed the skill of bringing a kind and gentle awareness to such patterns, with which she could both notice their onset at an earlier point and allow them to fade on their own accord. In addition, she ended the 8-week class with a detailed list of activities that she knew were important to maintaining a positive mood and responding effectively if her mood declined in the future. She had integrated a regular morning practice of mindful movement and the 3-minute breathing space, which she felt confident she would continue in the future. She also was very positive about the ways she was bringing mindful awareness to many of the regular daily activities of her life, including interacting with her coworkers and parenting her son. She ended the group with a sense of both gratitude and optimism.

SUMMARY AND CONCLUSIONS

MBCT is a brief group treatment that integrates the traditions of mindfulness meditation and CBT to help individuals with histories of depression develop practices that help prevent the relapse and recurrence of major depression. This chapter has reviewed the history of the development of MBCT, the basic theoretical model that guides the practice, the evidence base, and the clinical practice of MBCT. Distinguishing principles, strategies, and structural elements have been discussed, and key components have been illustrated by the case of a woman who completed the 8-week MBCT course.

Research addressing the key tenets of the MBCT model and its application to a wide array of clinical populations is emerging rapidly. Investigators are examining increasingly its application to individuals with current depressive symptomatology, as well as to subpopulations of depressed patients for whom extant treatment options are severely limited (e.g., pregnant and postpartum women). In addition, it will be important for future studies to examine in more detail the active ingredients of MBCT, parsing out the relative importance of the attentional components of mindfulness, the elements of compassion, the cognitive-behavioral skills, and the context of group support. Finally, as interest in MBCT expands, it may be important to explore novel methods with which to deliver core elements of the intervention. To date, little attention has been devoted to dissemination challenges that face MBCT and related interventions. As previously discussed, MBCT instructors are asked to develop a broad array of clinical competencies and to have a committed personal mindfulness practice. MBCT participants are asked to adhere to intensive demands for daily homework practice. It may be important to examine the ways these characteristics may limit the transportability of such approaches, what creative alternatives exist for disseminating MBCT (e.g., the telephone, the Internet, and self-guided print materials; Williams, Teasdale, Segal, & Kabat-Zinn, 2007), and whether the essential characteristics of MBCT can be retained in such formats. Each of these areas represents new and exciting frontiers for the investigation of MBCT and the potential value that its unique integration of mindfulness and cognitive-behavioral therapy may bring to individuals struggling with depression.

REFERENCES

American Psychiatric Association. (2000). Practice guideline for the treatment of patients with major depressive disorder (revision). *American Journal of Psychiatry, 157*(Suppl. 4).

Basco, M. R., & Rush, A. J. (1995). Compliance with pharmacology in mood disorders. *Psychiatric Annals, 25,* 269–275.

Beck, A. T. (1967). *Cognitive therapy and the emotional disorders.* New York: Meridian.

Beck, A. T., Rush, A. J., Shaw, B. F., & Emery, G. (1979). *Cognitive therapy of depression.* New York: Guilford Press.

Blackburn, I. M., Eunson, K. M., & Bishop, S. (1986). A two-year naturalistic follow-up of depressed patients treated with cognitive therapy, pharmacotherapy and a combination of both. *Journal of Affective Disorders, 10*(1), 67–75.

Coelho, H. F., Canter, P. H., & Ernst, E. (2007). Mindfulness-based cognitive therapy: Evaluating current evidence and informing future research. *Journal of Consulting and Clinical Psychology, 75*(6), 1000–1005.

Dobson, K. S., Hollon, S. D., Dimidjian, S., Schmaling, K. B., Kohlenberg, R. J., et al. (2008). Randomized trial of behavioral activation, cognitive therapy, and antidepressant medication in the prevention of relapse and recurrence in major depression. *Journal of Consulting and Clinical Psychology, 76*(3), 468–477.

Evans, M. D., Hollon, S. D., DeRubeis, R. J., Piasecki, J. M., Groe, W. M., Garvey, M. J., et al. (1992). Differential relapse following cognitive therapy and pharmacotherapy for depression. *Archives of General Psychiatry, 49,* 802–808.

Hollon, S. D., DeRubeis, R. J., Shelton, R. C., Amsterdam, J. D., Salomon, R. M., O'Reardon, J. P., et al. (2005). Prevention of relapse following cognitive therapy versus medications in moderate to severe depression. *Archives of General Psychiatry, 62,* 417–422.

Hollon, S. D., Thase, M. E., & Markowitz, J. C. (2002). Treatment and prevention of depression. *Psychological Science in the Public Interest, 3,* 39–77.

Judd, L. J. (1997). The clinical course of unipolar major depressive disorders. *Archives of General Psychiatry, 54,* 989–991.

Kabat-Zinn, J. (1990). *Full catastrophe living: Using the wisdom of your body and mind to face stress, pain, and illness.* New York: Dell.

Kenny, M. A., & Williams, J. M. G. (2007). Treatment-resistant depressed patients show a good response to mindfulness-based cognitive therapy. *Behaviour Research and Therapy, 45*(3), 617–625.

Kingston, T., Dooley, B., Bates, A., Lawlor, E., & Malone, K. (2007). Mindfulness-based cognitive therapy for residual depressive symptoms. *Psychology and Psychotherapy: Theory, Research and Practice, 80,* 193–203.

Kovacs, M., Rush, A., Beck, A. T., & Hollon, S. D. (1981). Depressed outpatients treated with cognitive therapy or pharmacotherapy: A one-year follow-up. *Archives of General Psychiatry, 38*(1), 33–39.

Ma, S. H., & Teasdale, J. D. (2004). Mindfulness-based cognitive therapy for depression: Replication and exploration of differential relapse prevention effects. *Journal of Consulting and Clinical Psychology, 72*(1), 31–40.

Nolen-Hoeksema, S. (1991). Responses to depression and their effects on the duration of depressive episodes. *Journal of Abnormal Psychology, 100,* 569–582.

Olfson, M., Marcus, S. C., Druss, B., Elinson, L., Tanielian, T., & Pincus, H. A. (2002). National trends in the outpatient treatment of depression. *Journal of the American Medical Association, 287,* 203–209.

Scher, C. D., Ingram, R. E., & Segal, Z. V. (2005). Cognitive reactivity and vulnerability: Empirical evaluation of construct activation and cognitive diatheses in unipolar depression. *Clinical Psychology Review, 25,* 487–510.

Segal, Z. V., Gemar, M. C., & Williams, S. (1999). Differential cognitive response to a mood challenge following successful cognitive therapy or pharmacotherapy for unipolar depression. *Journal of Abnormal Psychology, 108,* 3–10.

Segal, Z. V., Kennedy, S., Gemar, M., Hood, K., Pedersen, R., & Buis, T. (2006). Cognitive reactivity to sad mood provocation and the prediction of depressive relapse. *Archives of General Psychiatry, 63,* 750–755.

Segal, Z. V., Williams, J. M. G., & Teasdale, J. D. (2002). *Mindfulness-based cognitive therapy for depression.* New York: Guilford Press.

Shea, M. T., Elkin, I., Imber, S. D., Sotsky, F. M., Watkins, J. T., Collins, J. F., et al. (1992). Course of depressive symptoms over follow-up: Findings from the NIMH Treatment of Depression Collaborative Research Program. *Archives of General Psychiatry, 49,* 782–787.

Simons, A., Garfield, S. L., & Murphy, G. E. (1984). The process of change in cognitive therapy and pharmacotherapy for depression. *Archives of General Psychiatry, 41,* 45–51.

Simons, A. D., Murphy, G. E., Levine, J. L., & Wetzel, R. D. (1986). Cognitive therapy and pharmacotherapy for depression: Sustained improvement over one year. *Archives of General Psychiatry, 43*(1), 43–48.

Teasdale, J. D. (1988). Cognitive vulnerability to persistent depression. *Cognition and Emotion, 2,* 247–274.

Teasdale, J. D. (1999). Emotional processing, three modes of mind and the prevention of relapse in depression. *Behaviour Research and Therapy, 37,* S53–S77.

Teasdale, J. D., Moore, R. G., Hayhurst, H., Pope, M., Williams, S., & Segal, Z. V. (2002). Metacognitive awareness and prevention of relapse in depression: Empirical evidence. *Journal of Consulting and Clinical Psychology, 70,* 275–287.

Teasdale, J. D., Segal, Z. V., Williams, J. M. G., Ridgeway, V., Soulsby, J., & Lau, M. (2000). Prevention of relapse/recurrence in major depression by mindfulness-based cognitive therapy. *Journal of Consulting and Clinical Psychology, 68,* 615–623.

Teasdale, J. D., Taylor, M. J., Cooper, Z., Hayhurst, H., & Paykel, E. S. (1995). Depressive thinking: Shifts in construct accessibility or in schematic mental models? *Journal of Abnormal Psychology, 104*(3), 500–507.

Williams, J. M. G., Duggan, D., Taylor. S., Crane, C., & Fennell, M. J. (2006). Mindfulness-based cognitive therapy for prevention of recurrence of suicidal behavior. *Journal of Clinical Psychology, 62,* 201–210.

Williams, J. M. G., Russell, I., & Russell, D. (2008). Mindfulness-based cognitive therapy: Further issues in current evidence and future research. *Journal of Consulting and Clinical Psychology, 76*(3), 524–529.

Williams, M., Teasdale, J., Segal, Z., & Kabat-Zinn, J. (2007). *The mindful way through depression: Freeing yourself from chronic unhappiness.* New York: Guilford Press.

Wisner, K., Zarin, D. A., Holmboe, E. S., Applebaum, P. S., Gelenberg, A. J., Leonard, H. L., et al. (2000). Risk–benefit decision making for treatment of depression during pregnancy. *American Journal of Psychiatry, 157*, 1933–1940.

CHAPTER 11

Emotion-Focused/ Interpersonal Cognitive Therapy

Jeremy D. Safran
Catherine Eubanks-Carter
J. Christopher Muran

INTRODUCTION AND HISTORICAL BACKGROUND

Over the last two decades, Jeremy Safran and colleagues (e.g., Greenberg & Safran, 1987; Safran, 1998; Safran & Greenberg, 1986, 1991; Safran & Muran, 2000; Safran & Segal, 1990/1996) have endeavored to widen the scope of cognitive therapy by integrating principles from other theoretical traditions. In particular, our work has focused on the following three areas: the role of emotion in the change process, interpersonal processes in cognitive therapy, and ruptures in the therapeutic alliance (Safran, 1998). In this chapter, we summarize some of our contributions to these areas by discussing the theoretical basis of our work, presenting relevant empirical evidence, illustrating clinical applications, and exploring future directions.

Prior to the 1980s, cognitive therapy took an overly restrictive view of emotions. Emotions were regarded as a postcognitive phenomenon: it was assumed that faulty cognitive processes led to negative emotions, and that these cognitions must be changed to modify the negative emotions. The role of positive emotions was generally neglected in the cognitive therapy literature.

Beginning in the early 1980s, Leslie Greenberg and Jeremy Safran began a collaborative project aimed at articulating the role that various forms of affective experience can play in the change process (Greenberg & Safran, 1987, 1989; Safran & Greenberg, 1986, 1987, 1988, 1991). Greenberg and Safran (1987) synthesized relevant theory and research on the topic of emotion and advocated for the importance of delineating a variety of different affective change processes in psychotherapy. They argued that emotions play an essential role in human functioning, and that psychological problems are often the result of blocking or avoiding potentially adaptive emotional experiences. Greenberg and Safran described how resistance to emotions could be overcome in therapy to access underlying affective experience. In Safran and Greenberg (1991), they expanded upon the theoretical and therapeutic implications of their understanding of the role of emotions in human functioning by providing detailed descriptions of affective change events in different therapeutic orientations.

At about the same time, Safran also began to explore his interest in interpersonal processes in cognitive therapy. Influenced by the work of Harry Stack Sullivan, Donald Kiesler, and John Bowlby (among others), Safran began to develop a systemic framework for thinking about the therapeutic relationship in cognitive therapy (Safran, 1984, 1986, 1990a, 1990b). In *Interpersonal Process in Cognitive Therapy*, Safran and Segal (1990/1996) developed the notion of the *interpersonal schema*, an internal representation of self–other relationships that initially develops to maintain proximity to attachment figures. Interpersonal schemas guide the processing of interpersonal information and shape the individual's characteristic patterns of interaction with others. Safran and Segal noted that cognitive therapists tended to view relational factors as separate from the active ingredients of therapy—as a prerequisite for change rather than an intrinsic part of change. Safran and Segal argued that relational and technical factors are interdependent; therapeutic interventions can only be understood in the context of the relationship between the therapist and the patient. Safran and Segal also integrated Safran and Greenberg's work on emotion in psychotherapy by emphasizing the importance of accessing the patient's affective experience as a mechanism for change.

Safran and colleagues' third area of interest is the resolution of ruptures, or impasses, in the therapeutic alliance (Safran, 1993; Safran, Crocker, McMain, & Murray, 1990; Safran & Muran, 1996, 2000; Safran, Muran, & Samstag, 1994; Safran, Muran, Samstag, & Stevens, 2001). Our thinking in this area was influenced by a variety of sources, including Edward Bordin's (1979) conceptualization of the working alliance, mother–infant developmental research (Beebe & Lachman, 2002; Tronick, 1989), and Kohut's (1971, 1977, 1984) thinking on the topic of empathic failures. Beginning in the mid-1980s, Safran and colleagues, most notably J. Christopher Muran, have been conducting research on the role of the therapeutic relationship in the change process. Our work has focused on identifying impasses, or ruptures, in the therapeutic alliance, and developing models for resolving them. This work has helped to usher in a new generation of alliance research that moves beyond establishing the alliance as a predictor of outcome, and toward elucidating the processes involved in identifying and resolving deteriorations in the patient–therapist relationship (Safran & Muran, 1996; Safran et al., 2001).

Based on our research on alliance ruptures, we have developed a short-term therapy approach called *brief relational therapy* (BRT; Safran & Muran, 2000). BRT is an integrative treatment that builds on Safran's earlier work on emotion and interpersonal processes by synthesizing principles from humanistic and experiential psychotherapy and contemporary theories on cognition and emotion, as well as relational psychoanalysis. As we describe in greater detail later in this chapter, studies of the efficacy of BRT have found that it is as effective as cognitive therapy for the treatment of patients with Cluster C and personality disorder not otherwise specified (NOS) diagnoses (Muran, Safran, Samstag, & Winston, 2005). In addition, we have found preliminary evidence that BRT is more effective than cognitive therapy for patients with whom therapists have difficulty establishing therapeutic alliances (Safran, Muran, Samstag, & Winston, 2005). Currently, we are studying whether training cognitive therapists in the use of BRT rupture resolution strategies will lead to improvements in therapy process and outcome.

PHILOSOPHICAL AND THEORETICAL UNDERPINNINGS

As noted previously, early cognitive theory was based on the premise that emotion is a postcognitive phenomenon (Beck, 1976; Ellis, 1962). This conceptualization was influenced by the information-processing model in cognitive psychology (Dobson & Block, 1988) and its concept of the *schema*, a cognitive structure for organizing and processing information (Bartlett, 1932; Neisser, 1967; Singer & Salovey, 1991).

However, human beings do not process static information. Rather, we interact with our environment and acquire information through action (Shaw & Bransford, 1977). This link between cognition and action is captured by the *ecological model of perception* (Gibson, 1979). According to this model, human beings are biological organisms that live and operate in the context of specific environments and have adapted to our environmental niche through an evolutionary process. We actively perceive information from our environment concerning our adaptation to that environment. This evolutionary perspective is consistent with developments in contemporary emotion theory indicating that the emotional processing system evolved because it plays an adaptive role in human functioning (Greenberg & Safran, 1987; Safran & Greenberg, 1986, 1988). According to this perspective, emotions provide us with information about how we are interacting with and adapting to our environment. In particular, emotions give us feedback about the actions in which we are prepared to engage. Specific emotions correspond to specific self-protective behaviors. For example, when we perceive a situation as dangerous, we experience the emotion of fear, which gives us feedback that we are prepared to flee. Fear in a dangerous situation also leads us to value flight over other goals, such as eating and sleeping. In this way, emotions help us to prioritize goals in service of our survival.

Because emotions play an adaptive role in the survival of the species, the basic structure for emotional experience is considered to be neurologically hardwired (Izard, 1977; Plutchik, 1980; Tomkins, 1980). However, emotional responses can become elaborated through the process of learning. In particular, early experiences with attachment figures shape emotional responses. The infant's need to form an attachment with a caregiver is a crucial human drive (Bowlby, 1969, 1973, 1980). Maintaining contact and closeness with the caregiver is necessary for the infant's survival. Children learn to regulate their emotions in the process of maintaining relatedness to attachment figures. When the infant's relationship to his or her caregiver is disrupted, the infant experiences anxiety. This anxiety is a cue that alerts the infant to take whatever action is necessary to renew contact with the caregiver. For example, if parents respond to their daughter's anger with anger of their own, the child will learn that expressing her anger disrupts her relationship with her parents, which causes her anxiety. To reduce this anxiety and maintain proximity to her parents, the child will find other ways to regulate her own feelings of anger.

The child's experiences of regulating emotional expressions and other behaviors in interactions with attachment figures become incorporated into the child's long-term memory. Drawing on Tulving's (1983) distinction between episodic and semantic memory, Stern (1985) proposed that the infant encodes specific interactions with the caregiver in episodic memory. Interactions that are similar in nature become averaged in the child's memory over time, leading to the development of a generalized representation in semantic memory. This generalized, or prototypical, representation can be conceptualized as an interpersonal schema (Safran, 1986, 1990a; Safran & Segal, 1990/1996).

People develop interpersonal schemas that are adaptive in a developmental context because the schemas enable them to predict interactions with attachment figures. However, these schemas can become maladaptive if they are carried over into new interpersonal contexts. As an adult, the child who learned to avoid expressing her anger to her parents may have difficulty asserting herself in her relationship with a partner. She may avoid expressing dissatisfaction to her partner until she becomes so frustrated that she loses her temper. If her partner responds to her outburst negatively, then this reinforces her belief that anger is a dangerous emotion and strengthens her fear of asserting herself in the future. Thus, she will maintain her interpersonal expectations and her self-defeating pattern of unassertiveness. This process has been referred to as a *vicious circle* (Horney, 1950; Strachey, 1934; Wachtel, 1997) or a *cognitive-interpersonal cycle* (Safran, 1984, 1990a, 1990b; Safran & Segal, 1990/1996).

Individuals can become trapped in self-defeating cognitive-interpersonal cycles if they continue to adhere rigidly to interpersonal schemas that are no longer adaptive in their current interpersonal contexts. Individuals may fail to modify their schemas because they discount or dissociate schema-inconsistent information (Beck, 1976; Nisbett & Ross, 1980). Beginning with the infant's reaction to threats to the caregiver's proximity, behaviors and experiences that are associated with the disruption or disintegration of relationships come to be identified as dangerous and trigger anxiety. In an effort to cope with this anxiety, an individual may dissociate aspects of experience that elicit anxious feelings. However, dissociated aspects of experience are nonetheless expressed through nonverbal behavior and actions. The resulting incongruent communication results in characteristic responses from others that confirm one's expectations of self–other interactions. For example, an individual who has learned to associate her anger with the disruption of relationships may dissociate her own feelings of anger. However, despite the fact that she does not subjectively experience her anger, she may still behave aggressively and evoke aggression from others. This type of duplicitous communication (Kaiser, 1965) can play a role in psychopathology. Furthermore, by dissociating aspects of emotional experience, an individual is deprived of important information about his or her own goals and needs.

In addition, individuals have difficulty revising rigid schemas, because they have a restricted range of interpersonal behaviors (Carson, 1969, 1982; Kiesler, 1982a, 1982b; Leary, 1957). If an individual continues to pull for the same kinds of responses from others, he or she misses opportunities to have new experiences that would disconfirm his or her interpersonal schemas. For example, an individual who expects others to abandon him if he is vulnerable may take great pains to appear confident and self-reliant. However, this behavior may serve to keep others at a distance, which confirms his belief that vulnerable feelings are unacceptable. Thus, the individual misses the opportunity to have a positive experience of receiving support from others that could lead him to modify his interpersonal schemas.

Implications for Treatment

Cognitive and behavioral therapists have traditionally been critical of the psychoanalytic concept of transference. However, some theorists have argued that the client's behavior in therapy can offer a useful sample of his or her problem behavior (Arnkoff, 1983; Goldfried & Davison, 1976; Kohlenberg & Tsai, 1991; Leahy, 2003; Young, Klosko, & Weishaar, 2006). Safran and colleagues have argued that the therapeutic relationship is an important mechanism of change, and that therapeutic impasses can provide a particularly valuable source of information about the client's interpersonal schemas and opportunities to challenge and to modify them. Both therapist and patient contribute in conscious and unconscious ways to their interaction. *Ruptures* are deteriorations in the therapeutic relationship that emerge when both patient and therapist unwittingly participate in maladaptive cognitive-interpersonal cycles. If the therapist can become aware of the rupture, disengage from the cycle, and draw the patient's attention to what is transpiring between them, then this can lead to an opportunity to challenge the patient's rigid schemas and effect core structural change.

A primary technique for drawing the patient's attention to a rupture in the alliance is *metacommunication*. This term, originally used in a therapeutic context by Kiesler (1996), describes an attempt to increase awareness of each person's role in an interpersonal interaction by stepping out of the interaction and communicating directly about what is taking place between patient and therapist. Although transference interpretations are one form of metacommunication, in our work, metacommunications are not efforts to infer the patient's inner, unconscious experience. Rather, they are grounded in the therapist's immediate experience of the therapeutic relationship, which the therapist self-discloses. For example, the therapist might self-disclose his or her own emotional response to the client by saying, "I feel shut out by you" or "I feel like it would be easy to say something that would offend you." Or the therapist might provide feedback about the client's behavior (e.g., "I experience you as withdrawn right now") or about the therapist's sense of their interaction (e.g., "I have an image of the two of us fencing"). The objective of metacommunication is to articulate the therapist's implicit sense of what is happening in order to begin an explicit exploration of the patient–therapist interaction.

When therapist and patient begin to explore a rupture in the alliance, change can occur via two parallel processes: *decentering* and *disconfirmation* (Safran & Segal, 1990/1996). Decentering involves expanding patients' awareness of both their internal processes and how they interact with others. By attending to their experience with an open, curious, nonjudgmental attitude, patients learn to accept parts of themselves that they have tried to deny or disown. They become mindful of their anxiety and the situations that trigger it, and are able to acknowledge feelings and behaviors that they have dissociated. With greater awareness, patients are able to access a wider range of emotional experiences, which provide valuable feedback about their goals and their adaptation to their interpersonal environment. Through expanded awareness of their interpersonal schemas, patients can deautomate their self-defeating patterns. In addition, patients develop an increased sense of agency: Rather than viewing themselves as passive victims of circumstance, patients take greater responsibility for the choices they make.

As patients become more aware of their interpersonal schemas, the therapeutic relationship also provides an opportunity for the disconfirmation of these schemas. When the therapist does not respond to the patient in the complementary way that the patient expects (e.g., the therapist responds to hostility with compassion rather than counter hostility), this challenges the patient's maladaptive conception of his or her role in relationships. This experience provides the patient with the opportunity to develop more adaptive beliefs that will break the cognitive-interpersonal cycle and lead to behaviors that elicit more positive responses from others.

The therapist's ability to attune to the patient's painful emotions during a rupture, and to tolerate his or her own responses to the impasse, can also be transformative (Safran & Muran, 2000). This type of *containment*, to use Bion's term (1962, 1967, 1970), can help patients learn that neither they nor their relationships will necessarily be destroyed by painful, aggressive feelings. The role of emotional attunement in the therapeutic relationship may be similar to the process of attunement in early parent–child relationships. As Tronick (1989) and Beebe and Lachman (2002) have shown in their research on mother–infant dyads, there is an ongoing oscillation between periods in which mother and infant are affectively attuned, and periods in which they are miscoordinated. Healthy dyads are able to repair these moments of misattunement. Tronick (1989) suggests that this process of miscoordination and repair serves an important purpose: The baby learns to see the mother as potentially available, and to see the self as capable of establishing authentic emotional contact in the face of differences. In the same way, working through alliance ruptures may help the patient to develop healthier interpersonal schemas. The patient can gradually develop a schema that represents the other as potentially available, and the self as capable of negotiating relatedness, even in the context of ruptures (Safran, 1993; Safran & Segal, 1990/1996).

Current Challenges to the Theory

The attention to the role of emotion and interpersonal processes that has been the focus of Safran and colleagues' work is increasingly becoming incorporated into cognitive-behavioral therapy (CBT) treatments. Although CBT treatments have traditionally sought to decrease emotions, particularly negative emotions, a number of recently developed CBT approaches emphasize the value of increasing the client's awareness and acceptance of his or her internal emotional experience. For example, dialectical behavior therapy (DBT; Linehan, 1993), mindfulness-based cognitive therapy (Segal, Williams, & Teasdale, 2002), and acceptance and commitment therapy (Hayes, Strosahl, & Wilson, 1999) note the problems that arise when clients avoid and inhibit their emotional responses. These approaches encourage patients to attend to their emotional experience and allow it to inform and guide their behavior. CBT therapists have also begun to recognize that emotional arousal can be an important part of the change process (Burum & Goldfried, 2007), and that greater attention needs to be paid to the cultivation of positive emotions (Ehrenreich, Fairholme, Buzzella, Ellard, & Barlow, 2007). Samoilov and Goldfried (2000) have suggested that emotional arousal might be necessary to activate fully and change maladaptive belief structures. Barlow's (2002) treatment for panic attacks calls for therapists to induce panic-like symptoms during the session, so that clients can practice using deep breathing and relaxation techniques while their anxiety is activated. Foa and Kozak (1986) have shown that the presence of anxiety helps trauma patients to access and to modify maladaptive fear structures. Similarly, Castonguay, Newman, Borkovec, Holtforth, and Maramba (2005) have emphasized how emotional arousal helps clients with generalized anxiety disorder become more aware of their interpersonal needs.

Castonguay et al.'s (2005) treatment for anxious patients also points to the increasing emphasis on interpersonal processes in CBT treatments. Similarly, Kohlenberg, Kanter, and Bolling (2002) found that the efficacy of cognitive therapy is increased when integrated with elements of functional-analytic psychotherapy (Kohlenberg & Tsai, 1991), which employs principles of reinforcement to treat interpersonal problems. Cognitive-behavioral analysis system of psychotherapy (CBASP; McCullough, 2000), an empirically supported therapy for chronic depression (Keller et al., 2000), also focuses on understanding and changing interpersonal behaviors. Interpersonal effectiveness is a central component of DBT, which has been shown to be successful in improving interpersonal functioning in patients with borderline personality disorder (Linehan, Tutek, Heard, & Armstrong, 1994).

Increasing attention to the importance of emotion and interpersonal processes has expanded the ability of CBT treatments to reach more clients and has fostered more lasting changes. We believe that the effectiveness of CBT treatments can be further increased by placing greater emphasis on the therapeutic relationship. In particular, CBT approaches would benefit from incorporating the *two-person psychological perspective* (Safran & Muran, 2000), which emerges out of contemporary relational developments in psychoanalytic theory. This perspective is the result of a critical reaction to the traditional one-person psychology that emphasizes the individual experience of the patient, while regarding the therapist as a blank screen onto which the patient's fantasies are projected. In contrast to this focus on the patient in isolation, the two-person perspective views the patient–therapist relationship as the object of study, and sees the therapist as an engaged participant in the co-creation of the clinical situation (Aron, 1996; Benjamin, 1988; Mitchell, 1988, 2000; Safran & Muran, 2000).

The two-person perspective has several important clinical implications. First, it suggests that clinical formulations must be guided by and revised in light of information gleaned from an ongoing exploration of what is taking place in the relationship. Second, it is critical that the therapist explore his or her own contributions to the interaction with the patient. Third, the therapist cannot assume that the patient–therapist interaction parallels patterns in the patient's daily life. Because the therapist is also contributing to and shaping the interaction, the extent to which the interaction parallels the patient's other relationships must remain an open question.

Adopting the two-person perspective can draw CBT therapists' attention to the ways they contribute to their interactions with patients. In our current work using BRT with patients with Cluster C and personality disorder NOS diagnoses, the two-person perspective is reflected in our use of metacommunication, whereby the therapist may self-disclose his or her experience of and contribution to the interaction with the patient. However, we recognize that metacommunication is not the only way to incorporate a two-person perspective; furthermore, it may not be productive with certain patient populations. Patients with cognitive limitations may find particular metacommunications confusing, and may benefit from a more traditional, directive, and supportive approach. Patients with certain emotional and interpersonal limitations, who experience the subjectivity of the other person as intrusive, may respond poorly to metacommunications about the therapist's internal experience. For example, patients with severe borderline personality disorder, who have poor ability to mentalize, that is, to think about and understand their own and others' mental states (Allen, Fonagy, & Bateman, 2000; Fonagy, 1991, 2000), may have difficulty understanding and tolerating a therapist's self-disclosure about his or her own internal experience. Therapists working with such patients may make little use of metacommunication during the session. However, adopting a two-person perspective would nevertheless be helpful in guiding therapists' thinking about how their interaction with the patient is shaped by "the beliefs, commitments, hopes, fears, needs, and wishes of both participants" (J. Greenberg, 1995, p. 1).

EMPIRICAL EVIDENCE

Emotion in Psychotherapy

In their work on emotion, Safran and Greenberg hypothesized that interpersonal schemas are coded at both cognitive and affective levels. For this reason, it is important to access the affective level by working with clients in an emotionally alive fashion (Greenberg & Safran, 1987; Safran & Greenberg, 1987). Greenberg and his colleagues have built on these ideas in their research on the role of emotion in psychotherapy. They note that although emotional arousal is necessary for therapeutic progress, it is not sufficient: Emotional processing should also involve the integration of cognition and affect (Greenberg, 2002; Greenberg & Pascual-Leone, 1995). Once emotions are aroused, clients need to be able to reflect on and make sense of their emotions to change their maladaptive state.

Greenberg and colleagues have found empirical evidence of the value of emotional processing in their research on emotion-focused therapy (EFT). Studies of a manualized form of EFT for depression found that emotional processing in therapy predicted a reduction in symptoms and an increase in self-esteem (Goldman, Greenberg, & Pos, 2005; Pos, Greenberg, Goldman, & Korman, 2003). A study of EFT for clients with interpersonal problems and histories of childhood maltreatment found that increased emotional arousal during imagined contact with a significant other was related to good outcome (Greenberg & Malcolm, 2002). Given the centrality of emotional processing in EFT, clinical trials demonstrating the efficacy of EFT (e.g., Goldman, Greenberg, & Angus, 2006; Greenberg & Watson, 1998; Johnson, Hunsley, Greenberg, & Schindler, 1999; Paivio & Greenberg, 1995) offer further evidence of the importance of accessing patients' emotions in therapy.

Interpersonal Schemas

Safran and colleagues have conducted empirical investigations of the construct of interpersonal schemas, using the Interpersonal Schema Questionnaire (ISQ; for a detailed review, see Scarvalone, Fox, & Safran, 2005). Developed by Hill and Safran (1994), the ISQ evaluates individuals' expectations about the ways three different significant others (mother, father, and friend or romantic partner) would respond to a range of interpersonal behaviors. The 16 different interpersonal behaviors were derived from Kiesler's (1982b) interpersonal circle, with one behavior representing each of the 16 segments of the circumplex. Subjects are asked to indicate the type of expected response using a list of descriptors drawn from the octant version of the interpersonal circle (controlling, mistrustful, hostile, distant, submissive, trusting, friendly, or interested). Subjects also rate the desirability of the response.

According to interpersonal schema theory, maladaptive interpersonal schemas predispose individuals to psychopathology. Hill and Safran (1994) administered the ISQ to an undergraduate sample and obtained results consistent with this assertion: Participants with higher levels of symptoms expected more undesirable responses from significant others, whereas participants who reported low levels of psychological symptoms expected responses that were significantly more friendly, sociable, and trusting. In addition, less symptomatic participants expected more friendly responses to their own friendly behaviors, whereas participants with more symptoms expected more hostile responses to their hostile interpersonal behaviors. This finding of expectations of more complementary hostile responses in participants with greater symptomatology was replicated in a sample of Turkish university students (Soygut & Savasir, 2001). Similarly, Huebner, Thomas, and Berven (1999) found that students who used mental health services more frequently expected more hostility and inconsistency, and less satisfaction in their relationships than students who did not seek mental health services. Soygut, Nelson, and Safran (2001a) used the ISQ to identify maladaptive personality styles in patients with histrionic and schizotypal personality disorders. Mongrain (1998) used the ISQ to discriminate between dependent and self-critical personality styles in individuals at risk for depression. Cloitre, Cohen, and Scarvalone (2002) found that responses on the ISQ differed based on participants' trauma histories. Women without early abuse experiences expected warm and non-controlling responses from others. Women who were sexually abused in childhood but not in adulthood expected hostile but non-controlling responses from their parents, and warm and non-controlling responses from their current partners. Women who were sexually abused in both childhood and adulthood expected hostile and controlling responses from all others, even when they themselves were behaving in a warm and friendly manner.

Consistent with the Hill and Safran (1994) finding that participants with fewer symptoms had more positive expectations of others, Baldwin and Keelan (1999), in a study using the ISQ, found that individuals with high self-esteem were more confident of their ability to elicit affiliative response from others than were individuals with low self-esteem. Huebner and Thomas (1996) found that students studying to be rehabilitation counselors for individuals with disabilities were more likely than noncounselors to expect affiliative responses.

Studies using the ISQ have also provided support for the assertion that the patient's interactions with the therapist can provide a window into the patient's interpersonal schemas. Multon, Patton, and Kivlighan (1996) found that the more positive the patients' perceptions of their mothers, the more likely they were to develop a positive transference to the therapist. The converse was also found: The more negatively the mother was seen, the more likely a negative transference would develop. Soygut, Nelson, and Safran (2001b) found that patients who expected submissive behavior from others were more likely to agree with their therapists on the tasks and goals of therapy. Patients who expected and desired dominant responses from others were less likely to agree on goals.

In keeping with a two-person perspective of interpersonal schemas, the ISQ has also been used to highlight how the therapist's schemas impact the therapy relationship. Nelson (2002) administered the ISQ to a sample of 24 therapists and found that therapists who expected hostile responses from their fathers also tended to engage in hostile behaviors with their patients, as rated by the structural analysis of social behavior model (SASB; Benjamin, 1974). By linking ISQ ratings of relationships with early attachment figures to observed behaviors in the present, this study also provides evidence of how schemas based on previous relationships continue to structure interpersonal interactions and can become maladaptive when they are not revised to fit a new interpersonal context.

Resolving Alliance Ruptures

Our focus on identifying and addressing alliance ruptures builds on the strong consensus in the research literature that the quality of the alliance predicts outcome (Horvath & Symonds, 1991; Martin, Garske, & Davis, 2000; Samstag, Batchelder, Muran, Safran, & Winston, 1998; Tryon & Kane, 1990, 1993, 1995). Several studies have found that close attention to alliance ruptures in the session may play an important role in successful treatment. For example, Foreman and Marmar (1985) found that addressing the patient's problematic feelings in relation to the therapist was associated with good outcome in time-limited dynamic psychotherapy. Lansford (1986) found that successful efforts to address and repair alliance ruptures in short-term therapy were predictive of good outcome. Rhodes, Hill, Thompson, and Elliott (1994), in a study of patients' recall of rupture events, found that patients' willingness to assert their negative feelings about being misunderstood and therapists' ability to remain accepting and flexible typically led to rupture resolution, whereas therapists' unwillingness to discuss patients' assertions of being misunderstood and lack of awareness of patients' negative feelings often led to patients dropping out of treatment.

Our program of alliance rupture research is comprised of four recursive stages: model development, model testing, treatment development, and treatment evaluation (Muran, 2002; Safran & Muran, 1996; Safran et al., 2001). We have used task-analytic procedures (Greenberg, 1986) to develop and refine a model of the rupture repair process. In the first stage of the research program, we conducted a series of intensive analyses of therapy sessions in which alliance ruptures had reached some degree of resolution (Safran & Muran, 1996). Based on our observations, we proposed a stage process model of the resolution process. We also conducted a series of lag 1 sequential analyses to confirm the hypothesized sequences of events within resolution sessions and to demonstrate a difference between resolution and nonresolution sessions (Safran & Muran, 1996). This study confirmed that when therapists addressed alliance ruptures in a manner consistent with our model, this facilitated resolution of the rupture.

Over the years, we have conducted additional small-scale quantitative and qualitative studies to refine this model (Safran & Muran, 1996; Safran et al., 1990; Safran, Muran, & Samstag, 1994). Our process model now comprises five stages: (1) a rupture marker; (2) disembedding and attending to the rupture marker; (3) exploring the patient's experience of the rupture; (4) exploring the patient's avoidant behaviors; and (5) emergence of the patient's deep-seated wish or need.

In the development of this model, we have found it useful to draw on Harper's classification of challenge behaviors in therapy (Harper, 1989a, 1989b) to distinguish between two types of ruptures: withdrawals and confrontations. In a *withdrawal rupture*, the patient withdraws or partially disengages from the therapist, the patient's own emotions, or some aspect of the therapeutic process. In a *confrontation rupture*, the patient directly expresses anger, resentment, or dissatisfaction with the therapist, or some aspect of the therapy, or attempts to control the therapist. These two types of ruptures call for somewhat different resolution processes. In the process of resolving a withdrawal rupture, the patient usually moves through increasingly clearer articulations of discontent to self-assertion, in which the patient's need for agency is recognized and validated by the therapist. The resolution process for a confrontation rupture generally calls for the patient to progress through feelings of anger to feelings of disappointment and hurt over having been failed by the therapist, to contacting vulnerability and the wish to be taken care of and nurtured. For both types of ruptures, the avoidant behaviors that emerge in Stage 4 concern anxieties and self-doubts about the fear of being too aggressive or too vulnerable, associated with the expectation of retaliation or rejection by the therapist.

In the treatment development stage of our program, we drew on our findings from the model development and model testing stages, and developed a treatment that includes interventions that facilitate resolution (Safran, 2002a, 2002b; Safran & Muran, 2000). The BRT model has been manualized as a short-term treatment to facilitate clinical trial research, but it is not intrinisically a short-term model.

The treatment evaluation stage of our research program serves as both an evaluation of the efficacy of the treatment and a verification of the model. Muran et al. (2005) conducted a clinical trial comparing BRT with CBT and a short-term dynamic treatment in a sample of 128 patients with Cluster C and personality disorder NOS diagnoses. The majority (87%) of the patients in this sample were also comorbid for Axis I diagnoses. This study found evidence that BRT is possibly efficacious for Cluster C and personality disorder NOS diagnoses, according to the criteria established for empirically supported psychological therapies (Chambless & Hollon, 1998). Specifically, this study found that BRT was as effective as CBT and short-term dynamic psychotherapy on standard statistical analyses of change, including those conducted on repeated measures and residual gain scores. BRT was more successful than the other two treatments with respect to retention: BRT had significantly fewer dropouts than the short-term dynamic treatment (20 vs. 46%), and a difference approaching significance when compared to CBT (20 vs. 37%). This finding suggests that BRT's intensive focus on alliance ruptures may help to keep patients with personality disorders in treatment.

Drawing on a different sample of patients with Cluster C and personality disorder NOS diagnoses, Safran et al. (2005) conducted a pilot study to evaluate the feasibility of a research design for testing the efficacy of BRT for patients with whom it is difficult to establish a therapeutic alliance. This study also found evidence to suggest that BRT successfully keeps challenging patients engaged in therapy. In the first phase of the study, 60 patients were randomly assigned either to short-term dynamic therapy or short-term CBT, and their progress in the first eight sessions of treatment was monitored. On the basis of a number of empirically derived criteria, 18 potential treatment failures were identified. In the second phase of the study, these identified patients were offered the option of being reassigned to another treatment. The 10 patients who agreed to switch treatments were reassigned either to BRT or to a control condition. For patients coming from CBT, the control condition was the short-term dynamic treatment, and for patients coming from the dynamic therapy, the control condition was CBT. The study found that all five patients assigned to a control condition and seven of the eight patients who declined reassignment dropped out of treatment. By contrast, only one of the five patients in the BRT condition dropped out of treatment unilaterally. One additional BRT patient planned to end treatment early to accept a job offer in another country; this patient appeared to be progressing toward a good outcome at the time of the planned termination. The three BRT patients who completed the 30-session treatment were determined to be good outcome cases, with all three achieving a medium effect by follow-up. These results provide preliminary evidence supporting the potential value of BRT as a useful intervention in the context of alliance ruptures.

Limitations to Current Support

Empirical investigations of our resolution model and of BRT are limited by modest sample sizes, by a lack of racial/ethnic diversity among our predominantly European American patients and therapists, and by our focus on patients with Cluster C and personality disorder NOS diagnoses, although these are the most prevalent personality disorder classifications (Mattia & Zimmerman, 2001). The fact that our patients were highly comorbid for Axis I diagnoses, such as depression and anxiety, suggests that our model and treatment can be applied to these disorders. However, it is possible that our rupture resolution model and brief relational treatment would need to be modified to be effective with different patient populations.

An additional limitation of the feasibility study we discussed (Safran et al., 2005) was the failure to control for the nonspecific effects of being reassigned to a new therapist administering the same treatment. A new project that is currently under way addresses this concern by using a multiple baseline design, in which CBT therapists are taught to augment their standard treatment approach with alliance-focused interventions.

CLINICAL PRACTICE

BRT is an integrative treatment informed by our work on the use of emotion in psychotherapy, the cognitive interpersonal model, and our research on addressing ruptures in the therapeutic alliance. BRT assumes a two-person psychology and a dialectical or critical constructivist perspective (Hoffman, 1998; Mahoney, 1991): that is, both the therapist and the patient are regarded as contributing to the patient–therapist interaction, and each participant's experience and understanding of the interaction is understood to be constrained by his or her preconceptions and prejudices. In BRT, the focus is on both process and content. Specifically, aspects of sessions often emphasize a collaborative, accepting, nonjudgmental exploration of the patient's and therapist's experiences of their interaction. It is assumed that interventions can only be understood within the context of the patient–therapist relationship. Case formulations emerge over time, always informed by an evolving understanding of what is taking place in the therapeutic relationship in addition to any other information available to the therapist. The focus is often (but not always) on the here and now of the therapeutic relationship.

At the outset of treatment, BRT therapists help orient patients to the treatment by emphasizing the importance of developing the capacity to observe their internal processes and their actions in relationships with others. This capacity is a type of mindfulness or mentalizing ability (Allen, Fonagy, & Bateman, 2008). Increasing the patient's mindful awareness of his or her own internal experience may involve using experiential techniques to help the patient attend to bodily felt experience (Gendlin, 1981). The therapist may also carefully analyze the patient's manner of verbal and nonverbal expression as a source of information about affective states. The therapist can use sighs, gestures, and glances to focus the patient's attention on his or her emotions, and the information these emotional responses provide about the patient's goals and needs (Greenberg & Safran, 1989).

Throughout treatment, BRT therapists make extensive use of metacommunication as a means of increasing the patient's awareness of what is transpiring in the session. Some basic principles of metacommunication follow (for more detailed descriptions of these and other principles, see Safran and Muran, 2000):

1. *Start where you are.* Metacommunication should be based on the therapist's feelings and intuitions that emerge in the moment. What was true in one session may not be true in the next, and what was true at the beginning of a session may not be true later in that same session. Therapists should not simply apply supervisors' or colleagues' suggestions; rather, they should seek to become aware of their own experience of patients, and to accept and work through their feelings in the moment rather than trying to be somewhere they are not.

2. *Focus on the here and now.* The focus should be on the here and now of the therapeutic relationship rather than on events in prior sessions, or even earlier in the same session. Focusing on what is happening now helps patients become more mindful of their own experiences.

3. *Focus on the concrete and specific.* The focus should be concrete and specific rather than general. A concrete focus promotes patients' experiential awareness rather than abstract, intellectualized speculation. This focus also helps patients to make their own discoveries rather than buying into the therapist's version of reality.

4. *Do not assume a parallel with other relationship.* Although metacommunication serves as a means of disembedding from enactments, and over time modifies maladaptive relational schemas about self–other interactions, therapists should be cautious about prematurely attempting to establish a link between what is being enacted in the therapeutic relationship and other relationships in the patient's life.

5. *Explore with skillful tentativeness.* Communicate observations in

a tentative, exploratory manner, rather than making pronouncements as if they are indisputable facts. This tentativeness should be genuine, not simulated, and should communicate openness to collaboration rather than anxiety or lack of confidence on the part of the therapist.

6. *Establish a sense of collaboration and we-ness.* Patients often feel alone during a rupture. Frame the impasse as a shared dilemma that patient and therapist will explore collaboratively; acknowledge that "we are stuck together." In this way, instead of being yet one more in an endless succession of figures who do not understand the patient's struggle, the therapist can become an ally who joins the patient.

7. *Emphasize your own subjectivity.* The therapist should not speak as an authority figure with an objective view of the interaction. Rather, all metacommunications should emphasize the subjectivity of the therapist's perception. This helps to establish a collaborative, egalitarian environment, where the patient feels free to decide how to make use of the therapist's observation. In addition, emphasis on the subjectivity of the therapist's perception helps to reduce the patient's defensiveness and make the patient more open to questioning his or her own perceptions.

8. *Gauge intuitive sense of relatedness.* Therapists should continuously monitor their sense of emotional closeness or connection with patients. A greater sense of relatedness is a sign that the patient is in contact with his or her own inner experience. A decrease in relatedness is an indication that the therapist's intervention is hindering rather than facilitating the patient's efforts to access his or her inner experience.

9. *Evaluate and explore patients' responses to interventions.* If an intervention leads to a decrease in relatedness, as described previously, then the therapist needs to explore the patient's experience of the intervention. Close attention to patients' responses to interventions can help to clarify their interpersonal schemas. It can also help therapists to deepen their understanding of how they contribute to the interaction.

10. *Recognize that the situation is constantly changing.* It is important to keep moving—to use what is emerging in the moment as the point of departure for further metacommunication. Even the position of being stuck is workable once the therapist acknowledges and accepts it rather than trying to fight against it.

11. *Expect resolution attempts to lead to more ruptures, and expect to revisit ruptures.* Even the most thoughtfully and sensitively delivered metacommunication can exacerbate a rupture or lead to a new one. Metacommunication is not an ultimate intervention, but a step in the process of rupture resolution. In addition, therapists often find that the same impasse is revisited many times. Therapists should try to appreciate the ways in

which each occurrence is unique, and respond in the immediacy of the moment.

12. *Accept responsibility.* Therapists should accept responsibility for their contributions to the patient–therapist interaction in an open and non-defensive manner. This process can help patients become more aware of feelings that they have but are unable to articulate clearly, in part because they fear the therapist's response. For example, acknowledging that one has been critical can help patients articulate feelings of hurt and resentment. Accepting responsibility can validate patients' experience of the interaction and help them to trust their own judgment. Increasing patients' confidence in their judgment helps to decrease their need for defensiveness, which facilitates their exploration and acknowledgment of their own contribution to the interaction.

13. *Judiciously disclose and explore your own experience.* Therapists' feelings of being stuck or paralyzed often reflect their difficulty in acknowledging and articulating to themselves what they are currently experiencing. The process of articulating one's feelings to patients can free the therapist to intervene more effectively. It can also clarify the nature of the cognitive-interpersonal cycle in which the patient and therapist are caught. Another valuable intervention that is related to self-disclosure is inviting patients to suggest ways that the therapist might be contributing to the interaction, or to speculate about what the therapist might be experiencing internally. For example, a therapist might ask, "I wonder if you have any thoughts about what may be going on for me right now?" This invitation can help to clarify the patient's experience of the therapist and may lead to further elaboration of the patient's interpersonal schemas. It can also provide new insight into the therapist's contributions to the impasse. It is critical for the therapist to be open to accepting the patient's perception and to consider seriously its truth claim.

Case Illustration

This case study illustrates the theories and techniques that we have presented in this chapter. We present minimal information about the patient's diagnostic status, case history, and formulation, since it is not essential here for purposes of illustrating the principles of BRT or the process of change.

The patient Ruth contracted to receive 30 sessions of BRT. Ruth, a 52-year-old woman, had ended her marriage of 12 years, at the age of 36, because she felt that her husband was controlling, emotionally abusive, and generally unable or unwilling to be responsive to her emotional needs. Since her divorce, Ruth had engaged in a series of short-term affairs that she herself typically ended because of her dissatisfaction with them. At the beginning of treatment, she acknowledged that she desperately wanted to be in a "real relationship" but felt hopeless about the possibility. A second presenting problem revolved around her feelings of being "disempowered" and of not being treated respectfully by colleagues at work.

Although the therapist initially felt empathically engaged with Ruth, a pattern developed fairly rapidly in which he had difficulty maintaining a sense of emotional engagement with her and found himself biding time until the sessions ended. Ruth had a tendency to tell long stories with considerable obsessional detail, and to do so in an unemotional droning fashion, which left the therapist feeling distant and unengaged. In addition, she rarely paused to welcome any input or feedback. Although the therapist typically began sessions with a renewed intention of taking an interest in Ruth, he consistently ended up feeling bored and vaguely irritated.

R: How many sessions do we have left?

T: Ten more, including today.

R: OK ... OK ... so 10 more. Oh my God ...

T: So what's the "Oh my God?"

R: Well ... I certainly don't feel like everything's resolved ... you know ... and (clears throat) umm ... how can we speed it up (laughs)? Well, you know, I don't know if just coming here and complaining and being teary ... if that's really the more productive thing.

T: It sounds like you're feeling kind of frustrated. Can you say any more?

R: Well ... I guess I feel like asking you for an evaluation ... or how we should proceed or something.

T: I don't want to sound evasive ... but I'm not sure how to answer your question at this moment. Maybe we'll be able to come back to it later, and I'll be able to answer it in a way that feels helpful. But I'm wondering how you're feeling about what's going on between us in this moment?

R: Well ... I mean ... I don't feel like I'm blaming you in any way. I just think that it's easy for me to get sidetracked ... and I may need help being reined in a little. I just feel like I need to have some concrete ... not direction ... I don't know ... I feel like I need help being brought back on topic. And as we've discussed, when I don't know what the other person is thinking, I tend to go on and keep throwing lines out in an attempt to get a response.

T: So part of it is that you want me to help you keep focused.... And are you also saying that you'd feel more comfortable if I were more forthcoming about what's going on for me?

R: Well, I guess so. I mean sometimes I feel like there's some kind of real connection that goes on, and then other times I think I'm totally spinning this yarn, and you know ... you're just waiting for me to come back or something.

T: It sounds like your sense of how connected we are ... how engaged I am and how much I'm there for you ... fluctuates.

R: Uh huh. I mean ... I don't think that you don't like me, but I think this has been hard work. And hard work for you too. And I know from working with people ... you like them the best when they make you feel good about what you're doing. And I don't know if I've been a success story.

T: Uh huh.

R: So you know ... when somebody ... when I'm feeling like embraced ... you know ... totally accepted ... like purely and unconditionally ... then I'm more relaxed in a way.

T: Right ... and you haven't always gotten that sense from me.

R: Right. Yeah.

T: That at some fundamental level ... that I'm here for you feeling deeply accepting and caring.

R: Right. There's a reservation. And I think I'm always trying to figure out where the other person is ... like feeling their pulse in a way.

This session contains many of the features of the resolution process for withdrawal ruptures. Ruth begins the session by partly withdrawing from the interaction as she anxiously considers how little time she has left in treatment (Stage 1 of the withdrawal resolution model). When the therapist attempts to explore Ruth's feelings (Stage 2), she expresses her negative feelings and concerns but in a qualified, avoidant way (Stage 3). She conceptualizes the problem as resulting from her own lack of focus but implicitly blames the therapist for not helping her to be more focused. The therapist acknowledges her request for help with focusing but highlights her concerns about his opaqueness. Whereas Ruth expresses her concerns in a diffuse or self-blaming fashion, the therapist highlights his contribution ("It sounds like your sense of how connected we are ... how engaged I am and how much I'm there for you ... fluctuates"). This leads to the emergence of Ruth's deeper concerns about his not really caring about her.

T: So ... how am I doing right now?

R: I think that you're receptive ... but I also want to know about my perceptions so far. I want you to tell me if I'm right or not. Are my perceptions accurate or distorted?

T: Well ... I think you're right that my feeling of engagement fluctuates.... We've talked about this before to some extent. But also, it feels to me that I've been feeling increasingly more disengaged over the last few sessions.

R: And your feeling disengaged relates to my wandering and losing focus?

T: I'm not completely sure ... but I think so ...

R: Well, then in the time we have left, I want you to help me stay focused. And I also want to know why I drift away. OK? So where do we go from here?

T: I'm not sure ... but I'm wondering if you can say anything about how my feedback felt for you ... and also when you say "Where do we go from here?", what you're feeling?

When the therapist validates Ruth's perception by acknowledging his responsibility for contributing to the impasse ("I think you're right that my feeling of engagement fluctuates"), she responds by continuing to place the ball in his court ("So where do we go from here?") The therapist senses the angry feelings underlying her words and attempts to explore her reaction to his feedback.

R: It's like ... I'm not going to take all the responsibility.

T: So ... is there a sense maybe ... that it feels like I've been blaming you?

R: Yeah ... I guess so. It's like I've really sincerely tried to get to important things ... and it's like ... I guess I'm asking for your help.

T: OK ... so that sounds important.

R: Yeah ...

T: It's like you're saying, "I'm really doing everything I can."

R: Right. It's not like you have to keep prodding me to get me to say what I feel. You might in a certain way ... but I think I've been very forthcoming about my feelings as far as I know them.

T: Right. And you're basically saying, "I need help. I want more from you."

R: Right.

T: What does that feel like, to say "I want more from you"?

R: Well, I immediately want to qualify it. I mean ... I need more from you because we only have 10 sessions ... so we need to work faster.

By empathizing with the feelings and wishes that are implicit in what Ruth is saying, the therapist facilitates Ruth's self-assertion of her underlying wish for more help from the therapist (Stage 5). However, when the therapist begins to explore the feelings associated with acknowledging this wish, Ruth begins to contact her avoidance (Stage 4). An ongoing alternation between exploring the rupture experience (Stage 3) and exploring the patient's avoidance (Stage 4) is common in resolution processes.

T: So it sounds like it's uncomfortable to ask for what you want from me.

R: Yeah.

T: Can you say anything more about your discomfort?

R: Well ... it's like I'm being unreasonable and expecting too much ... but still ... I have a tendency to blame myself when things aren't going well in a relationship. And I don't want to do that here.

T: Yeah. It's not really fair for you to have to take all the blame if things don't work out for you here ...

R: If I'm not to blame. I'm asking you to be really honest and tell me if I go off and start talking about a crack in the ceiling or whatever. Actually, as I'm saying that, I'm feeling stronger.

T: Uh huh ... and the essence of what you're saying in feeling stronger ... is that you want me to take some of the responsibility for what's going on ... and you don't want to feel blamed for something that's not your fault ...

R: Yeah ... and I just had a thought, "I want this time to be about me."

T: Uh huh.

R: I don't want this to be a kind of academic observation ... and I'm demanding that you be engaged in whatever problems I have ... as mundane as they may be, as repetitive as they may be.

T: That sounds important. What does it feel like to say that?

R: Well ... I feel like I'm stamping my feet in a way. You know ... like "Goddamn it!" (Laughs) You know ... like "Give me that!"

T: Right.

R: But you know ... it feels OK to say it ... and actually I don't know that I thought this consciously at all ...

T: Uh huh.

R: But I guess a momentum is building, and I'm becoming more self-centered in it, like I want this to be about me and it should be.

T: Right.

R: And then the defensive part of me thinks, "It has to be about me ... the person that I am ... I can't try to be a more interesting person for you to be more engaged."

T: I don't see how that's defensive. Basically, you're saying "I want to be accepted on my own terms ... for who I am."

R: Yeah ... yeah ...

T: And that sounds important. You know ... I think part of what you're saying is that when I tell you that my attention is wandering, you're feeling, "The hell with you! I want you to accept me for who I am."

R: Yeah. Exactly.

The exploration of Ruth's avoidance helps her to articulate and recognize the self-criticism that blocks the direct expression of her underlying wish. This helps her to bypass the self-criticism and move once again toward expressing feelings and wishes that have been avoided (Stage 5).

There were times in this session when the therapist felt strongly chastised, pressured, and momentarily at a loss as to how to respond to Ruth's pressure. At the same time, Ruth's ability to express her need for more emotional engagement helped the therapist to empathize more fully with Ruth's experience of not feeling accepted and validated by him. The process of metacommunicating about his difficulty in staying engaged helped the therapist to make explicit that which was already implicit—that is, his difficulty in being there for Ruth in a present and attuned fashion on a consistent basis. At the same time, however, the therapist's metacommunication did not constitute a complete disembedding from the cognitive-interpersonal cycle that was being enacted; rather, it was a new step in the dance that was already taking place. By encouraging Ruth to tell him about the impact of his metacommunication on her, and by being receptive to her feedback, the therapist was able to develop a greater empathic appreciation of her dilemma, in part as a result of his increased experiential appreciation of the way he had become a perpetrator in a victim–abuser cycle. The experience of challenging the therapist, and seeing that their relationship was able to survive this challenge, enabled Ruth subsequently to bring her feelings of despair, as well as her vulnerability and dependency, more fully into the relationship.

SUMMARY AND CONCLUSIONS

Over the past 20 years, Safran and colleagues have helped to push the boundaries of cognitive therapy in the areas of emotion, interpersonal process, and alliance ruptures. Safran and Greenberg's work on the role of emotion in psychotherapy was an important correction to cognitive therapy's overly restricted view of emotion. They highlighted the adaptive role of emotions in helping individuals to identify and prioritize goals and needs. They noted that engaging a patient's emotions in the therapy session is an important part of the change process; indeed, the patient's emotions must be aroused to access the patient's full internal experience. Empirical studies by Greenberg and colleagues provide evidence of the therapeutic value of activating emotions in the therapy session and helping patients to reflect on, and make sense of, their affective states.

With the concept of the interpersonal schema, Safran and colleagues highlighted the interdependence of cognitive and interpersonal processes. Interpersonal schemas shape the way that people relate to both their inner and outer worlds on an ongoing basis. They represent the bases for the cognitive-interpersonal cycles that structure our relationships with others. Rigid, maladaptive interpersonal schemas can lead to interpersonal problems. Safran and colleagues' work with the ISQ provides support for the link between maladaptive schemas and forms of psychopathology.

Ruptures in the therapeutic alliance provide a window into the patient's (and the therapist's) maladaptive interpersonal schemas. By attending to and exploring a rupture in a nondefensive fashion, therapists can help patients to decenter and observe the interaction, and to become more aware of their own self-defeating interpersonal patterns. By providing a new experience of being in a relationship, the therapeutic encounter can also help to disconfirm patients' interpersonal schemas, which can lead to core structural change. Our research on strategies for addressing and resolving alliance ruptures offers evidence of the value of paying close attention to impasses in therapy, particularly with patients with personality disorders, who often have difficulty forming strong alliances.

Challenges that remain include expanding our work on alliance ruptures to more diverse patient populations, and exploring whether our rupture resolution strategies need to be revised in these new interpersonal contexts. Presently, our focus is on the challenge of how to effectively teach CBT therapists to use rupture resolution strategies when ruptures arise. An important component of successfully negotiating alliance ruptures is for the therapist to be mindful (Safran & Reading, 2008). To disembed from a cognitive-interpersonal cycle and to explore with the patient how each is contributing to the impasse, therapists must be able to acknowledge undesirable feelings, such as anger or jealousy. Mindfulness allows the therapist to refine his or her attentional skills to become more aware of internal experience, including his or her emotions and underlying wishes and needs. Once therapists become aware of their difficult feelings, they need to regulate these feelings in a constructive fashion to be able to provide affect regulation or containment for the patient. Mindfulness is a valuable skill in this regard as well, because it allows the therapist to cultivate a sense of internal space by decreasing attachment to any particular feeling. The increased awareness that comes with mindfulness can also help therapists to better recognize how their own interpersonal schemas are shaping their interactions with patients.

An important question is how to inculcate mindfulness in therapists in training. Psychoanalysts have long maintained that managing difficult countertransference feelings is a critical therapeutic skill that one develops through personal treatment. Similarly, we believe that the cultivation of an ongoing mindfulness practice can play a valuable role in the development of mindfulness in therapists. In addition, the technique of metacommunication can be seen as a form of mindfulness in action (Safran & Maran, 2000). Developing the skill of mindfulness can potentially enhance therapists' ability to metacommunicate in a skillful manner—and conversely an ongoing process of skillful metacommunication can potentially enhance the therapist's (and patient's) capacity for mindfulness. Future directions for our work include greater exploration of how to encourage and support therapists in the development of a mindfulness practice, and empirical investigations of whether this does positively impact therapeutic process and outcome. We hope that our efforts to understand better how to expand therapists' awareness of their role in the patient–therapist interaction will help both to broaden the perspective and enhance the effectiveness of cognitive therapists.

REFERENCES

Allen, J. G., Fonagy, P., & Bateman, A. (2008). *Mentalizing in clinical process.* Arlington, VA: American Psychiatric Publishing.

Arnkoff, D. (1983). Common and specific factors in cognitive therapy. In M. J. Lambert (Ed.), *Psychotherapy and patient relationships* (pp. 85–125). Belmont, CA: Dorsey Press.

Aron, L. (1996). *A meeting of minds: Mutuality in psychoanalysis.* Hillsdale, NJ: Analytic Press.

Baldwin, M. W., & Keelan, J. P. R. (1999). Interpersonal expectations as a function of self-esteem and sex. *Journal of Social and Personal Relationships, 16,* 822–833.

Barlow, D. H. (2002). *Anxiety and its disorders: The nature and treatment of anxiety and panic* (2nd ed.). New York: Guilford Press.

Bartlett, F. C. (1932). *Remembering.* Cambridge, UK: Cambridge University Press.

Beck, A. T. (1976). *Cognitive therapy and the emotional disorders.* New York: International Universities Press.

Beebe, B., & Lachman, F. M. (2002). *Infant research and adult treatment.* Hillsdale, NJ: Analytic Press.

Benjamin, J. (1988). *The bonds of love.* New York: Pantheon Books.

Benjamin, L. S. (1974). Structural analysis of social behavior. *Psychological Review, 81,* 392–425.

Bion, W. R. (1962). *Learning from experience.* New York: Basic Books.

Bion, W. R. (1967). Notes on memory and desire. In E. B. Spillius (Ed.), *Melanie Klein today* (Vol. 2, pp. 17–21). London: Routledge.

Bion, W. R. (1970). *Attention and interpretation.* London: Heinemann.

Bordin, E. (1979). The generalizability of the psychoanalytic concept of the working alliance. *Psychotherapy: Theory, Research, and Practice, 16,* 252–260.

Bowlby, J. (1969). *Attachment and loss: Vol. 1. Attachment.* New York: Basic Books.

Bowlby, J. (1973). *Attachment and loss: Vol. 2. Separation, anxiety, and anger.* New York: Basic Books.

Bowlby, J. (1980). *Attachment and loss: Vol. 3. Loss: Sadness and depression.* New York: Basic Books.

Burum, B. A., & Goldfried, M. R. (2007). The centrality of emotion to psychological change. *Clinical Psychology: Science and Practice, 14,* 407–413.

Carson, R. C. (1969). *Interaction concepts of personality.* Hawthorne, NY: Aldine.

Carson, R. C. (1982). Self-fulfilling prophecy, maladaptive behavior, and psychotherapy. In J. C. Anchin & D. J. Kiesler (Eds.), *Handbook of interpersonal psychotherapy* (pp. 64–77). New York: Pergamon Press.

Castonguay, L. G., Newman, M. G., Borkovec, T. D., Holtforth, M. G., & Maramba, G. G. (2005). Cognitive-behavioral assimilative integration. In J. C. Norcross & M. R. Goldfried (Eds.), *Handbook of psychotherapy integration* (2nd ed., pp. 241–260). New York: Oxford University Press.

Chambless, D. L., & Hollon, S. D. (1998). Defining empirically supported therapies. *Journal of Consulting and Clinical Psychology, 66,* 7–18.

Cloitre, M., Cohen, L., & Scarvalone, P. (2002). Understanding revictimization among childhood sexual abuse survivors: An interpersonal schema approach. *Journal of Cognitive Psychotherapy, 16,* 91–111.

Dobson, K. S., & Block, L. (1988). Historical and philosophical bases of the cognitive-behavioral therapies. In K. S. Dobson (Ed.), *Handbook of cognitive-behavioral therapies* (pp. 3–38). New York: Guilford Press.

Ehrenreich, J. T., Fairholme, C. P., Buzzella, B. A., Ellard, K. K., & Barlow, D. H. (2007). The role of emotion in psychological therapy. *Clinical Psychology: Science and Practice, 14,* 422–428.

Ellis, A. (1962). *Reason and emotion in psychotherapy.* New York: Stuart.

Foa, E. B., & Kozak, M. J. (1986). Emotional processing of fear: Exposure to corrective information. *Psychological Bulletin, 99,* 20–35.

Fonagy, P. (1991). Thinking about thinking: Some clinical and theoretical considerations in the treatment of a borderline patient. *International Journal of Psycho-Analysis, 72,* 1–18.

Fonagy, P. (2000). Attachment and borderline personality disorder. *Journal of the American Psychoanalytic Association, 48,* 1129–1146.

Foreman, S. A., & Marmar, C. R. (1985). Therapist actions that address initially poor therapeutic alliances in psychotherapy. *American Journal of Psychiatry, 142,* 922–926.

Gendlin, E. T. (1981). *Focusing.* New York: Bantam Books.

Gibson, J. J. (1979). *The ecological approach to visual perception.* Boston: Houghton Mifflin.

Goldfried, M. R., & Davison, G. C. (1976). *Clinical behavior therapy.* New York: Holt, Rinehart & Winston.

Goldman, R. N., Greenberg, L. S., & Angus, L. (2006). The effects of adding emotion-focused interventions to the client-centered relationship conditions in the treatment of depression. *Psychotherapy Research, 16,* 536–546.

Goldman, R. N., Greenberg, L. S., & Pos, A. E. (2005). Depth of emotional experience and outcome. *Psychotherapy Research, 15,* 248–260.

Greenberg, J. (1995). Psychoanalytic technique and the interactive matrix. *Psychoanalytic Quarterly, 64,* 1–22.

Greenberg, L. S. (1986). Change process research. *Journal of Consulting and Clinical Psychology, 54,* 4–11.

Greenberg, L. S. (2002). *Emotion-focused therapy: Coaching clients to work through their feelings.* Washington, DC: American Psychological Association.

Greenberg, L. S., & Malcolm, W. (2002). Resolving unfinished business: Relating process to outcome. *Journal of Consulting and Clinical Psychology, 70,* 406–416.

Greenberg, L. S., & Pascual-Leone, J. (1995). A dialectical constructivist approach to experiential change. In R. A. Neimeyer & M. J. Mahoney (Eds.), *Constructivism in psychotherapy* (pp. 169–191). Washington, DC: American Psychological Association.

Greenberg, L. S., & Safran, J. D. (1987). *Emotion in psychotherapy.* New York: Guilford Press.

Greenberg, L. S., & Safran, J. D. (1989). Emotion in psychotherapy. *American Psychologist, 44,* 19–29.

Greenberg, L. S., & Watson, J. (1998). Experiential therapy of depression: Differential effects of client-centered relationship conditions and process experiential interventions. *Psychotherapy Research, 8,* 210–224.

Harper, H. (1989a). *Coding Guide I: Identification of confrontation challenges in exploratory therapy.* Sheffield, UK: University of Sheffield.

Harper, H. (1989b). *Coding Guide II: Identification of withdrawal challenges in exploratory therapy.* Sheffield, UK: University of Sheffield.

Hayes, S. C., Strosahl, K. D., & Wilson, K. G. (1999). *Acceptance and commitment therapy: An experiential approach to behavior change.* New York: Guilford Press.

Hill, C., & Safran, J. D. (1994). Assessing interpersonal schemas: Anticipated responses of significant others. *Journal of Social and Clinical Psychology, 13,* 366–379.

Hoffman, I. Z. (1998). *Ritual and spontaneity in the psychoanalytic process: A dialectical–constructivist view.* Hillsdale, NJ: Analytic Press.

Horney, K. (1950). *Neurosis and human growth.* New York: Norton.

Horvath, A. O., & Symonds, B. D. (1991). Relation between working alliance and outcome in psychotherapy: A meta-analysis. *Journal of Counseling Psychology, 38,* 139–149.

Huebner, R. A., & Thomas, K. R. (1996). The relationship between attachment, psychopathology, and childhood disability. *Rehabilitation Psychology, 40,* 111–124.

Huebner, R. A., Thomas, K. R., & Berven, N. L. (1999). Attachment and interpersonal characteristics of college students with and without disabilities. *Rehabilitation Psychology, 44,* 85–103.

Izard, C. E. (1977). *Human emotions.* New York: Plenum Press.

Johnson, S. M., Hunsley, J., Greenberg, L., & Schindler, D. (1999). Emotionally focused couples therapy: Status and challenges. *Clinical Psychology: Science and Practice, 6,* 67–79.

Kaiser, H. (1965). The problem of responsibility in psychotherapy. In L. B. Fierman (Ed.), *Effective psychotherapy: The contribution of Hellmuth Kaiser* (pp. 1–13). New York: Free Press.

Keller, M. B., McCullough, J. P., Klein, D. N., Arnow, B., Duner, D. L., Gelenberg, A. J., et al. (2000). A comparison of nefazodone, the cognitive behavioral analysis system of psychotherapy, and their combination for the treatment of chronic depression. *New England Journal of Medicine, 342,* 1462–1470.

Kiesler, D. J. (1982a). Interpersonal theory for personality and psychotherapy. In J. C. Anchin & D. J. Kiesler (Eds.), *Handbook of interpersonal psychotherapy* (pp. 3–24). New York: Pergamon.

Kiesler, D. J. (1982b). Confronting the client–therapist relationship in psychotherapy. In J. C. Anchin & D. J. Kiesler (Eds.), *Handbook of interpersonal psychotherapy* (pp. 274–295). New York: Pergamon.

Kiesler, D. J. (1996). *Contemporary interpersonal theory and research: Personality, psychopathology, and psychotherapy.* New York: Wiley.

Kohlenberg, R. H., Kanter, J. W., & Bolling, M. Y. (2002). Enhancing cognitive therapy for depression with functional analytic psychotherapy: Treatment guidelines and empirical findings. *Cognitive and Behavioral Practice, 9,* 213–229.

Kohlenberg, R. H., & Tsai, M. (1991). *Functional analytic psychotherapy: Creating intense and curative therapeutic relationships.* New York: Plenum Press.

Kohut, H. (1971). *The analysis of the self.* New York: International Universities Press.

Kohut, H. (1977). *The restoration of the self.* New York: International Universities Press.

Kohut, H. (1984). *How does analysis cure?* Chicago: University of Chicago Press.

Lansford, E. (1986). Weakenings and repairs of the working alliance in short-term psychotherapy. *Professional Psychology: Research and Practice, 17,* 364–366.

Leahy, R. L. (2003). *Overcoming resistance in cognitive therapy.* New York: Guilford Press.

Leary, T. (1957). *Interpersonal diagnosis of personality.* New York: Ronald.

Linehan, M. (1993). *Cognitive behavioral treatment of borderline personality disorder: The dialectics of effective treatment.* New York: Guilford Press.

Linehan, M., Tutek, D., Heard, H. J. L., & Armstrong, H. E. (1994). Interpersonal outcome of cognitive behavioral therapy for chronically suicidal borderline patients. *American Journal of Psychiatry, 151,* 1771–1775.

Mahoney, M. J. (1991). *Human change processes.* New York: Basic Books.

Martin, D. J., Garske, J. P., & Davis, M. K. (2000). Relation of the therapeutic alliance with outcome and other variables: A meta-analytic review. *Journal of Consulting and Clinical Psychology, 68,* 438–450.

Mattia, J. I., & Zimmerman, M. (2001). Epidemiology. In J. W. Livesley (Ed.), *Handbook of personality disorders: Theory, research, and treatment* (pp. 107–123). New York:Guilford Press.

McCullough, J. P. (2000). *Treatment for chronic depression: Cognitive Behavioral Analysis System of Psychotherapy (CBASP).* New York: Guilford Press.

Mitchell, S. A. (1988). *Relational concepts in psychoanalysis.* Cambridge, MA: Harvard University Press.

Mitchell, S. A. (2000). *Relationality: From attachment to intersubjectivity.* Hillsdale, NJ: Analytic Press.

Mongrain, M. (1998). Parental representations and support-seeking behavior related to dependency and self-criticism. *Journal of Personality, 66,* 151–173.

Multon, K. D., Patton, M. J., & Kivlighan, D. M. (1996). Development of the Missouri Identifying Transference Scale. *Journal of Counseling Psychology, 43,* 243–252.

Muran, J. C. (2002). A relational approach to understanding change: Plurality and contextualismin a psychotherapy research program. *Psychotherapy Research, 12,* 113–138.

Muran, J. C., Safran, J. D., Samstag, L. W., & Winston, A. (2005). Evaluating an alliance-focused treatment for personality disorders. *Psychotherapy: Theory, Research, Practice, Training, 42,* 532–545.

Neisser, U. (1967). *Cognitive psychology.* East Norwalk, CT: Appleton & Lange.

Nelson, L. (2002). *Predicting therapist hostility.* Unpublished doctoral dissertation, New School University, New York.

Nisbett, R., & Ross, L. (1980). *Human inference: Strategies and shortcomings of social judgement.* Englewood Cliffs, NJ: Prentice-Hall.

Paivio, S. C., & Greenberg, L. S. (1995). Resolving "unfinished business": Efficacy of experiential therapy using empty-chair dialogue. *Journal of Clinical and Consulting Psychology, 63,* 419–425.

Plutchik, R. (1980). *Emotion: A psychoevolutionary synthesis.* New York: HarperCollins.

Pos, A. E., Greenberg, L. S., Goldman, R. N., & Korman, L. M. (2003). Emotional processing during experiential treatment of depression. *Journal of Consulting and Clinical Psychology, 71,* 1007–1016.

Rhodes, R., Hill, C., Thompson, B., & Elliott, R. (1994). Client retrospective recall of resolved and unresolved misunderstanding events. *Counseling Psychology, 41,* 473–483.

Safran, J. D. (1984). Some implications of Sullivan's interpersonal theory for cognitive therapy. In M. A. Reda & M. J. Mahoney (Eds.), *Cognitive psychotherapies: Recent developments in theory, research, and practice* (pp. 251–272). Cambridge, MA: Ballinger.

Safran, J. D. (1986, June). *A critical evaluation of the schema construct in psychotherapy research.* Paper presented at the annual meeting of the Society for Psychotherapy Research Conference, Boston, MA.

Safran, J. D. (1990a). Towards a refinement of cognitive therapy in light of interpersonal theory: I. Theory. *Clinical Psychology Review, 10,* 87–105.

Safran, J. D. (1990b). Towards a refinement of cognitive therapy in light of interpersonal theory: II. Practice. *Clinical Psychology Review, 10,* 107–121.

Safran, J. D. (1993). Breaches in the therapeutic alliance: An arena for negotiating authentic relatedness. *Psychotherapy: Theory, Research, Practice, Training, 30,* 11–24.

Safran, J. D. (1998). *Widening the scope of cognitive therapy: The therapeutic relationship, emotion, and the process of change.* Northvale, NJ: Aronson.

Safran, J. D. (2002a). Brief relational psychoanalytic treatment. *Psychoanalytic Dialogues, 12,* 171–195.

Safran, J. D. (2002b). Reply to commentaries by Warren, Wachtel, and Rosica. *Psychoanalytic Dialogues, 12,* 235–258.

Safran, J. D., Crocker, P., McMain, S., & Murray, P. (1990). Therapeutic alliance rupture as a therapy event for empirical investigation. *Psychotherapy: Theory, Research, and Practice, 27,* 154–165.

Safran, J. D., & Greenberg, L. S. (1986). Hot cognition and psychotherapy process: An information processing/ecological approach. In P. C. Kendall (Ed.), *Advances in cognitive-behavioral research and therapy* (Vol. 5, pp. 143–177). San Diego, CA: Academic Press.

Safran, J. D., & Greenberg, L. S. (1987). Affect and the unconscious: A cognitive perspective. In R. Stern (Ed.), *Theories of the unconscious and theories of the self* (pp. 191–212). Hillsdale, NJ: Analytic Press.

Safran, J. D., & Greenberg, L. S. (1988). Feeling, thinking, and acting: A cognitive framework for psychotherapy integration. *Journal of Cognitive Psychotherapy: An International Quarterly, 2,* 109–131.

Safran, J. D., & Greenberg, L. S. (Eds.). (1991). *Emotion, psychotherapy, and change.* New York: Guilford Press.

Safran, J. D., & Muran, J. C. (1996). The resolution of ruptures in the therapeutic alliance. *Journal of Consulting and Clinical Psychology, 64,* 447–458.

Safran, J. D., & Muran, J. C. (2000). *Negotiating the therapeutic alliance: A relational treatment guide.* New York: Guilford Press.

Safran, J. D., Muran, J. C., & Samstag, L. W. (1994). Resolving therapeutic alliance ruptures: A task analytic investigation. In A. O. Horvath & L. S. Greenberg (Eds.), *The working alliance: Theory, research, and practice* (pp. 225–255). New York: Wiley.

Safran, J. D., Muran, J. C., Samstag, L. W., & Stevens, C. (2001). Repairing alliance ruptures. *Psychotherapy: Theory, Research, Practice, Training, 38,* 406–412.

Safran, J. D., Muran, J. C., Samstag, L. W., & Winston, A. (2005). Evaluating alliance-focused intervention for potential treatment failures: A feasibility study and descriptive analysis. *Psychotherapy: Theory, Research, Practice, Training, 42,* 512–531.

Safran, J. D., & Reading, R. (2008). Mindfulness, metacommunication, and affect regulation in psychoanalytic treatment. In S. Hick & T. Bien (Eds.), *Mindfulness and the therapeutic relationship* (pp. 122–140). New York: Guilford Press.

Safran, J. D., & Segal, Z. V. (1990/1996). *Interpersonal process in cognitive therapy.* New York: Basic Books. (Original work published 1990)

Samoilov, A., & Goldfried, M. R. (2000). Role of emotion in cognitive-behavior therapy. *Clinical Psychology: Science and Practice, 7,* 373–385.

Samstag, L. W., Batchelder, S. T., Muran, J. C., Safran, J. D., & Winston, A. (1998). Early identification of treatment failures in short-term psychotherapy: An assessment of therapeutic alliance and interpersonal behavior. *Journal of Psychotherapy Practice and Research, 7,* 126–143.

Scarvalone, P., Fox, M., & Safran, J. D. (2005). Interpersonal schemas: Clinical theory, research, and implications. In M. W. Baldwin (Ed.), *Interpersonal cognition* (pp. 359–387). New York: Guilford Press.

Segal, Z. V., Williams, J. M. G., & Teasdale, J. D. (2002). *Mindfulness-based cognitive therapy for depression: A new approach to preventing relapse.* New York: Guilford Press.

Shaw, R., & Bransford, J. (Eds.). (1977). *Perceiving, acting, and knowing: Toward an ecological psychology.* Hillsdale, NJ: Erlbaum.

Singer, J. L., & Salovey, P. (1991). Organized knowledge structures and personality. In M. Horowitz (Ed.), *Person schemas and maladaptive interpersonal patterns* (pp. 33–80). Chicago: University of Chicago Press.

Soygut, G,. Nelson, L., & Safran, J. D. (2001a). The relationship between interpersonal schemas and personality characteristics. *Journal of Cognitive Psychotherapy, 15,* 99–108.

Soygut, G., Nelson, L., & Safran, J. D. (2001b). The relationship between pretreatment interpersonal schemas and therapeutic alliance in short-term cognitive therapy. *Journal of Cognitive Psychotherapy, 15,* 59–66.

Soygut, G., & Savasir, I. (2001). The relationship between interpersonal schemas and depressive symptomatology. *Journal of Counseling Psychology, 48,* 359–364.

Stern, D. N. (1985). *The interpersonal world of the infant.* New York: Basic Books.

Strachey, J. (1934). The nature of the therapeutic action of psychoanalysis. *International Journal of Psycho-Analysis, 15,* 127–159.

Tomkins, S. S. (1980). Affect as amplification: Some modifications in theory. In R. Plutchik & H. Kellerman (Eds.), *Emotion: Theory, research, and experience* (Vol. 1, pp. 141–164). San Diego: Academic Press.

Tronick, E. (1989). Emotions and emotional communications in infants. *American Psychologist, 44,* 112–119.

Tryon, G. S., & Kane, A. S. (1990). The helping alliance and premature termination. *Counselling Psychology Quarterly, 3,* 233–238.

Tryon, G. S., & Kane, A. S. (1993). Relationship of working alliance to mutual and unilateral termination. *Journal of Counseling Psychology, 40,* 33–36.

Tryon, G. S., & Kane, A. S. (1995). Client involvement, working alliance, and type of therapy termination. *Psychotherapy Research, 5,* 189–198.

Tulving, E. (1983). *Elements of episodic memory.* Oxford, UK: Oxford University Press.

Wachtel, P. L. (1997). *Psychoanalysis, behavior therapy, and the relational world.* Washington, DC: American Psychological Association.

Young, J. E., Klosko, J. S., & Weishaar, M. E. (2006). *Schema therapy: A practitioner's guide.* New York: Guilford Press.

CHAPTER 12

Concluding Remarks

Nikolaos Kazantzis
Mark A. Reinecke
Arthur Freeman

It is easier to produce ten volumes of philosophical writing than
to put one principle into practice.
—Leo Nikolayevich Tolstoy

This book has presented contemporary behavioral and cognitive-behavioral
models and their applications in clinical practice. Our aim was to showcase
the diversity of approaches through case examples that link theory with
practice. Theoretical models thread our formulations of the cognitive, emotional, behavioral, and physiological factors involved in our patients' problems. They help us to frame the patients' views of themselves, the world,
and their future, and ultimately to guide the development of a treatment
plan that can meet their therapeutic needs and goals. Each chapter provides
for the reader a succinct overview of the theoretical basis for the approach,
including its history, philosophical and theoretical foundations, the state of
the empirical evidence, and a demonstration of the clinical application using
specific case material.

A BASIC REQUIREMENT FOR COMPETENT PRACTICE

Understanding the theoretical underpinnings of psychotherapy is a basis
and context for competent therapeutic practice. Theoretical models help us
to appreciate patients' belief systems, emotions, and behaviors as a gestalt

363

rather than as a series of component parts. This capacity to develop cohesive formulations to explain the development and maintenance of patients' problems enables us to tailor and adjust therapy. Patients are likely to engage in those therapies that seem relevant and helpful to them, and to disengage from those that do not.

The case conceptualization (or formulation) is the operationalization of theory in practice. *Case conceptualization* is a framework for formulating hypotheses about the etiology and maintenance of patient problems, and provides a map for planning therapy. Whether based within a single model or an integration of models, the skill of using case conceptualization is the true test of mastering theory in a clinical context. Of course, once the conceptualization is developed, there is a need for the clinician to continue to develop a working alliance in a manner consistent with (or required by) the theoretical model (e.g., some therapies require a collaborative empiricism). To further facilitate therapy's progress, the discussion of attainable therapeutic goals for the individual patient and integration of relevant and timely interventions are important. Thus, the integration of theory starts at the point of assessment and formulation but extends through the entire delivery of psychotherapy.

The models represented in this book emphasize pragmatic, present-oriented therapies that focus on problematic behaviors and thoughts. Many emphasize skills building and learning to empower patients to cope better with the inevitable challenges of life. Others draw from insight-oriented approaches and contextualize the individual as part of a system that also requires intervention and support. There are many roads to Rome, many ways to cook spaghetti and meatballs, and many ways to develop an effective therapy for a given patient. Several resources in our professional literature show how the problems described by the same patient might be effectively addressed in different ways by practitioners of different therapies. There is simply no "one" right way to develop treatment. However, the effectiveness of any given approach depends on practitioners' understanding and adherence to the model(s) they are practicing.

Some readers might have expected that an edited volume of this nature would have prompted the development of a unified theory or system for psychotherapy. We have specifically avoided such thinking, because we applaud diversity in approaches to working with patients, and see it as necessary if we are to respond to the diversity of individuals who seek therapy. As our understanding of affective states, anxiety, impulsivity, and interpersonal relations evolves, so too will our theories, science, and practices. But our goal should not be simply to reduce the number of theoretical models; it is more useful to encourage new ideas and practices than to restrict them.

INTERVENTIONS DO NOT DEFINE THE THERAPY

The contents of this book illustrate that interventions do not necessarily define therapy. Practitioners would be mistaken to believe they are practicing Beckian cognitive therapy simply because they use thought records. Others would be mistaken to believe that they are *not* practicing behavioral activation therapy simply because a patient planned a mindful or meditative exercise as part of activity scheduling. In all instances, it is not the surface description of what patients are doing, but *why* they are engaging in the task, that is important. It is the therapist's responsibility to explain how any given intervention will lead to productive gains toward achieving patients' therapeutic goals. Thus, a competent clinician applies theoretical knowledge to clinical skills. It is this combination that defines competence. Without the ability to integrate practice with theory, practice is likely to be poor.

ADHERENCE AND FLEXIBILITY IN GROUNDING PRACTICE IN THEORY

Clinical researchers have significantly contributed to our understanding of the effectiveness of psychotherapy. Decades of research have been devoted to demonstrating the effectiveness of "talk" therapies in ameliorating symptoms and improving patient functioning.

Systematization of interventions in research trials often requires that the clinical trial clinician adopts a one-size-fits-all, diagnosis-specific treatment plan. Treatment selection based on disorder is simply too rigid to be responsive to the individual needs of patients in practice. Authors have demonstrated that some research trial participants have greater symptom severity than do many patients presenting in outpatient clinics. However, the procedures required to conduct sound clinical research often result in data that lack broader generalizability.

Manualization of interventions may have led to *less* effective service delivery in research trials. Through the real (or perceived) restriction of the interventions that the therapists are able to integrate into practice, some studies may have weakened or underestimated the effects of the therapy under investigation. For instance, there are real theoretical limitations in extracting and attempting to contrast the "behavioral" and "cognitive" components of Beckian cognitive therapy. The limitation would be that each condition reflects a therapy that differs from the system of psychotherapy developed by Aaron T. Beck.

Research may inadvertently encourage consumers of research to focus on the "intervention packages" rather than to base their practices flexibly within a model. Two case conceptualizations of the same patient, within the same therapeutic model, may yield different therapeutic interventions—yet these different approaches may be beneficial. Clinical work based firmly on a theoretical understanding is flexible; it allows the practitioner to tailor interventions to patient idiosyncrasies, thus making them more potent and relevant. Flexible adherence to a model (or combination of models) is a basic requirement for competence in the practice of behavioral and cognitive therapies (see Figure 12.1). There is simply no "cookbook" approach that turns all therapists into effective chefs producing al dente pasta every time.

It is our hope that readers of this volume will gain a broad perspective of the state of the art for behavioral and cognitive therapies in clinical practice. Clinicians who practice the models articulated in these chapters will discover the depth and breadth of application of the various approaches. Researchers are called to link theoretical models to the flexible use of interventions and, specifically, to target hypothesized mechanisms of change in future research.

Much of psychotherapy research has been preoccupied with demonstrating effectiveness in relation to medication and waiting-list controls. Comparatively few data are available on the extent to which therapies achieve their benefits through the hypothesized mechanisms of change. As our science evolves, it is likely there will be a synchronicity between our reliance on patient self-report and more objective measures of therapeutic benefit. We are currently challenged to demonstrate the extent of generalization of adaptive skills, the extent of belief change, and long-lasting benefits in interpersonal and other areas of functioning due to therapy. We also have few data on therapists' competence in case conceptualizations, and how such conceptualizations can be integrated into sessions and guide the direction of interventions used in therapy. Some of the therapies presented in this book need first to operationalize the mechanisms of change before such research can be carried out.

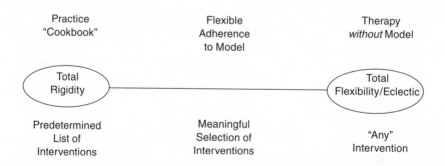

FIGURE 12.1. Aspects of rigidity and flexibility in integrating theory into practice.

We caution against using techniques simply because they are new, fashionable, or a favorite of the therapist. We advocate for *adherence* to a guiding theoretical model, or a cohesive integration of models. If we have done our job, this volume will serve as a valuable contribution in demystifying the role of cognitive and behavioral theories in clinical practice—and facilitate a more cohesive bond between the two.

ACKNOWLEDGMENT

We thank Frank Dattilio, Jim Nageotte, and Kevin Ronan for comments on a previous version of this chapter.

Index

Page numbers followed by an *f* or *t* indicate figures or tables